An Experiential Approach to Psychopathology

Giovanni Stanghellini •
Massimiliano Aragona
Editors

An Experiential Approach to Psychopathology

What is it like to Suffer from Mental Disorders?

Springer

Editors
Giovanni Stanghellini
Department of Psychological, Humanistic and Territorial Sciences
'G. d'Annunzio' University
Chieti, Italy

'D. Portales' University
Santiago, Chile

Massimiliano Aragona
Sapienza University and Crossing Dialogues Association
Rome, Italy

ISBN 978-3-319-80691-4 ISBN 978-3-319-29945-7 (eBook)
DOI 10.1007/978-3-319-29945-7

Printed on acid-free paper

This Springer imprint is published by Springer Nature
The registered company is Springer International Publishing AG Switzerland

Contents

Phenomenological Psychopathology: Toward a Person-Centered Hermeneutic Approach in the Clinical Encounter

1

Giovanni Stanghellini and Massimiliano Aragona

This introduction is an overall outlook of the methods used in phenomenological psychopathology. The several meanings of the term 'psychopathology' are differentiated, together with a brief overview of the main ideas in philosophical phenomenology. Then, the principal methodological concepts in use in phenomenological psychopathology are discussed: form and content, explaining and understanding, static and genetic understanding, *epoché* and *eidos*, the existentialia exploring the basic way human beings exist in the world. Finally, the hermeneutic approach in psychopathology is discussed at three levels: the hermeneutics of mental symptoms, the hermeneutic circle in the relationship between symptoms and diagnosis, and the hermeneutics of the deep subjective structure on which the previous levels are grounded.

1.1 Psychopathology as the Basic Science for Mental Health Care

A book of phenomenological psychopathology firstly needs to define exactly how the two key terms ("phenomenology" and "psychopathology") will be intended. This is because scholars use them differently in different contexts. Accordingly,

G. Stanghellini
Department of Psychological, Humanistic and Territorial Sciences, 'G. d'Annunzio' University, Chieti, Italy

"D. Portales" University, Santiago, Chile
e-mail: giostan@libero.it

M. Aragona (✉)
'D. Portales' University, Santiago, Chile
e-mail: massimiliano.aragona@uniroma1.it

G. Stanghellini, M. Aragona (eds.), *An Experiential Approach to Psychopathology*,
DOI 10.1007/978-3-319-29945-7_1

some terminological clarification is useful to avoid possible misunderstandings. So the first question is: *What is Psychopathology?*

In many instances, this word is used as a synonym for "mental symptom," "mental syndrome," "mental disorder," and the like. For example, the reader of a paper entitled "Psychopathology in Multiple Sclerosis" can reasonably expect to find there the assessment (usually by means of "rating scales") of a more or less large array of mental symptoms, like depression, anxiety, and so on. This use of the word psychopathology is very general and, although acceptable, adds nothing to the information transmitted by the use of more specific names for individual mental symptoms and/or disorders.

In contrast to this very general use, in which psychopathology is defined by its focus on some "pathological" mental contents and abnormal expressions and behaviors, in all other cases psychopathology is conceived as a method or a discipline. Such a shift from content to method is best illustrated by the focus on methodological awareness in Karl Jaspers' *General Psychopathology* (1963, p. 5): "If we wish to raise our statements and discoveries to firm ground, above the daily flood of psychological notions, we shall almost always be forced to reflect on our methodology." Starting from this common ground, different emphases explain further variation in the use of the same word.

In a second, very common usage, the term "psychopathology" refers to the purely descriptive study of mental symptoms. More specifically, the method employed to study mental symptoms, their formal features allowing a distinction from similar phenomena. Descriptive psychopathology is the common language or *koiné* that allows specialists each speaking their own dialect or jargon to understand each other. Its "breeding ground" is the work of Karl Jaspers and the Heidelberg School (Janzarik 1976). Descriptive psychopathology gives a concrete description of the psychic states which patients actually experience; it delineates and differentiates them as sharply as possible; and it creates a suitable terminology (Jaspers 1963, p. 55). It is quintessential in recognizing and naming the abnormal or pathological phenomena that affect the human mind. The main objects of descriptive psychopathology are the patients' experiences. The form in which these experiences are presented is considered more significant than their contents. Perceptions, ideas, judgments, feelings, drives, and self-awareness are all forms of psychic phenomena, denoting the particular mode of existence in which a content is presented to us.

A third psychopathological approach derives directly from such a descriptive psychopathology, considering the significance of the enucleated phenomena within the psychiatric diagnosis and classification. In this context, the study of isolated symptoms shall allow the *identification of specific diagnostic entities* that, in turn, enable prediction of natural history and response to treatment. This use of psychopathology as the tool for nosographic diagnosis is well illustrated by Kurt Schneider's *Clinical Psychopathology* (1975), where the thorough descriptive characterization of mental symptoms makes possible the differential diagnosis between mental pathologies.

It should be stressed that although psychopathology is about all that, it is not just about that. In fact, the focus on a purely descriptive psychopathology is *prima facie* in line with the biomedical approach that looks for the formalization of good *explananda*, i.e., symptoms and diagnoses intended as natural entities to be reduced and reconceived as *effects* of some supposed underlying (neuro)biological dysfunction which explains them. A psychopathological approach does not exclude seeing mental symptoms and disorders as caused by possible dysfunctions to be cured (Jaspers himself clearly wrote that the use of the explanatory method is admissible, coherent, and potentially unlimited: Jaspers 1963). However, the psychopathologist is also well aware that by reducing a complaint to a symptom of a dysfunction, we unavoidably overshadow the fact that a complaint has a meaning for the individual sufferer. Moreover, if psychopathology is conflated with nosography, only those symptoms that are supposed to have diagnostic value will be investigated, thus loosing relevant information that is not already classified. Accordingly, the focus on the explanation of mental symptoms and on diagnosis discourages attention to real people's experiences. Whereas symptomatology and nosology are strictly illness oriented, psychopathology is also *person* oriented, since it attempts to describe the patient's experience and his/her relationship to himself/herself and to the world. This leads us to the last two ways to intend the term psychopathology.

The fourth way to use the world psychopathology takes into account the subjective experience of the patient as it can be re-experienced by an empathic listener. This roughly corresponds to Jaspers' use of the word "phenomenology." This is, first and foremost, the meaning of psychopathology that inspires this book—the exploration of the experiential or personal dimension of mental pathology or "what is it like" to suffer for a given mental disorder. Its principal purpose is *understanding*. The patients' subjective experience is the "object" of this practice. Mental disorders are apparent in the realm of human subjectivity as abnormal, skewed, or constrained experiences, expressions, and behaviors. This is how mental disorder is presented to us. Mental disorders are first of all *mental*. A pathology of the psyche constitutes an experienced condition and a family of behaviors, feelings, and conscious contents, the peculiar significance of which emerges within a personal existence and history, and a sociocultural context. Such a kind of pathology is, therefore, completely on view only because of what has been called "the personal level of analysis" (Hornsby 2000; Gabbani & Stanghellini 2008). Only at this level, indeed, the real correlates of a psychopathological condition can be understood in their peculiar feel, meaning, and value for the subjects affected by them (Stanghellini 2007). The comprehension of the pathological significance of a psychic state (i.e., its meaning in a personal life) requires a kind of analysis which exceeds the range of a naturalistic approach. What one sees physically may be changes in receptor function, neurotransmitter metabolism, or whatever. But such changes cannot be diagnosed as "disordered" in and of themselves: they require mental abnormalities to be detected. The norm at play here is first and foremost at the mental level. The point here is that mental disorders appear on the personal level. Subpersonal abnormalities are only picked out as such by the person-level experience of disorder. The altered level of dopamine release would not be seen without the person already having been given a diagnosis of schizophrenia. And even if this should happen, an altered level of dopamine release in itself is not a mental disorder.

Finally, in a fifth meaning, psychopathology refers to a more global exploration of the patients' experiences. Here the exploration of the patient's subjective experiences is more hermeneutical than simply descriptive and focused on personal experiences as they appear in the patient's field of consciousness and can be re-experienced by an empathic listener. At play at this level is the search for a deep structure of subjectivity that makes possible the emergence of abnormal experiences and their organization in mental disorders. This level of inquiry builds on and extends the work of Minkowski, von Gebsattel, Straus, Binswanger, Tellenbach, Tatossian, Lanteri Laura, Blankenburg, and many others. Phenomenological investigation of abnormal human experience suggests a shift of attention from mere symptoms (i.e., state-like indexes for nosographical diagnosis) to a broader range of experiential phenomena that are indicative of trait-like features of a subject's experience of itself and its world—the life-world. A life-world is the province of reality inhabited by a given person, having its own *style* of subjective experience. The exploration of patients' experience and their life-worlds involves two distinct steps. The first—called *phenomenal* exploration—is the gathering of qualitative descriptions of a person's lived experiences. For instance, a patient may describe his thoughts as alien ("thoughts are intruding into my head") and the world surrounding him as fragmented ("the world is a series of snapshots"). The result is a rich and detailed collection of the patients' self-descriptions (Stanghellini and Rossi 2014). In this way, we detect the critical points where the constitution of experience is vulnerable and open to derailments reflecting the "phenomenal features" of patients' subjective experiences of specific contents, e.g., objects and events, in themselves and the world. In short, phenomenal exploration as first step focuses on contents; experience is considered here in a content-based way.

The second step aims to shift to phenomenology proper in that it seeks the underlying or basic structures or existential dimensions of the life-worlds patients live in. Abnormal phenomena are here viewed as the outcome of a profound modification of human subjectivity within the world. Phenomenology is committed to attempting to discover the common source that ties the seemingly heterogeneous individual experiences or phenomena related to contents together, thus targeting its underlying constitutive structures. This is done by finding similarities among the manifold phenomena and, possibly, the basic and underlying change in what we describe as *trans-phenomenal*. The term *trans*-phenomenal, rather than merely "phenomenal," refers to the fact that what is investigated at this level is not directly experienced. The concept of "trans-phenomenal" targets those features that underlie and, even more important, *constitute* subjective experience prior to and independent of the contents, e.g., events and objects. This second step of phenomenological analysis, then, aims to recover the underlying structures that usually recede into the background and remain implicit yet operative in our subjective self- and world experience.

The fourth and fifth meanings of psychopathology best illustrate what we mean by a "phenomenological approach" to psychopathology and will be discussed in detail in the following sections.

Now we shall briefly discuss why, in our view, psychopathology is so important for nowadays psychiatry. According to Stanghellini and Broome (2014), there are at least six reasons for psychopathology to be at the heart of psychiatry.

1. Psychiatry being a heterogeneous discipline, it needs a common ground and a joint language. Patients' lived experience being prioritized, psychopathology can be understood as a shared language that allows clinicians with different theoretical backgrounds to understand each other when dealing with mental disorders.
2. Psychopathology is useful to establish rigorous diagnoses in fields like psychiatry where the major disorders cannot be neuroscientifically defined as disease entities, but are exclusively syndromes defined according to characterizing symptoms, such as abnormal subjective experiences.
3. Psychopathology functions as a bridge between the human and clinical sciences, providing the basic tools to make sense of mental suffering.
4. Psychiatry addresses abnormal human subjectivity. Psychopathology attempts to define what is abnormal (rather than taking for granted commonsense views) and to grasp which elements of mental life remain normal in the context of illness.
5. Psychopathology connects understanding with caring and makes an effort to establish a methodological as well as ethical framework for this.
6. Psychopathology is about bridging understanding (meaningfulness of first-person subjective experience) and explanation (neurobiological causality) in research and clinical settings. Accordingly, basic psychopathological knowledge is a prerequisite for research addressing subpersonal mechanisms.

In conclusion, psychopathology is not one of numerous approaches aiming at conceptualizing mental disorders or illuminating their pathogenesis from a specific theoretical perspective. With its emphasis on systematic assessment of human subjectivity, it represents the basic study of mental phenomena, which is presupposed to any clinical and research enterprise.

1.2 Phenomenology: A Rigorous Method to Study Phenomena of Consciousness

What is phenomenology? As a concept, i.e., the study of phenomena as they appear to us, its historical roots are very old. On the contrary, the word "phenomenology" is more recent. Apparently it was coined in 1764, when J.H. Lambert combined two Greek stems (*phainomenon*, to appear and *logia*, discourse, science) into the German word *Phänomenologie*. Here the word phenomenology was used in the context of a theory of illusion or appearance in optics. Kant was probably influenced by Lambert's ideas when, in the *Critique of Pure Reason*, he traced the distinction between what appears (the *phenomenon*) and the unknowable "thing in itself" (the *noumenon*). Later, Hegel, Whewell, Hamilton, and Mach made use of the word "phenomenology" to describe views of their own. Thus, at the end of the nineteenth century, the term "phenomenology" was largely used by many writers with different nuances depending on the theoretical context. It is at the turn of the century that the word phenomenology acquires its specific meaning, referring to the philosophical inquiry intended as a rigorous method to study phenomena of consciousness. Drawing on ideas of the empiricists (the importance of experience), Descartes (the methodological doubt bracketing commonsense beliefs), Kant (the foundation of the transcendental Self), Brentano (the intentionality of mental acts), and Bolzano (the characterization of propositions as pure logical entities not implying a subjectivity thinking about them), Edmund Husserl founded *phenomenology* as a philosophical method whose motto was *we must go back to the "things themselves"* (Husserl 2001, p. 168). It is hard to summarize Husserl's work in a brief text, mainly because "Husserl himself found difficult to recognize himself in a finished and printed work because his thought developed as a work in progress during all his life, [. . .] Husserl's focusing on phenomenological themes cannot be reduced to single writings and does not follow a strict chronological order" (Farina 2014, p. 51). However, we can try to summarize at least those basic concepts we need for the discussion:

1. Husserl's phenomenology is mainly an epistemological enterprise, i.e., it focuses on how we do know what we know; however, it is also an ontology, because from the way things are given to our knowledge, we can say something about their nature.
2. Whatever we know, we know it from the vantage point of our own state of consciousness. Only what is given to our consciousness is knowable, so rigorous knowledge must be based on it.
3. We shall suspend our obvious trust in naturalistic beliefs regarding both the certainty of science and the objectivity of the commonsense world (Husserl calls this preliminary act *epochè*). Such active bracketing is necessary because the beliefs in the obvious existence of the objects are prejudices that distort pure knowledge.
4. Consciousness is not a space filled with representations but an active process. Hence, objects of knowledge are not independent, objective facts. They are the result of the intentional act of knowing, i.e., they exist as objects of knowledge only in relation to a subjective pole that knows them.
5. By focusing on our act of knowing, we discover that the object as we see it in its entirety is the result of a complex process of synthesis (often "passive" and unaware of itself) grounded on manifold partial perspectives.
6. We can perform imaginative successive subtraction of all those points of view that can be eliminated without affecting the object (e.g., of a chair we are seeing, we can progressively change the color, the material of which it is made, etc., and we still have a chair). By consistently applying this "imaginative variation," we finally arrive at one point when the subtraction of the last feature lets the object

itself to disappear. This characteristic that cannot be eliminated, otherwise the object is no more itself, is the "essential" feature, which Husserl calls the *eidos*.

There are many other concepts that could be remembered here (e.g., the distinction between *noesis* and *noema*, the distinction between physical (Körper) and experienced (*Leib*) body, the characterization of the "life-world," the process of intersubjective reciprocal recognition, etc.). However, here it was important to give the reader at least the basic concepts to understand in which sense Husserl's phenomenology is a rigorous enquiry into the way things present themselves to consciousness.

In conclusion, Husserl's phenomenology is the careful study of the manifestation of the things themselves in their full evidence in experience. It aims to explore the way phenomena appear and the relation between what appears and the one to whom something appears, abstracting from already acquired knowledge. We'll see below how this rigorous method solicited psychopathologists to rely on it in order to make possible a rigorous description of the otherwise ineffable abnormal mental phenomena.

Starting from Husserl, the history of phenomenology undertook different and unexpected developments which in some cases were far away from Husserl's original thought. There is no space here to describe them in detail; however, at least the main trends and variations shall be outlined.

Probably the most important figure is represented by Martin Heidegger, who was Husserl's strict collaborator in Freiburg. The history of the divergence between Husserl and Heidegger's understanding of phenomenology significantly involves personal issues, on the background of the Nazi's raising power in Germany. However, there were also key theoretical differences. In *Being and Time*, Heidegger (1927) denies the importance for phenomenology of the reduction to the essences (the *eidetic* method), discards a significant part of Husserl's approach for having improperly retained the centrality of the transcendental self (in Heidegger's view, Being is already and always a "Being-with-others" [*Mit-Dasein*]), and more heavily than Husserl he emphasizes the ontology of the phenomenon in opposition to its epistemology. Accordingly, in Heidegger the phenomenon is no more the *appearance*, as in the empiricist and Kantian traditions, of which a relic was also to be found in Husserl (although in Husserl there was a positive "ontological" part as well: i.e., the way phenomena were given in knowledge also says something on the *things themselves*). In Heidegger, the phenomenon is, according to its etymology, a positive manifestation of the thing itself, or, better, a manifestation of the *Being*. Here the metaphysical question about the Being, and the metaphysical inquiry in general, returns after being eclipsed for almost one century. This metaphysical turn is probably of minor importance for psychopathology, but in doing so, Heidegger starts his analysis from the being that poses the question of Being and for whom the answer is relevant: that being is the human being (the *Dasein* in Heidegger's terms), and this is why his philosophy can also be read as an anthropology whose key concepts are relevant for psychopathology. The original coexistence of subject and object before any differentiation takes place; the world as a character of the *Dasein* and the object as something defined by its use for human beings; the fact that the presence of other human beings doesn't need to be justified, because we are originally together, the *Dasein* being always and already *mit-Dasein*; the "existentialia" (*Existenzialen*) as general categories indicating the fundamental ways of being in the world; all these are fundamental anthropological contributions by Heidegger, strongly inspiring generations of phenomenologically oriented psychopathologists.

We will discuss in detail some of these concepts later. Here it is important to highlight that Heidegger's *Being and Time* also represents a shift of emphasis from phenomenology strictu sensu to hermeneutics and that within hermeneutics itself, it is a move from *understanding* conceived as the interpreter's reliving (*nacherleben*) the author's intention (as it was in the romantic tradition), to *understanding* as the *Dasein* that understands himself in his being situated in his world, i.e., as the progressive clarification of a self-comprehension which is already a pre-comprehension (something which is originally given and awaits to be better articulated in the hermeneutical circle by means of the interpretation). Later, H.G. Gadamer (1960) will further expand this stance by stressing that historical work is important for us because it changes our own horizon, history mainly being the history of the effects (*Wirkungsgeschichte*). With this, the shift of interpretation from the author's mind to the effects the text has on the reader is completed, and such a European hermeneutical position will have as its counterpart American pragmatism.

Returning to the phenomenological/hermeneutical movement, it undertook manifold developments in several countries, deeply influencing several research fields, e.g., historiography, metaphysics, logics, linguistics, philosophical anthropology, psychology, theology, ethics, esthetics, etc.

In France, Sartre's existentialism was profoundly influenced by Jaspers, Husserl, and Heidegger. Among the key concepts he borrowed from phenomenology, there was *intentionality*, "interpreted in a personal way to deconstruct the substantiality of consciousness and to free it from any form of interiority" (Farina 2014, p. 60). In Sartre's (2004, p. 186) own words: "consciousness is always 'in situation' because it is always free, there is always and at every moment the concrete possibility for it to produce the unreal."

A few years later, building on Husserl's distinction between the physical and the living body, Merleau-Ponty was highlighting that perceiving is an active process performed by an embodied consciousness entering in a vital relationship with a lived world. Hence, a dualism between body and psyche was rejected because "Taken concretely, man is not a psyche joined to an organism, but rather this back-and-forth of existence that sometimes allows itself to exist as a body and sometimes carries itself into personal acts. [. . .] It is never a question of the incomprehensible encounter of two causalities, nor a collision between the order of causes and the order of ends" (Merleau-Ponty 2013, p. 90).

This fundamental issue of the relationship between natural causes and human motives (reasons, meanings, values, ends) will find in Ricoeur (1969) one of the most interesting hermeneutical efforts, trying to reconcile the naturalistic drives hypothesized by Freud and the teleonomy assumed by Hegel.

For reasons of space, we have to stop here our description of the phenomenological/hermeneutical/existential contributions, assuming that we have succeeded in showing at least the basic ideas useful to understand phenomenological psychopathology.

To conclude this section, we have seen that *phenomenology* is a term used in different contexts with important differences in meaning. Leaving aside its early use in esthetics and metaphysics, sensu strictu "phenomenology" refers to the method elaborated by its recognized father, Edmund Husserl. However, many other important thinkers are credited to be part of the phenomenological movement, irrespective of so many significant differences. Hence, sensu lato, we may consider as phenomenological all those contribution, in Europe as well as in several other countries, dealing with the experiential analysis of the acts of consciousness, with hermeneutics and with existential issues. To sum up, the phenomenological movement is not a close and self-referential school, but the manifold contribution of several thinkers sharing a family resemblance.

1.3 The Birth of Phenomenological Psychopathology: The State of the Art in Jaspers' Time and His Solutions

There is some debate about the real importance of Jaspers' *General Psychopathology* for both psychopathology, in general, and phenomenological psychopathology, in particular. According to Berrios (2013a), the young Jaspers is not particularly original in its foundation of psychopathology, both the name psychopathology and its basic contents (the careful description of mental symptoms) being already established in nineteenth-century alienism, in Germany and especially in France. Moreover, to talk of Jaspers' approach as an instance of phenomenology is misleading because he used the term to apply to the study of mental phenomena in a way that is largely inconsistent with that of Husserl; hence, Jaspers' quotation of Husserl's *Logical investigations* should be considered more as a marriage of convenience than as a real example of phenomenological analysis (Berrios 1993). We may agree, and nevertheless we would like to stress that it is not a case if the centennial of Jaspers' *General Psychopathology* was celebrated so widely in the world (e.g., Stanghellini and Fuchs, 2013), while Emminghaus[1] is known only by a few historically minded psychiatrists. The point is that Jaspers' book can be considered the *veritable foundation* of psychopathology as a specific discipline studying abnormal mental phenomena, a discipline which is practically connected

[1] Hermann Emminghaus (1845–1904) was a German psychiatrist, author of an 1878 book on psychopathology entitled *Allgemeine Psychopathologie zur Einführung in das Studium der Geistesstörungen*. Jaspers was surely aware of this book, as well as the contributions of Störring and Morselli.

but theoretically clearly distinguishable from both psychiatry and clinical psychology (of which it represents the foundation, a sort of "basic science") and a discipline with its own methodological rules and, above all, self-aware of its own methods and specificities.

So, it is true that the young Jaspers had found in the Heidelberg's clinic a fully developed and already available knowledge about mental symptoms and their connection to psychiatric diagnosis, mainly following the ideas of Kraepelin. And he had also found there significant incentives to consider more in depth the humanistic side of our discipline (particularly under the influence of Grühle). But all this material was largely *not systematized*, and Jaspers was asked to write the *General Psychopathology* expressly in order to *secure* such a psychopathological knowledge in a systematic and (as far as possible) coherent system. This is the main reason for writing that book, and thus it was a sort of methodological foundation of a specific discipline whose knowledge was beforehand unsystematically dispersed in psychiatric textbooks. The young Jaspers was the right man for this job, primarily due to his philosophical/methodological knowledge and critical attitude—and also because his healthy problems were preventing him from a fuller involvement in clinical activities, leaving space for study.

When Jaspers started working on it, some alternative views on mental illness were competing. At one side, there was Kraepelin's system of classification, aimed at enucleating real natural entities (the mental diseases) starting from course and phenomenal presentation and looking for a convergence with anatomical and other neurobiological findings. On the other side, there were neurological constructions starting from the known functioning of the nervous system and trying to derive from this possible mental dysfunctions (at least this is the picture Jaspers gives us of systems like those of Meynert and Wernicke, which following Janet he considers "mythologies of the brain"). Finally, still peripheral respect to the academic environment but in rapid growth, there was the psychoanalytic explanation of mental symptoms as symbolic representation of unconscious causes [Jaspers will dispute this approach more directly in the following years: see on Rossi-Monti (2013)].

In short, Jaspers added to previous "psychopathologies" his relevant contribution on the following.

First, a major enhancement was surely methodological. As seen, Jaspers clearly claims that if we have to avoid to be continuously displaced by the emergence of new and unstable fashions, so common in psychiatry, we have to ground our psychopathological research on clear methodological reflections. On this regard, there are three important consequences (Rosini et al. 2013):

1. Man cannot be fully known through a unique, overarching, and dominant point of view. On the contrary, many points of view, many different approaches, and many methods of inquiry are needed. Every method has its own domain of application and its own results. But every method should be aware of its own limitations, thus avoiding to illicitly transcend them. This is Jaspers' *methodological pluralism*.

2. We cannot avoid to carry with us our preconceptions when approaching the study of psychopathology. However, we must always try to enhance our insight on our preconceptions, thus transforming our *prejudices* (which operate tacitly, hence being at risk of introducing into the research unnoticed conflicting and contradictory assumptions) into *presuppositions*. The latter are the conscious methodological assumptions that guide and also constrain our empirical research.[2]
3. We must refuse all radical reductionisms, either neurobiological (Jaspers' abovementioned criticism to "the mythologics of the brain") or psychological (the assumption that every psychopathological phenomenon can be understood psychologically). In Jaspers' view, reductionism is not contradictory per se, but it is not satisfying because it excludes from the field of inquiry those features of the phenomena that do not fit into the model. Because many excluded features are relevant to psychopathology, a model that a priori leaves out them is not satisfying.

The second important contribution of Jaspers' *General Psychopathology* is his phenomenology. Above we acknowledged Berrios' critique to Jaspers' use of the term "phenomenology." We agree that there are relevant differences in the way Jaspers uses that term. However, there are also similarities; for example, his claim that we should "bracket" already made theoretical systems in order to go directly to our patients' lived experience clearly echoes Husserl's "bracketing" of theoretical as well as commonsense knowledge in the so-called epochè.[3] Similarly, the importance given to the acts of consciousness, the self-confinement of psychopathology to the study of conscious experiences as the unavoidable starting point of any further sort of inquiry about the mind, and the emphasis on a full description of phenomena as they are given in consciousness bear a resemblance to Husserl's phenomenological approach.

Despite this, Jaspers' phenomenology differs from Husserl's because (a) while Husserl's phenomenology applies to every object of knowledge (his examples being often concrete objects seen from different perspectives), Jaspers' phenomenology applies to a much more restricted domain, i.e., that of subjective symptoms (the lived experiences, or *Erlebnisse*), and (b) Jaspers intends the phenomenological method as a rigorous form of descriptive psychology, rejecting Husserl's eidetic research. As far as we know, at the beginning, Jaspers believed he was strictly

[2] It should be stressed that this distinction between prejudices and presuppositions is not yet clearly expressed in the 1913 first edition of the *General Psychopathology*, although the critique of prejudices is somehow already there. Probably the 1913 edition was more confident on the possibility of an approach free of prejudices (today it would be called atheoretical) than later, philosophically more mature editions.

[3] Of course both Husserl and Jaspers inherit this issue from the antimetaphysical spirit which was quite diffused in the philosophical debate of the last part of the nineteen century; i.e., a post-Kantian legacy arguing against all-comprehensive theoretical systems (like Hegel's) and proposing a return to lived experience.

following Husserl's method, interpreted as a descriptive psychology; it is only later that he acknowledges the difference, but then, in a footnote added to a later edition of his *General Psychopathology*, he explicitly rejected eidetic phenomenology by stressing that its own phenomenology had to be intended as a descriptive enterprise.

Hence, Jaspers usage of the term "phenomenology" is heterodox respect to Husserl's usage of this word sensu strictu. However, a family resemblance and a general influence of Husserl's stance are apparent, and in any case, there are at least three key positive contributions of Jaspers' phenomenology to psychiatry and clinical psychology (Rosini et al. 2013):

1. First, the main function of Jaspers' phenomenology is to stress the importance of subjective experiences in psychopathological research. It is noteworthy that in the same years many psychologists were rejecting the study of mental phenomena to self-confine their research on the analysis of behaviors. On the contrary, Jaspers claims that subjective experiences are essential and must be studied scientifically. What he calls phenomenology is a rigorous description of the subjective psychopathological phenomena. We think that subjective experiences are an essential part of the psychopathological inquiry today as they were one century ago (Aragona 2012).
2. In order to be scientific, such an assessment of the patient's subjective experiences must be grounded on what is effectively present in his/her communication. Accordingly, in Jaspers' view, both neurobiological and psychoanalytic theories were foreign to phenomenology.

   The neurobiological approaches were responsible of a prejudice in that they pretended to deduce from putative neurobiological mechanisms the consequent mental phenomena; as Jaspers suggests, they failed because they postulated mental phenomena that the patients never reported, while they did not predict mental phenomena effectively complained by the patients.

   Psychoanalysis was responsible of a methodological mistake because it explained mental phenomena by means of a "mythological entity" (the unconscious) that was unsuitable to be studied scientifically. Indeed, only conscious phenomena are open to Jaspers' phenomenological study.
3. Finally, one of the most important contributions of Jaspers' phenomenology is the very insightful and rigorous description of the empathic act that Jaspers calls (following the romantic usage) the act of "understanding" (*Verstehen*). We will return on this in a following section.

1.4 The Need of Phenomenological Psychopathology Nowadays: The Current Crisis of Psychiatry

Psychiatry is periodically said to be in crisis, and during its history, there was always someone proposing a radical reformation based on neurobiology, sociology, etc. Moreover, in some periods, it was argued that psychiatry had to be completely thrown out because mental diagnoses were not pathologies at all but just different ways of communication; hence, as a medical discipline, psychiatry was a nonsense. Such a continuous attack and request of radical change is unusual in other scientific disciplines, and it is mainly due to the fact that (in Kuhnian terms) psychiatry is not a mature science but a pre-paradigmatic discipline with many distinct and irreconcilable schools of thought. According to Kuhn (1970), in such a state of the art, it is normal that scholars write books devoted to justify their philosophical/theoretical grounds and to attack other views proposing their own alternative solutions to the problems of the discipline. If this is the general state of psychiatry as a discipline, one of us (Aragona 2009a, b) argued that psychiatric nosology after 1980 had displayed a paradigmatic dynamic (a shared view of the matter, a specialized language and method, the publication of results on specialized journals, focusing on research details without the typical pre-paradigmatic need to rediscuss in any occasion the fundamental tenets of the ideas involved). In particular, it was emphasized that with the birth of the DSM-III, we had assisted to a disappearing of the infinite local nosographies that had characterized earlier psychiatry, to the rise of a shared nosographic language, and to a strong influence on epidemiology, research, education, and clinical activity (e.g., almost all new manuals of psychiatry, almost all clinical research trials, etiological researches, and epidemiological surveys are based on the DSM diagnostic criteria).

A historical study showed that from Kraepelin to the DSM-5 there was a line of continuity that involved all versions of the DSM (Aragona 2014a), and nevertheless something radically new is maybe happening nowadays, suggesting that psychiatric nosology is a paradigm involved in a state of scientific crisis whose most powerful proposal of solution is currently based on neurobiology (Aragona 2014b).

In this section, we will discuss the reasons for the current state of crisis, asking if this is only a superficial problem that can be amended within the nosographic system, or a more radical crisis forcing us to put in question our views on psychiatry in general (its image largely depending on the view on what kind of entities are mental disorders, a view largely conveyed by the implicit theoretical assumptions of the classification systems). If this is the case, the proposed shift to the neurobiological approach is itself problematic. It has been stressed that the "recent growth of neuroscientific paradigms in psychiatry has led to renewed challenges for clinicians and researchers in combining objective knowledge of brain functioning with the subjective experiences [of the patients, and that s]imilar challenges in the early years of the twentieth century, during psychiatry's 'first biological phase', led Karl Jaspers to insist on the importance of meanings as well as causes in psychopathology" (Stanghellini et al. 2013, p. 287).

To sum up, this section discusses the main problems involved in the current crisis of psychiatry and defends the idea that neuroscience alone is not sufficient to solve them, because many psychiatric challenges are rooted in descriptive and hermeneutic issues pertaining to the psychopathological inquiry. Hence, a renewed phenomenological psychopathology is needed in order to put our discipline on a solid ground.

1.4.1 The Unintended Side Effect: Persons Lost in Diagnostic Criteria and Rating Scales

Current psychiatry is largely dominated by procedures involving the application of operative diagnostic criteria and the "measurement" of mental symptoms by means of rating scales and structured interviews, whose main aim is to increase inter-rater reliability. Such an approach to mental disorders derives from the work started in the 1970s by the so-called "neo-Kraepelinian" school, with the subsequent fundamental aid of the leader of the DSM-III project, R. Spitzer. In short, their main idea was that psychiatry had lost credibility mainly because psychiatrists had radically different views on mental diseases. As a consequence, this was responsible of scarce terminological and procedural precision. Psychoanalysis, which was the leading school of thought in the American psychiatry of the time, was considered largely responsible for this state of affairs, due to its subjectivist stance, its lack of standardized diagnostic procedures, and its use of obscure and unverifiable concepts.

A return to its own medical roots was then proposed as the solution for psychiatry's discredit, and Kraepelin's rigorous classification was seen as the best historical example for what was needed in psychiatry: a meticulous description of mental symptoms and illness course in order to enucleate reliable disease entities that further research could prove to be based on altered neurobiological mechanisms.

Years ago a well-known paper lamented that, after several years of rigorous application of this approach, American psychiatrists had to acknowledge that unintended side effects were emerged (Andreasen 2007). The author was the pupil of one of the leaders of the neo-Kraepelinian school, and for many years, she had followed that model trying to integrate it with new available methods and knowledge. For example, in an editorial celebrating one of the most important publications of the neo-Kraepelinian school, she commented that "25 years after that groundbreaking article, psychiatry is not only founded on diagnoses that are validated by clinical description and epidemiological criteria, but it is challenged by the opportunity to probe more deeply into mechanisms and perhaps to reach very fundamental levels of knowledge about etiology that will have profound implications for treatment and prevention" (Andreasen 1995, p. 161). However, with time the expected results did not come, and Andreasen realized that such a failure was related to unintended consequences deriving from the worldwide application of the neo-Kraepelinian DSM: "the study of phenomenology and nosology that was so treasured by the Mid-Atlantics[4] who created DSM is no longer seen as important or relevant. Research in psychopathology is a dying (or dead) enterprise" (Andreasen 2007, p. 111). Perhaps the most striking limitation of a psychiatric praxis reducing the diagnostic process to the administration of rating scales and the application of diagnostic criteria is its intrinsic

[4] The universities teaching the neo-Kraepelinian approach in the 1970s.

dehumanization: "DSM has had a dehumanizing impact on the practice of psychiatry. History taking—the central evaluation tool in psychiatry—has frequently been reduced to the use of DSM checklists. DSM discourages clinicians from getting to know the patient as an individual person because of its dryly empirical approach" (Andreasen 2007, p. 111). A resource against such a dehumanizing approach is the acknowledgment that besides impersonal diagnostic criteria and brain mechanisms, psychiatry is and must essentially be focused on people. Hence, it has to be concerned with the patients' subjective experiences and the personal meanings the individuals attribute to their psychopathological experiences, being aware that the personal idioms of distress and the active interplay between the person and his/her abnormal experiences (personal elaboration) significantly mold the clinical picture, the illness course, and the therapeutic trajectory. Accordingly, we support a *person-centered approach* in psychiatry, considering "patients as active and meaning-making entities rather than as passive individuals and their attempts at self-understanding as potentially adaptive. This is important in contemporary practice at a number of levels. Crucially, it helps improve understanding of the unique personal values and beliefs by which each individual's experiences [...] are shaped, thus enhancing insight and improving the quality of the clinician-patient relationship" (Stanghellini et al. 2013, p. 292).

1.4.2 The Scientific Failure: Reliability Without Validity

The DSM-5 (American Psychiatric Association 2013) has been published in the midst of unusual controversy. Criticisms had always been advanced, but in the past, the DSM system was the dominant paradigm and criticisms were mainly the unheard complaints of the looser schools of thought. Today it's different, because it is the credibility of the DSM itself that is in question. For example, Maj commented that since the publication of the DSM-IV: "Only a couple of decades have passed, but those already seem 'good old days'. Much of that enthusiasm and faith has now vanished [...] the questions I am now receiving from journalists [...] focus not so much on 'new developments in the manual' (the most common question when the DSM-IV was launched) as on [...] 'why we produce this classification at all, since we do not have a solid ground on which to base it'" (Maj 2012, p. 161). Why such a dramatic change of view?

The present crisis of the DSM was not unexpected. From the very beginning of the revision process, the editors of the DSM-5 had clearly presented the demoralizing state of the art resulting from research evidences. DSM-IV psychiatric diagnoses were largely:

1. Unspecific, allowing no prediction about prognosis and therapeutic outcomes
2. Heterogeneous, including within the same concept individuals presenting with different clinical pictures
3. Instable, the same patient fulfilling the criteria for different diagnoses at different times

4. Plagued by excessively high comorbidity
5. Without external validators, laboratory tests and/or neurobiological findings being not available to confirm the phenomenally based diagnosis

Their conclusion was that "research exclusively focused on refining DSM-defined syndromes may never be successful in uncovering their underlying etiologies" (Kupfer et al. 2002, p. xix). In other words, although the DSM-III was credited to have improved the inter-rater reliability (i.e., the agreement between independent clinicians looking at the same psychiatric interview), Spitzer's prediction that with more reliable diagnoses validity research would have consequently advanced was not confirmed.

Subsequent epistemological research claimed that the abovementioned problems deriving from the application of the DSM diagnostic criteria were not just "empirical" results that could find a resolution by extensive application of evidence-based methods. Rather, it was suggested that they could be better understood if they were reconceived as Kuhnian "anomalies," i.e., apparently empirical outputs largely dependent upon the way the classification system is internally structured (Aragona 2009a, b). A few of such problems, i.e., the DSM scarce phenomenal determination of mental symptoms and the basic belief that they can be objectively described, are relevant for the present discussion and will be discussed below. Here it is sufficient to highlight that we are in a particular historical period coinciding with the end of the neo-Kraepelinian long-lasting dominance in psychiatry, and in the next years, the survivors of such a nosographic overemphasis will need to reorganize the discipline on firmer grounds, paying more attention to the specific qualities of the patients' experiences. In conclusion, according to Zachar and Jablensky (2014, pp. 9–10), "the neo-Kraepelinian paradigm established by Robins and Guze and institutionalized in the DSM has resulted in so many problems and inconsistencies that a crisis of confidence has become widespread [and this drives] a transition from a period of normal science (where the paradigm serves as an integrating framework in which questions are asked and answered) to a period of *extraordinary science*. The defining features of the fragmented periods called extraordinary science include: (a) lack of agreement on what are the most appropriate methodologies, (b) magnification of the problems that define the crisis into the most important problems of the discipline, (c) the generation of speculative new theories, and (d) a dramatic increase of interest in exploring the philosophical assumptions of the discipline."

1.4.3 Lack of Phenomenal Determination

A widely acknowledged problem with current classification systems and the assessment instruments derived from them is their insufficient attention to the qualitative specificities of the assessed mental phenomena. We will see why the definition of symptoms "as oversimplified phenomenal variants" (Stanghellini and Rossi 2014, p. 237) is inappropriate. But firstly, why is it so?

Two intertwined major aims of the DSM-III significantly influenced the approach on this issue: the diagnosis of any mental disorder had to be based on reliable observation, and clinicians from different schools of psychiatry had to feel comfortable when using the same terms. Because most source of disagreement was thought to depend from the fact that qualitative nuances were more difficult to detect and that different schools tended to highlight different qualitative features of mental phenomena, the architects of the DSM-III chose to use lists of symptoms whose definition was commonsensical and detection was simple as much as possible. Moreover, because in the diagnostic procedure different schools tended to give different weights to this or that symptom, the diagnostic criteria were organized as quantitative lists with diagnostic thresholds, without a hierarchical organization of symptoms depending on their possible importance. Examples of this are the DSM-5 definitions of euthymic mood as "mood in the 'normal' range" (tautology), "bizarre" schizophrenic delusion defined as a delusion involving "a phenomenon that the person's culture would regard as physically impossible" (vagueness), the same weight of antithetical symptoms in the same diagnosis (e.g., weight loss or gain, and decrease or increase in appetite, in major depression), and so on.

Such a choice to prefer a quantitative and commonsensical approach was responsible (together with other choices) of many current anomalies in the application of the diagnostic criteria to the clinical and research populations. For example:

1. Lack of distinction between the once called "endogenous" or "vital" depression (typical of melancholics), and the dysphoric "depression" in borderlines reacting to a disillusion can improperly increase the chance to make a diagnosis of major depression and borderline personality disorder in comorbidity.
2. Lack of distinction between Jaspers' primary and secondary delusions can magnify the impression of continuity of mixed cases between schizophrenia and affective disorders and also increase the internal heterogeneity of samples of patients selected for research.
3. Lack of distinction between fundamental and accessory symptoms increases the inclusion in the same sample of non-prototypical patients, hence internal diagnostic heterogeneity and consequent poor prognostic and treatment specificities.

Examples of this kind could be multiplied, but here is sufficient to stress one key point: starting from heterogeneous samples is practically very difficult to point to possible underlying neurobiological dysfunctions. Hence (as stated in Sect. 1.4.2), the failure of the neo-Kraepelinian approach is mainly a problem of lack of validity, and it cannot be solved by simply increasing neurobiological research, because it is the phenomenal characterization of the samples to be studied that is primarily in question. As we will see in this book, European psychopathology has always been concerned with a careful qualitative distinction and delimitation of psychopathological phenomena, in order to grasp their essential features independently from nonspecific or derivative symptoms. For example, several chapters of this book will show that schizophrenic people are not simply carriers of delusions, voices, and other incoherent symptoms in a number sufficient to make diagnosis.

Rather, essential self-disorders specifying a general specific *Gestalt* are nuclear disturbances that lie beneath superficial paranoid phenomena. Accordingly, although diagnostic criteria (nosographic organizers) may be useful for simple communication, understanding persons with mental disorders also requires a more fine-grained competence in detecting nuanced but fundamental phenomena representing the core of the phenomenal picture. Independently from strict nosographic usages, at this core level, psychopathological concepts organize a complex array of psychopathological phenomena in unities based on meaningful structures (psychopathological organizers) (Rossi-Monti and Stanghellini 1996). This is the task of the so-called structural psychopathology, which "assumes that the manifold of phenomena of a given mental disorder is a meaningful whole, i.e., a structure. The symptoms of a syndrome are supposed to have a meaningful coherence" (Stanghellini 2010, p. 320); hence, the phenomenal specificities and the internal links between the parts of the structure should be thoroughly investigated.

1.4.4 The Promised Neurocognitive Revolution (The RDoC Project)

It has been argued that psychiatry is in a scientific crisis and that today the most powerful revolutionary proposal comes from the neurocognitive field (Aragona 2014b).

Early proposals (Murphy 2006; Sirgiovanni 2009) had suggested to ground psychiatric diagnoses neither on the microlevel (the genes or other molecular/biochemical features) nor on the macro-level of behavior and personality; rather, cognitive scientists were invited to focus on an intermediate level, that of the cognitive computational modules, mental disorders being conceived as "breakdowns of neurocomputational mechanisms" (Sirgiovanni 2009, p. 47).

More recently, the US National Institute of Mental Health launched an ambitious research plan called "Research Domain Criteria (RDoC) project" (Insel et al. 2010; Cuthbert and Insel 2013). Although the DSM-5 presented itself as a "bridge" between the old model and the RDoC project, the RDoC project proposes a radical change in psychiatric research. In fact, its aim is "to shift researchers away from focusing on the traditional diagnostic categories as an organizing principle for selecting study populations towards a focus on dysregulated neurobiological systems" (First 2012, p. 15). We do not consider here the many criticisms against this model, confining our discussion on the basic features of the RDoC project and on its continuity and differences compared to the usual DSM-based approach. Only then we will raise some critical concerns whose discussion might be useful in this context.

Firstly, the RDoC proposal is not a diagnostic system in its classical sense but a matrix based on basic areas of psychological (cognitive) functioning to be correlated to corresponding brain circuits. That is, it focuses on cognitive domains as the key constructs around which available evidence (from different sources, from genes to self-observation) should be trans-nosographically organized (First 2012; Cuthbert and Insel 2013). As such, it has no immediate concrete effects on psychiatric nosography; it is just in a future, when/if the expected research findings will be sufficient, that it will be possible to build on these bases a new, radically different nosography, grounded on a neurocognitive paradigm. Epistemological research suggested that such a model is revolutionary because it radically changes the direction of the validation process: while in the traditional approach researchers are "expected to proceed from phenomenally defined disorders *back* to the discovery of their etiology, in the etiopathogenic approaches the direction is expected to be from "subpersonal" dysfunctions (of genes, brain processes, or cognitive mechanisms) *ahead* to the resulting phenomenal picture" (Aragona 2014a, p. 40). However, despite its recognized revolutionary potential, the RDoC project remains largely continuous with the traditional reductionist ideal of validation intended as the discovery of the neurobiological processes responsible for mental disturbances.

Hence, some basic problems remain: how are the cognitive disturbances to be investigated phenomenally characterized? Why are they limited to those already enlisted? Can other cognitive domains be added in the future or is it a close system? Are they independent or interconnected functions? Are they homogeneous or heterogeneous? It can be predicted that questions like these will be part of the debate on the RDoC system as they were in the case of mental symptoms and disorders.

Here it is sufficient to stress that the RDoC model is interesting but with some possible problems. One of them is that, more or less explicitly, it conveys a reductionist idea assuming that what really matters is neurobiological explanation in terms of neurocircuits, chemistry, and genes, while the space dedicated to the experiential and relational features is at best marginal. Once again, as it was the case with reductionist models of the past, the risk is to transform psychiatry in a neurological activity where the sufferer as a person is lost.

1.5 Toward a Person-Centered, Multidisciplinary, Empathic, Human- and Value-Friendly Psychopathology

In the previous sections, we discussed the limitations of old and new mainstream approaches in psychiatry. We showed that what remains quite the same in different ages is the basic idea that the study of mental illnesses should focus on the underlying neurobiological dysfunction of which they are supposed to be the expressions. In such a context, in order to go further, psychiatry should increase its "objectivity," that is it should look at diseased deanimated bodies whose abnormal cognitions and behaviors should be seen as dysfunctional mechanisms to be normalized. This should be done preferably by means of direct intervention through pharmacological modulation, physical neurostimulation or neuroinhibition (e.g., transcranial magnetic stimulation and electrical devices), and when psychotherapy is considered, its role is admitted only because it is a nonphysical activity that nevertheless changes the brain. As stated above, in such a perspective, the individual sufferer and his/her world made of meaningful connections, significant relationships and values are completely lost. This is not to deny that people have a brain and that the brain is the organ to be studied to explain people's perceptions, emotions, cognitions, and actions, including both normal and abnormal ones. Yet, is this satisfying? Somehow ironically, although the model described above pretends to be medically oriented, nowadays medicine is deeply involved in a critical self-evaluation. From such self-criticism arises the idea that disconnecting the whole sufferer and dispersing its body parts under the aegida of different unconnected specialties was responsible of worse treatments, increased costs, and poorer compliance. Accordingly, "as medicine has become more powerfully scientific, it has also become increasingly depersonalised, so that within many areas of clinical practice it has been possible to witness the substitution of scientific medicine for scientistic medicine and to see an accompanying collapse of humanistic values in the principles and practice of medicine. [. . .] now that we can 'cure', we no longer retain any responsibility to 'care'—thus exacerbating [. . .] a crisis of knowledge, compassion, care and costs—and which risks a grave outcome for patients and clinicians alike" (Miles and Mezzich 2011, p. 208).

In psychopathology, a person-centered approach draws attention to the patient as a human being who has an active role in interacting with his/her basic disturbances and in the shaping of the psychopathological syndrome. Thus, in this context, the patient is seen as a meaning-making individual, a self-interpreting agent engaged in a world shared with other persons and whose individual values and experiences are key aspects of his/her self-understanding (Stanghellini et al. 2013).

Some key concepts are important here because they are part of a necessary general stance that psychiatrists (above all, those psychiatrists and psychologists who have clinical responsibilities) shall share independently from their respective schools of thought. Being phenomenology a humanistic contribution to the psychopathological science, it has a significant role in promoting such key notions. However, we believe that their importance largely transcends the phenomenological school and shall be part of a more basic common ground for any human being curing and caring for mental sufferers.

1.5.1 A Person-Centered Approach

As seen, the entire medicine is facing a radical challenge: while it is and has to be continuously more scientifically informed, technological, and evidence-based, in doing so it risks (and unfortunately this already happened) to lose the human contact with the sufferer, reduced to a dysfunctional body or part, de-individualized, and transformed in the "carrier" of a disease. We saw that this has negative effects on crucial issues like the therapeutic alliance and compliance, which are important in internal medicine as they are in psychiatry. Moreover, today's biological medicine is also reconsidering the primacy given to the disease with respect to its "carrier": in fact, individual differences promise to be key features for future individualized therapies; e.g., persons with different metabolism may respond differently to the same drug, despite having the same disease. The study of individual genetic differences is another case in point. If this is particularly relevant in internal medicine, it is at least equally important in psychopathology, where the patient is never the simple "carrier" of an independent disease. In fact, each individual, with his/her unique strengths and resources as well as needs and difficulties, plays a central role in actively shaping his/her disorder, its course, manifestation, outcome, etc. (Stanghellini et al. 2013). As said by Strauss (1992), the person is never peripheral, merely as a passive victim of a disease; rather, persons are "goal-directed" beings with an active role in shaping their own symptoms and guiding the evolution of the phases of their disorder. Accordingly, any clinical approach to mental sufferers has to be strictly individualized, because different persons have different needs and resources.

1.5.2 A Multidisciplinary Approach

One of the major limitations of current medicine is when different disciplinary approaches do not communicate in the individual case. However, in medicine the opposite case is often available, e.g., when physics, biologists, engineers, nurses, and clinicians with different specialties (internal medicine, radiology, surgery) coordinate themselves in a unique staff for the treatment of complex cases by means of technologically advanced devices. Psychiatry should be constitutively open to a multidisciplinary approach, because the biopsychosocial model of mental illness has significantly shaped its organization in the twentieth century. However, in many instances, it was organized totally independently from internal medicine, and for this reason in the last decade, the World Psychiatric Association increased its efforts to promote the importance of general medicine in the management of mental disorders. On the other side, there are examples of service organization where psychiatrists self-limited their activity to diagnostic assessment (largely using neuroimaging and laboratory analyses, although both provide unspecific results, the diagnosis being phenomenally based) and psychopharmacological intervention, without the necessary integration of the psychological and social level. Today the treatment of complex eating disorders, which so heavily involve the physiopathology of the body, was the occasion for the organization of multidisciplinary and integrated services where psychiatrists, psychologists, nurses, rehabilitators, and physicians expert in nutrition work together and coordinate their activities. However, while efforts were done for the integration of psychiatry and internal medicine, a lot remains to do for an improved dialogue between the schools of psychiatry and psychology. In fact, different schools are often in opposition to each other, showing the above discussed pre-paradigmatic state of the art well described by Kuhn.

A philosophical approach to psychiatry is here particularly important because it shows that most difference between schools is due to their acceptance of different philosophical basic tenets. Being aprioristically accepted, such basic claims often act as Jaspersian prejudices, and their explicit discussion and clarification is often very useful in order to increase collaboration between clinicians holding different views.

Moreover, a phenomenological approach that focuses on phenomena as they give themselves to consciousness in all of their concrete and distinctive features further increases the possibility of a reliable agreement. In fact, here "the primary object of inquiry is the patient's subjectivity, focusing on patient's states of mind as they are experienced and narrated by them [...]. Theoretical assumption are minimized and the structures of the patient's experience are prioritized" (Stanghellini and Rossi 2014, p. 238). This increases the possibility of a shared agreement on the phenomena themselves, independently from (and prior to) causal accounts addressing etiological explanations and subpersonal mechanisms. It should be stressed that although there are apparent similarities between this approach and the DSM-III's atheoretical claim, one significant difference is that phenomenology brackets theoretical preknowledge by means of a conscious, deliberate, and philosophically informed technical act of judgment suspension (the *epoché*), while the DSM suggests a naïve atheoretical stance based on a covert neopositivist assumption that symptoms are real entities which are directly observable without the need of any inference (Aragona 2013). This last atheoretical implicit belief contrasts the acknowledgement that mental symptoms are observed from the point of view of the observer (theory-ladenness) and are the product of a hermeneutical process taking place within the patient as well as in the dialogical exchange between patient and fellows, the clinician included (Berrios 2013b; Aragona and Marková 2015). Neglecting the intrinsic hermeneutics of mental symptoms leads to ineffectiveness, for clinical practice, of standard interviews molded on research-objectifying procedures, because it overlooks that the assessment of a mental state involves two kinds of reductions. According to one of us (Stanghellini 2013, p. 326), the first "is performed by the speaker who tries to find the propositional correlate of a given mental state, or the 'right words' to communicate it. The other reduction is performed by the listener who must sometimes interpret the speaker's meaning by asking the speaker and himself 'what does he mean by that?' This problem, which plagues psychopathological research and clinical practice, becomes even more acute in using standardized assessment, since when interviewees respond to questionnaires, they might have very different understandings of the questions, and this may lead to the inaccurate conclusion that different individuals or groups have similar experiences or beliefs."

Finally, a value-based sensibility (see below) is also helpful in reducing conflicts between the members of a service, thus promoting the interdisciplinary dialogue (Fulford and Stanghellini 2008).

1.5.3 An Empathic, Human- and Value-Friendly Approach

The phenomenological stance promotes the importance of empathy, humanities, and values in the approach to mental sufferers. Empathy is a complex, multifaceted, and polysemic concept. We will discuss it in detail in the following section, because it is a key concept in phenomenological and hermeneutic psychopathology. Here we briefly concentrate on the basic empathy in the therapeutic relationship, which is simply a general stance of "openness" and "attunement" to the other human being and his world of meanings. In this sense, an empathic relationship is defined as "other-oriented feelings of concern, compassion, and tenderness experienced as a result of witnessing another person's suffering" (Batson et al. 1990), and in psychiatry and psychology, it is also seen as a way of "putting the patient and yourself at ease" (Othmer and Othmer 2002), as well as a special technique to elicit trust in order to achieve rapport and relevant information (Turner and Hersen 2003). Of course, an empathic openness to the other human being in the therapeutic relationship is not a specific feature of phenomenological psychopathology, because it is the common basis for the vast majority of psychotherapies and it should be considered fundamental also in biological psychiatry. So, phenomenological psychopathology shares with many other approaches an emphasis on the importance of a general empathic stance in the therapeutic relationship, but it is much more than this. We will see later that in psychopathology empathy is not only a mere precursor to the genuine article of psychopathological understanding. Rather, it is the medium itself where understanding takes place, and psychopathological empathy can be additionally differentiated along the lines of the debate on the concept of "understanding" (*Verstehen*), from Jaspers to post-Heideggerian developments.

To this basic openness, phenomenological psychopathology adds a specific philosophical expertise that brings to psychiatry and clinical psychology a methodologically rigorous defense of complexity and anti-reductionism views. According to Fulford et al. (2004), a philosophical stance gives psychiatry a more complete picture of its structure, promoting a better characterization of the psychiatrist's role in crucial areas including the role of patients (philosophy puts patients first) and research (where philosophy reconnects minds with brains).

Finally, the work in values-based practice (VBP) is based not only in philosophical value theory but also in the contribution of phenomenological psychopathology. The specific contributions of VBP include:

1. Raising awareness of the role of values even in categorical psychiatric diagnostic systems.
2. Providing a clear theoretical explanation for the relative prominence of values in psychiatric diagnostic classifications (derived from the relative complexity of human values in the areas with which psychiatry is concerned).
3. Through the policy frameworks and training methods already established for values-based practice (Fulford and Stanghellini 2008). It is noteworthy that phenomenological psychopathology is interconnected with VBP, at the same time being one of its theoretical sources and a field of application of its principles.

1.6 The Phenomenological Analysis of Suffering

This section will explore in detail the main concepts, i.e., the categories of thought that inform the experiential encounter in clinical and research activity performed with a phenomenological approach. As we will see, the utilization of such concepts in practice is manifold, paralleling the multiple phenomenological views that influenced psychopathologists in different ways. Hence, the following concepts are not held by all phenomenologically oriented psychopathologists in the same way; some of them put more emphasis on some terms and reject others and vice versa. What is common is a general family resemblance and a deep involvement in human meaningful relationships.

1.6.1 Bracketing Theoretical Preknowledge

One of the key methodological steps in phenomenology is the so-called epoché which is an active and rigorous bracketing of our obvious as well as scientific/theoretical preknowledge, in order to go directly "to the things themselves" as they appear to consciousness. We stressed above that Husserl's *epoché* differs from more recent naïve atheoretical stances because the latter do not bracket obvious preknowledge but implicitly assume it in the form of a covert neopositivist trust in the description of mental symptoms viewed as mere objects (Aragona 2013). On the contrary, the phenomenological *epoché* assumes that objects of knowledge are not mere facts but are intentionally constituted in consciousness activity. Binswanger (1923) directly refers to Husserl's phenomenology as science of the pure essence of phenomena as they give themselves in the categorical intuition. He stresses that Husserl's essences are beyond the gnoseological distinction between real and ideal, because phenomenology is against *all* theories, gnoseological theories included. Hence, in Binswanger's view, Husserl would leave these problems aside. Although in this 1923 work he does not mention explicitly the word *epoché*, this "atheoretical" claim is Binswanger's way to describe it. However, he also stresses some differences between philosophical and psychological phenomenology, because while in the former the suspension of judgment is radical, in psychology such "bracketing" is only relative because its object (e.g., the perceptive act) is still considered as a real act, really occurring in a real men. A similar position is accurately carried on by Tatossian (1997, p. 10) who stresses the phenomenological "change of attitude, which is abandonment of the natural and «naive» attitude, that is to say [abandonment] of that attitude where, being either psychiatrists or not, we apprehend what we encounter as objective realities existing independently from us, being them psychical or material realities. Phenomenology is not interested in realities as such but in their conditions of possibility, hence it doesn't start before having practiced, in one or the other form, the *phenomenological reduction*, which suspends the natural attitude and its claims, or better its implicit or explicit theses about reality. This reduction or *epoché* is the foundational act of Husserl's phenomenology—what poses the problem of the relationships between philosophical phenomenology and psychiatric phenomenology."

Jaspers discussed this issue in a quite different vein. As discussed above, the founder of *General Psychopathology* can be considered a phenomenologist only in a broad sense, because his phenomenology differs from Husserl's eidetic research. However, also in Jaspers there is the need of bracketing preknowledge in order to go to the psychopathological phenomena themselves. The main difference is that Jaspers conceives his position as an empiricist one; he writes unambiguously that his aim is to describe mental pathological phenomena as they *really* are, intending as they effectively present themselves in the clinical encounter. Here the philosophical roots are not in phenomenology (although Jaspers quotes with admiration Husserl as a significant influence in his psychopathology) but in the post-Kantian views characterizing the late nineteenth-century "dispute on methods" in human sciences. There Jaspers finds an anti-metaphysic spirit that rejects a priori theoretical systems in favor of a *new* empiricist approach focused on the direct analysis of the lived experience (*Erlebnis*). The debate between Dilthey and the neo-Kantians is illustrative of this basic issue. It is from this, as well as from a rejection of some neurobiological systems of the time (particularly those of Meynert and Wernicke), that Jaspers moves in suggesting the need to make explicit and scrutinize the prejudices influencing our appraisal of mental phenomena. It is just after bracketing prejudices that we can approach mental phenomena in order to study them as they really present to our consciousness. In different words, "Avoiding all theoretical prejudices is the quintessential methodological as well as ethical (i.e., maximum respect for the person as a subject of experience) prerequisite of descriptive psychopathology. Descriptive psychopathology is not concerned with any subsidiary speculations, psychological constructions, interpretations or evaluations, but solely with the phenomena that are present to the patient's consciousness" (Stanghellini 2013, p. 341).

Finally, a few words are needed on Heidegger's view on the matter, because in general his ideas strongly influenced (and still influence) phenomenological psychopathology. Heidegger is very clear in tracing a sharp distinction between Husserl's and his own concept of the phenomenological reduction as a method to bracket the natural attitude and commonsense assumptions that accompany it. In Heidegger's account, for Husserl "phenomenological reduction [...] is the method of leading phenomenological vision from the natural attitude of the human being whose life is involved in the world of things and persons back to the transcendental life of consciousness and its noetic-noematic experiences, in which objects are constituted as correlates of consciousness. For us phenomenological reduction means leading phenomenological vision back from the apprehension of a being [...] to the understanding of the being of this being" (Heidegger 1982, p. 21). Hence, for Heidegger we always start our analysis from some concrete being, and at this level Husserl's *epoché* applies; but the essence of Heidegger's method is to go beyond that being in order to go back to its being. In his words, "[a]pprehension of being, ontological investigation, always turns, at first and necessarily, to some being; but then, *in a precise way, it is led away from that being and led back to its being*. We call this basic component of phenomenological method—the leading back or re-duction of investigative vision from a naively apprehended being to being *phenomenological reduction*" (Heidegger 1982, p. 21).

In conclusion, phenomenological psychopathology shares a common view on the importance of the *epoché* and phenomenological reduction for the sake of its analysis of psychopathological phenomena. However, under this commonality, there are interesting nuances: Jaspers appears at least partially independent from Husserl's account, while Binswanger and the majority of those following a Daseins-analytic perspective, although in general clearly indebted to Heidegger's ideas, on this particular point (phenomenological reduction) follow Husserl's view and (at least to our knowledge) substantially neglect Heidegger's alternative account.

1.6.2 The Distinction Between Form and Content

According to Berrios (2013c), "[i]t is customary to talk about the 'form' and the 'content' of mental symptoms: indeed, this distinction is central to the so-called 'phenomenological' approach. In spite of this, both concepts are not very well defined in the specific context of psychopathology." The history of the form/content distinction (Berrios 2013c) and the Kantian influence on Jaspers' usage of it (Walker 2013) are beyond the purposes of this introduction. Here we will focus on Jaspers' distinction for the aims of his *General Psychopathology* and on subsequent developments.

Jaspers describes three different ways to trace the distinction between form and content. The first is the most important for him, and we will discuss it in detail later. The other two are the following: one (the second case he describes) is the divide between the form as the general syndrome as a whole ("periodic phases of dysphoria" in Jaspers' example) and contents as the particular symptoms that may be part of the syndrome (in this example, dipsomania, wandering, suicide). As far as we know, Jaspers did not further elaborate on this, implicitly suggesting that this second meaning was not very important in his conception. The other distinction (the third case) is between the form as a very general, global change of the entire personality, as in the schizophrenic or hysteric experience (Jaspers' examples), and the content as every "variety of human drive and desire, every variety of thought and fantasy, [which] can appear as content in such forms and find a mode of realisation (schizophrenic, for instance, or hysteric) in them" (Jaspers 1963, p. 59). On this, interpretations slightly diverge: Berrios (2013c) suggests that according to this definition, "the psychological modality itself becomes the 'content' and is subordinated to the higher concept of diagnosis that becomes the 'form'." On the contrary, Aragona (2009c) does not emphasize the diagnosis (which is the focus of the second case) but the global change of the person's existence (of the way of Being in the World, we may say phenomenologically) and interprets it as part of Jaspers' confrontation with Binswanger's *Daseinsanalyse*.

In any case, it is the first distinction between form and content that is central in Jaspers' *General Psychopathology*, because the main objects of descriptive psychopathology are the patients' experiences and particularly the form in which these experiences is presented (Stanghellini 2010). In Jaspers' words, "form must be kept distinct from content which may change from time to time, e.g. the fact of a hallucination is to be distinguished from its content, whether this is a man or a tree, threatening figures or peaceful landscapes. Perceptions, ideas, judgments, feelings, drive, self-awareness, are all forms of psychic phenomena; they denote a particular mode of existence in which content is presented to us" (Jaspers 1963, pp. 58–59). It is noteworthy that here there is a minor but interesting ambiguity in Jaspers sentence, because it swings between form as formal characteristics of a given psychopathological phenomenon (e.g., hallucination) and form as type of intentional act (to use Brentano's terminology): in the example, perceptions, ideas, judgments, etc. Considering that a major aim of Jaspers' psychopathology is to scientifically describe and differentiate psychopathological phenomena, the emphasis should be on specific formal features of single phenomena, and this also explains why Jaspers adds that "from the phenomenological point of view it is only the form of the phenomenon which interests us" (Jaspers 1963, p. 59). This is because it is only through the form that we can give enough stability to the phenomenal description, in order to generalize our observation to any phenomenon of the same type (e.g., all hallucinations should share the same basic formal characteristics), while content is idiosyncratic, strongly depending on the life history of the patient. In other words, contents may be idiosyncratic, whereas forms reflect transpersonal generalizable aspects of the acts of consciousness (Stanghellini 2010, p. 323). But of course our patients' life history is fundamental in the psychotherapeutic relationship, and this is why Jaspers adds that although form is the most important for phenomenology, "the psychologist who looks for meaning will find content essential" (Jaspers 1963, p. 59).

Subsequent developments focused on the global way of being of the patient in his/her world. According to Stanghellini (2010, p. 321), a good case in point is Minkowski's structural psychopathology: in order to reconstruct the patient's life-world (which in his view is far more important than simply counting his symptoms), Minkowski "methodically brackets or suspends all the 'ideo-affective' (cognitive and affective) contents of experience, and focuses on formal aspects or the spatio-temporal configurations that are implicit in the patient's experiences. The main guidelines for this are lived space and time, but the way the patient experiences his own body, self and other persons are also included in Minkowski's inquiries. The depressive patient's experiences, examined from this angle, manifest profound anomalies as compared to the common-sense world we all live in. Following this path, to a certain extent it is possible to feel or imagine what it is like to live in that world. However, at this stage of reconstruction the lived world still lacks a core that keeps its parts meaningfully interconnected." So the next step is to look for grasping "the structural nexus that lend coherence and continuity to them, because each phenomenon in a psychopathological structure carries the traces of the underlying formal alterations of subjectivity" (Stanghellini 2013, p. 344). Accordingly, it is through the import of Heidegger's *existentialia* in phenomenological psychopathology that this is systematically addressed. We will discuss this in a section below. In the meanwhile it is enough to stress that this is important for the present discussion of the form/content distinction, because the aim of such a systematic analysis is the reconstruction of the other's lived world by grasping the *form* in which his experience is set in time and space, the *mode* in which he experiences his own body and others, and the *way* the physiognomy of material things appears to his senses (Stanghellini 2013, p. 339).

1.6.3 The Distinction Between Explaining and Understanding

The late nineteenth century saw the emergence of an epistemological dispute concerning the most appropriate methods for the emerging human sciences (sociology, history, jurisprudence, economy, and the like), as well as the proper place of psychology (is it a natural or a human science?). Comte's positivism had proposed to extend the methods of natural sciences to human sciences (e.g., the newborn sociology), while those disciplines that did not fit those methods had to be considered nonscientific at all (in Comte's view, psychology was a case in point). Despite disagreements on the place of psychology in their classification, both neo-Kantians and Dilthey agreed that human sciences (their name for them was *Geisteswissenschaften*: sciences of the spirit) were scientific but that their methods were different from those applied in natural sciences. There was additional disagreement regarding the defining features of human sciences, but this is beyond our present aim.

One important contribution was Dilthey's rejection of experimental psychology in order to support a "descriptive and analytic psychology" which should start from the phenomenal wholeness as it presents itself in the stream of consciousness (Dilthey 1977). There Dilthey pronounce his famous aphorism "We explain nature, we understand the spirit." There is some debate on the real importance of Dilthey's dichotomy for psychopathology, and in later occasions, Dilthey himself seemed to suggest that psychology could use and integrate both experimental and comprehensive methods. In any case, the distinction between causal explanation and empathic understanding is the distinctive feature of Jaspers' contribution to the birth of psychopathology as a scientific discipline.

In Jaspers' view, psychopathology uses both methods in order to find relationships between subsequent phenomena. At one side, we can causally explain any psychopathological phenomenon as the effect of an (known or hypothesized) underlying cause. Here the epistemological model is that of a chain of causes and effects explaining the functioning of a mechanism. Transposed into medicine, this is the chain from etiology to final symptoms via pathophysiological changes. In Jaspers' words, "the appreciation of objective causal connections [...] seen 'from without'" (Jaspers 1963, p. 28). It is noteworthy that Jaspers adds that we can *always* hypothesize causal brain mechanisms underlying psychopathological phenomena; hence, in psychopathology this approach finds *no limits*. But Jaspers adds that, although possible, causal explanation is not always satisfying for the needs of psychopathology. Psychopathology is not only a science of nature, but it is also a human science (see above Jaspers' methodological pluralism). In many instances, we are not satisfied to know that somebody acted as he did because some parts of his brain were activated, while others were inhibited. If we want to know why he did so, we need to understand his reasons, his motivations, and his purposes. This is a different level that can be grasped only by means of a totally different method. This method is *understanding* (Jaspers' *Verstehen*); it consists in reproducing (*nachbilden*) in ourselves a representation of what is actually taking place in the mind of that person. In Jaspers' psychopathology, such understanding was mainly an empathic understanding, an emotional reliving (*Nacherleben*, *Nachgefühl*). We will discuss it in the next section. Now it needs to be stressed that Jaspers clearly admitted that by means of this method we can understand those phenomena which are similar to what we might have experienced in similar circumstances. However, there are many phenomena that, despite our efforts, we are unable to understand empathically. Among the examples given, it is typical the case of primary delusions, which in Jaspers' terms are underivable and un-understandable phenomena. Hence, in Jaspers' view, the act of understanding is fundamental for psychopathology, but unfortunately it is a *limited* method: it can apply well in some circumstances, allowing for a humanistic study of mental phenomena, but it cannot apply in other cases, where it must be substituted by other methods.

We will see later that many psychopathologists returned on this problem trying to find a different method in order to understand our patients' way of being in the world. Here is enough to stress that despite relevant differences, psychopathologists agree at least on the need to find a method in order to grasp the patients' existential world, thus preserving a humanistic access to their own way to conceive, feel, and value their experiences.

Before concluding this section, we would like to emphasize that the parallel questions explaining/understanding and causes/reasons have been and still are extensively debated in epistemology. However, even a summary of this debate would be too long to find space in this introduction.

1.6.4 Characteristics and Limitations of Jaspers' Empathic Understanding

The literature on this issue is huge; here we limit our discussion to the main features of Jaspers' concept of understanding (*Verstehen*), to those points that although only implicit in his text need to be openly discussed, and the main epistemological limitations of such an approach.

In the first part of his *General Psychopathology*, Jaspers starts describing as much rigorously as possible the pathological mental phenomena. There he sharply distinguishes between those phenomena which are objectively given to our observation (e.g., behaviors) and subjective experiences (*Erlebnisse*) that, being part of the private world, are not directly observable from the exterior. Here the question is:

how is it possible to scientifically grasp, describe, differentiate, and univocally denominate such phenomena if they are not directly observable? Jaspers proposes his "phenomenological" method called "static understanding." Although we do not observe directly the subjective experiences of our patients, we can make them present in our consciousness by means of a sort of transposition, of reliving in ourselves what the other is actually living. This is an empathic act which gives us the material for the appraisal of such subjective, private experiences, in order to use them scientifically. Technically, such an empathic understanding requires a preliminary bracketing of our prejudices in order to grasp the phenomenon as it presents itself in our consciousness: "The first step, then, is to make some representation of what is really happening in our patients, what they are actually going through, how it strikes them, how they feel. We are not concerned at this stage [...] with any subsidiary speculations, fundamental theory or basic postulates. [...] Conventional theories, psychological constructions, interpretations and evaluations must be left aside. [...] We refuse to prejudge when studying our phenomena, and this openmindedness, so characteristic of phenomenology, [...] must be acquired painfully through much critical effort and frequent failure. [...] Phenomenological orientation is something we have to attain to again and again and involves a continual onslaught on our prejudices" (Jaspers 1963, p. 56).

Once this basic material is grasped by means of such an act of static understanding, the next question is how mental phenomena are interrelated. This is the second part of Jaspers' *General Psychopathology*, where he traces the abovementioned distinction between explaining and understanding. While, at least in principle, all phenomena can be part of an explanatory chain of mechanistic causes and effects, some psychopathological phenomena need to be viewed as typically human in order to preserve their specificity. In Jaspers' own words: "Phenomenology presents us with a series of isolated fragments broken out from a person's total psychic *experience*. [...] How are all these various data to be related? In some cases the meaning is clear and we understand directly *how one psychic event emerges from another*. This mode of understanding is only possible with psychic events. In this way we can be said to understand the anger of someone attacked, the jealousy of a man made cuckold, the acts and decisions that spring from motive. In phenomenology we scrutinize a number of qualities or states and the understanding that accompanies this has a *static* quality. But in this question of connectedness, we grasp a psychic perturbation, a psyche in motion, a psychic connection, the actual emergence of one thing from another. Here our understanding has a *genetic* quality" (Jaspers 1963, p. 27).

Jaspers' concept of "understanding" has distinctive features that shall be briefly considered.

First of all, it is an empathic, emotional understanding (*ein fühlendes*). He clearly stresses that rational understanding of the meaning of a sentence is not his concept of understanding, because what he has in mind is understanding the person through his phrase, not simply the sentence in itself: "where we understand how certain thoughts rise from moods, wishes or fears, we are understanding the connections in the true psychological sense, that is by empathy (we understand the speaker). Rational understanding always leads to the statement that the psychic content was simply a rational connection, understandable without the help of any psychology. Empathic understanding, on the other hand, always leads directly into the psychic connection itself. Rational understanding is merely an aid to psychology, empathic understanding brings us to psychology itself" (Jaspers 1963, p. 304).

The second feature is what has been called "the problem of the right distance" (Villareal and Aragona 2014). Empathic understanding is neither emotional fusion nor cold distance; it is something in between, where the "sympathetic tremulation of one psyche with the experiences of another" coexists with scientific objectification of "such experience critically" (Jaspers 1963, p. 22). According to Ballerini (2003), an important issue for the psychopathologist is his need to modulate the distance between himself and the patient. In his view, the therapist and patient continuously change their interpersonal distance, with a continuous oscillation between the extremes of a fusional and a sidereal distance, i.e., between general objective categorization and individual existential subjectivity.

Third, genetic understanding is asymmetric (Villareal and Aragona 2014). In the case of causal explanation, we move from the phenomenon to be explained to the causes that produced him. Once the causal chain is known, and we realize it conforms causal laws, we can invert the direction of the inferential process and assert that, if the cause is present and all other circumstances are the same, the effect is produced by necessity. Hence, causal explanation is symmetric and allows law-like predictions as well as post hoc reconstructions. On the contrary, genetic understanding allows us, by empathy, to grasp the motivations that led the person to perceive, feel, or act as he did, but this knowledge cannot be subsumed under a law. Hence, while in that occasion he did something, he could also have done something else (here the concept of *freedom* applies), so we can at best realize that a general tendency occurred, but we can never be sure that in similar circumstances the person in question will do the same again.

Fourth, the possibility of understanding is limited. We cannot always relive in ourselves what is happening in our interlocutor. We can understand phenomena that at least in principle we can or could reexperience ourselves, and this means that understanding is based on a common ground between human beings, a shared world of meanings that make it possible. Thus, we can understand phenomena that we already know in a first-person perspective (e.g., we can understand the other's sadness because we know how is it like to be sad), or that we can know in principle (e.g., I can project myself into the other's life and circumstances and feel that if I was at his place, I would have felt as he did), or that we can feel as meaningful although exaggerated (e.g., we may say that at his place we would have not reacted as he did, but also feel that although such a reaction is quantitatively exaggerated, nevertheless it is qualitatively congruent with circumstances and personal features of the person in question). Famously, Jaspers' claim that schizophrenic primary delusions are un-understandable raised several critiques and was used by Binswanger and many others as a starting point to explore different ways to "understand" psychotic experiences (we will discuss this later). Here it shall be briefly remarked that some critiques were unfair to Jaspers, because what he really asserted was not that schizophrenic primary delusions had to be necessarily explained looking for neurobiological causes but simply that his method was limited and that psychopathologists had to be aware of such an intrinsic limitation. Jaspers himself mentions philosophical clarification as well as other forms of interpretation (not necessarily psychoanalytic) as other possible ways to transcend the limits of understanding.

Fifth, the limits of understanding are not fixed once for all. Interestingly, Ballerini (2003, p. 40) stressed that the limits of our ability to understand depend on "consistency, deepness, and duration" of the therapeutic relationship. Drawing on this concept, it was emphasized (Villareal and Aragona 2014) that there are at least four basic features influencing the possibility of understanding:

1. The characteristics of the clinical setting, which may be more or less favorable to self-disclosure
2. The duration of the therapeutic relationship
3. The personal characteristics of the patient
4. The personal characteristics of the clinician

Accordingly, the limits of understanding are not fixed but movable and changeable, and understandability itself shall not be conceived as an intrinsic characteristic of psychopathological phenomena but as an *emerging relational property* within the clinical encounter.

As seen, the analysis of the main features of Jaspers' concept of understanding raises several problems, the most important being epistemological: empathic understanding entails an implicit twofold movement, i.e., I must have a direct access to my own emotions, and I shall recognize that what I'm feeling is how the person in front of me actually feels. Here two epistemological problems are involved, the first being the more general problem of introspection (do we have any direct access to our own mental states?) and the second being the more specific problem of empathy ("how do I know that I am not projecting my own experiences onto the other?" Stanghellini 2013, p. 338). An analysis of these questions is far beyond the possibilities of this introduction, but the reader shall be aware of them as well as of other epistemological shortcomings (Oulis 2014) that make Jaspers' understanding an approach to psychopathology which is still useful and important, but also in need of revision.

1.6.5 Looking for the Essence (Eidetic Research)

We already introduced words like "eidos" and "eidetic research," which are the technical terms used by Husserl to describe the aim of phenomenological analysis after bracketing pre-given ordinary and theoretical knowledge. In the intentional act of exploring phenomena as they give themselves to consciousness, the aim is to progressively remove unessential properties and perspective views in order to grasp the essence of the thing itself. Roughly, if the thing remains itself after progressively removing several features (e.g., color, shape, and so on) but finally vanishes when a feature is eliminated, then that feature is its essence. Farina (2014, p. 55) stresses the intuitive nature of Husserl's essences: "This knowledge of the essence of things is what Husserl calls "eidetic intuition", which takes place not by abstraction or comparison of similar things, as erroneously believed the empiricists, but by a direct intuition of what is universal". This emphasizes a possible contrast between an intuitional and an empirical understanding of Husserl, which maybe explains similar interpretative fluctuations in the reception of Husserl's "rigorous method" (as Husserl himself was used to call it) by clinicians.

Binswanger imported Husserl's essences in the psychopathological debate. In an early methodological paper (Binswanger 1923), he claims that psychopathologists should advance, step by step, from the particular empirical and individual facts toward the meta-empirical, general pure essences described by Husserl. Binswanger appears well aware of the meaning Husserl had given to the word "essence" and to his eidetic research. In fact, he clearly writes that when we consider perceptive acts, we acknowledge that we can perceive the same object (a key, in his example) from an endless series of possible points of view, but we see a unique object (this description conforming to Husserl's concept of "synthesis"). Moreover, he rightly defines Husserl's phenomenology as a discipline describing the essence of the immanent products of consciousness. Hence, it is sure that in 1923 Binswanger has a good knowledge not only of Husserl's *logical researches* but also of his further eidetic development in the *ideas*. Despite this fact, there are some significant differences in Binswanger's own way to conceive essences. In fact, his essences are more akin to immediate artistic intuitions than Husserl's rigorous derivation from subsequent and systematic acts of eidetic variation. For example, Binswanger writes that when we see Marc's colored horses, the painter clearly forces nature by representing a blue or a red horse, and nevertheless he has seen and expressed the proper "essence" of the horse. This seeing is not through the eyes, but it is an immediate awareness that looks inside, which has nothing to envy to sensorial knowledge and yet it is maybe more reliable. In the same article, Binswanger returns on this point and specifies that such an intuitive vision of essences in scientific phenomenology should not be confused with the artistic intuition, but also that the two forms of intuition have "undoubtful and strict relationships" which are beyond the contraposition between science and art. Therefore, a significant space for interpretation remains here, so that in psychopathology phenomenological reduction and eidetic appraisal tend to fluctuate between scientific dissection of phenomenal appearances at one side and a more global and intuitive vision of essential themes on the other side. Binswanger's famous clinical cases may be read as examples of the second type.

Finally, in a recent article, Stanghellini and Rossi (2014) contrast both superficial mental symptoms (like those described in diagnostic manuals) and endophenotypes to a new level of analysis that they call the "pheno-phenotypes paradigm." In this view, mental symptoms are not accidental meaningless disturbances occurring to a patient. Rather they are the manifestation of some implicit quintessential "core" change in the fundamental structures of the patient's subjectivity.

It is this fundamental global "core" of human subjectivity which transpires through the single symptoms and gives to the whole syndrome a specific and characteristic *Gestalt* that many psychopathologists call "phenomenological essence."

1.6.6 A Hermeneutic Framework for Psychopathology

The primary "object" of inquiry of phenomenological psychopathology "is the patient's subjectivity, focusing on patients' states of mind as they are experienced and narrated by them" (Stanghellini and Rossi 2014, p. 238). At this level, it aims at "a systematic knowledge of patients' experiences, so that the features of a pathological condition emerge in their peculiar feel, meaning, and value for a patient" (Stanghellini and Rossi 2014, p. 238). It is noteworthy that here is already at play a hermeneutic approach, because subjective experiences are not simply "given"; they are not objects that can be simply itemized in operative diagnostic criteria. Mental symptoms are the product of a complex hermeneutic process involving a recursive interpretation between two poles: the patient's self-interpretation of what he/she is feeling and the clinician's interpretation of what the patient is trying to communicate. Due to different personal, familial, and sociocultural conceptual categories and idioms of distress, the patient may perceive, interpret, and express differently what he/she is experiencing (cp. Berrios 2013b; Aragona and Marková 2015). Similarly, another interpretative act "is performed by the listener who must sometimes interpret the speaker's meaning by asking the speaker and himself "what does he mean by that?" This problem, which plagues psychopathological research and clinical practice, becomes even more acute in using standardized assessment, since when interviewees respond to questionnaires, they might have very different understandings of the questions, and this may lead to the inaccurate conclusion that different individuals or groups have similar experiences or beliefs. An interview is a linguistic event. It is not a behavioral-verbal interchange simply *mediated by* language. Rather, it happens *in* language" (Stanghellini 2013, p. 326). Accordingly, subjective mental states may be opaque to its owner and *errors in translation* may always occur; nevertheless, this hermeneutic status of mental symptoms is constitutive, and for this reason a hermeneutic approach to psychopathology is not a philosophical surplus but a necessary requirement in psychiatric and psychological trainings. In fact, the acknowledgment of the hermeneutic co-construction of mental symptoms "implies, in practice, that the coding of each item of an interview always requires an (often laborious) process of interpretation—rather than a pseudo-objective simple 'ticking'" (Stanghellini 2013, p. 326).

If this applies to the hermeneutics of any individual symptom, it should also be stressed that phenomenological psychopathology considers the assessment of symptoms as part of a more general diagnostic "hermeneutic circle" where symptoms are recognized because they are part of a whole picture, the latter being more than a mere sum of items in a list (Aragona 2013). In other words, it "goes beyond the description of isolated symptoms and the use of some of those symptoms to establish a diagnosis. It aims to understand the meaning of a given world of experiences and actions grasping the underlying characteristic modification that keeps the symptoms meaningfully interconnected" (Stanghellini 2010, p. 320). Hence, the manifold of (abnormal) phenomena in a syndrome is interconnected, and the internal links between them are not etiological (i.e., based on causal relationships) but phenomenological (based on meaningful relationships). Stanghellini (2010) proposed the concept of structure to enlighten such a meaningful interconnection of apparently manifold phenomena. Meaningfulness shall be found in the structure itself, without involving elements that do not belong to the structure. Hence, meaningfulness emerges from the internal links between the elements of the structure, which are not juxtaposed but interrelated. Let's consider the following examples: Bleuler's acknowledgment of a meaningful interplay between the experience of primary symptoms and the reaction of the personality leading to secondary symptoms, Minkowski's *trouble générateur*, the phenomenological *eidos* which in a single phenomenon summarizes what is characteristic of the entire picture, the search of a common *Gestalt* characterizing the entire syndrome, and Huber and Klosterkoetter's description of a meaningful development from basic symptoms to full-blown mental disturbances. Even though they are the fruit of partly different perspectives, they exemplify the common view, in phenomenological psychopathology, that mental phenomena pertaining to a given syndrome are neither the result of a merely statistical association nor the product of a purely biological common pathophysiology. Rather, they are part of a meaningful whole where possible outputs of neurocognitive basic disturbances may trigger the person's "top-down" reaction seeking to make sense of such basic changes. This highlights the patient's active role in interacting with his/her distressing experiences and in the shaping of his/her symptoms, course, and outcome (Stanghellini et al. 2013). It is this self-hermeneutic process that makes understandable the meaningful link between apparently manifold symptoms in a given patient, i.e., the common structure of the whole clinical picture.

The process described above introduces a third point which is fundamental in phenomenological psychopathology: the central "active role that the person, as a self-interpreting agent or "goal-directed being" engaged in a world shared with other persons, has in interacting with his/her basic disorder and in the shaping of psychopathological syndromes" (Stanghellini et al. 2013, p. 289). This entails a shift of attention from apparent symptoms to the deeper level of the person's life-world or, as it is often said, the way the human presence (*Dasein*) is in the world and with others (*in-der-Welt mit-Dasein*). Here the single symptoms as well as their meaningful interconnection in the syndrome's structure are seen as the phenomena through which the hidden dimension of existence is made manifest. Accordingly, it was proposed that in psychopathology a phenomenological motto should be "making the invisible visible" (Stanghellini 2013, p. 333), meaning that through the *text* produced in the clinical encounter between patient and clinician, the deep architecture of the life-world inhabited by the person shall emerge.

Such a deep structure is particularly emphasized by Cargnello (2010), who remarks that the primary "object" of the phenomenological inquiry is neither the mental phenomenon as natural object nor the mere subjectivity of the sufferer or the examiner. On the contrary, it is a non-derivable primum, i.e., how the human presence projects himself/herself in the world and at the same time reveals himself/herself in expressing it in his/her original *exsistere*.

The phenomenological search for a deep structure of subjectivity, which makes possible the emergence of abnormal experiences and their organization in mental disorders, builds on and extends the work of Minkowski, von Gebsattel, Straus, Binswanger, Tellenbach, Tatossian, Lanteri Laura, Blankenburg, and many others. The way they approach the matter is interrelated but also different on some points. Here we will focus on a representative example, i.e., Binswanger's *Daseinsanalyse*. According to Needleman (1963), it can be generally considered as a transposition of Heidegger's *Daseinsanalytik* to the problems of psychiatry, although we shall stress that Binswanger does not simply import Heidegger's concepts but actively reinterprets them. We have already introduced some key concepts of Heidegger's philosophy, so we can focus only on those notions which play a major role in the analysis of the way the human being projects his existence in the world and with the other human fellows. We just remember that Heidegger's *Sein und Zeit* was conceived as a metaphysical inquiry on the Being and an anthropological use of it is possible only because the human being (*Dasein*) is the being that poses the question of the Being. Binswanger's anthropological analysis of the human presence is clearly a misinterpretation of Heidegger's ontological intentions, and nevertheless it has been heuristically fruitful, not only in psychopathology.

The image of man which is suggested by this "implicit" Heideggerian anthropology is that while natural objects are mere presence (*Vorhandenheit*), i.e., objects that can be observed from outside and subdivided in their properties, human beings are open projects displaying their potentialities.

They are already and constitutively in the world, and for the human beings the objects of the world are originally known not as mere objects but as possible tools to be used, as something "at-hand"; accordingly, the pragmatic context is primary, and cognitive objectification (what we now call representationalism) is a secondary and derived modality.

Humans are already together, in mutual relationship with their human fellows (*mit-Dasein*); accordingly, we are originally part of a human community and the problem of solipsism can only arise in a secondary reflective stance, having already severed the knowing subject and the objects of knowledge.

Humans are intrinsically hermeneutic entities, implicitly self-interpreting their position in the world, in their own context, and attuning to it; accordingly, self-interpretation before being a reflective introspectionism is a pre-reflective accordance within the situation, which usually appears obvious because of such pre-reflective attunement.

Humans are also in a given emotional basic attitude, in a given time and space, and so on.

All these concepts can be heuristically imported in psychopathology, opening the possibility to study the basic structure of our patients through the analysis of the so-called existentials, and in effect this is Binswanger's project: "The intention governing Binswanger's *Daseinsanalyse* was to understand psychiatric symptoms as the expression of an alteration of the structural components of one's basic being-in-the-world. To do this, he had to take the ontologically determined existentials[5] of Heidegger and bring them into the frame of concrete human existence (that is, applying the ontological a prioris to the concrete individual)" (Kraus 2010, p. 3).[6]

According to Needleman (1963), the existential a prioris function in a manner analogous to the Kantian categories, in that they are the forms through which ontic reality can manifest itself to the *Dasein*. And Kraus (2010) adds that because Heidegger's *Existentialien* are the fundamental structures of *Dasein*, and because the openness of *Dasein* makes the being-in-the-world of the person possible, the existentials can be conceived as different kinds of possible-being (*Sein-können*). In other words, they are basic possible ways to be, allowing a study and a comparison of the different ways of being-in-the-world characterizing psychopathological conditions.

According to Stanghellini (2013, p. 344), "The guidelines for reconstructing the life-world a person lives in are the so called *existentialia*, namely, lived time, space, body, otherness, materiality, and so on. [...] In this way we can trace back this transformation of the life-world to a specific configuration of the embodied self as the origin of a given mode of inhabiting the world, perceiving, manipulating, and making sense of it." In this way, the phenomenological analysis of the basic existential dimensions of human existence aims at disclosing and grasping the conditions that make possible the emergence of surface symptoms. In this vein, Heidegger's *existentialia* are the implicit, tacit, and pre-reflexive core structures of experience or, using different words, the way subjectivity must be structured to make phenomena appear as they appear to the experiencing human subject.

1.7 Conclusions

This book is structured in two parts. The individual chapters represent the second part and are organized with a progressively abstracting structure that should lead the reader from the living material of concrete case histories to the theoretical

[5] Existentials, existentialia, and existential a prioris are different translations of the same term, i.e., Heidegger's *Existenzialien*.

[6] This last sentence introduces another fundamental distinction between the ontological level, which is the study of the Being, pertaining to the metaphysics (the level of analysis in Heidegger's Being and Time), and the ontic level, which is the level of concrete existence of this or that being. Needleman labels Binswanger's approach as "meta-ontic," as something lying in between the ontological and the ontic level. To avoid unnecessary complications, it is enough to consider that the ontic level is the level of concrete existence and that psychopathological analyses, dealing with the way of being in the world of real persons, can be conceived as ontic analyses.

implications for clinical practice and research in psychiatry, clinical psychology, and psychotherapy. Written by leading phenomenologists, these chapters are concrete examples of the importance and usefulness of a phenomenological approach to persons experiencing mental sufferance. This introduction represents the first part of the book and should provide the reader with an overall picture of the methods used in phenomenological psychopathology. In doing so, we tried to be sensitive to historical development of the ideas and philosophical influences, although the main focus was to draw a comprehensive (and hopefully understandable) schema of the main methods and concepts used in phenomenological psychopathology. Focusing on theoretical issues, this *Introduction* is abstract compared to the living relationships between patients and healers that were at the basis of these theoretical concepts. We consider this as the necessary price to be paid in order to give the reader a general idea of the matter in a synthetic text. We are confident that the concrete examples flourishing in the following chapters will provide the reader of the necessary exemplars to concretely visualize the issue in its full complexity and comprehensiveness.

A few final remarks are needed in order to stress the main points discussed in this Introduction.

First, we argued that phenomenological psychopathology is important per se in order to give clinicians the needed skills to understand and appropriately take care of persons experiencing mental sufferance. However, we also stressed that this is even more important in this particular period of scientific crisis of psychiatry, when the general *Zeitgeist* and the consonant proposals to solve the crisis are strongly oriented toward reductionist neurocognitive models, with the concrete risk to see patients as deanimated bodies. At the opposite, phenomenological psychopathology focuses on persons. It is a person-centered, empathic, and value-friendly approach to mental sufferers which are seen more as companions of a common experience aimed at the empowerment than as mere carriers of broken mechanisms. Hence, phenomenological psychopathology stresses the importance of taking care of persons as a whole, not just of some dysfunctional parts of their bodies.

Second, we tried to show the main methods and theoretical commitments underlying the phenomenological approach. We stressed that phenomenological psychopathology is not a monolith but a method partly shared by original thinkers holding a family resemblance. Accordingly, not all distinctions and concepts are assumed by all thinkers, and free thinking and possibility to dissent are values that phenomenological psychopathology endorse. On this respect, its approach is very far from some "parochial" approaches pervading many schools of thought in psychiatry and psychology. In phenomenological psychopathology, there is not an orthodox knowledge to be strictly followed and defended. In general, positive knowledge on single issues is important but not as much as the ability to cultivate doubts and methodological self-criticism, in line with the Kantian epistemology where reason criticizes itself in order to respect its own limits. Phenomenological psychopathology respects other points of view, suggesting that many different perspectives can contribute to knowledge, provided that they do not pretend to have a total and absolute knowledge (see on this Jaspers' critique of prejudices).

Hence, phenomenological psychopathology is not to be intended as a humanistic view against scientific and neurocognitive programs, but as a methodological stance rejecting absolutist thinking in general.

Third, we discussed the different meanings of the term "psychopathology," suggesting that we conceive it (with Jaspers) as a scientific discipline studying the phenomena presented by psychiatric patients with the aid of several methods of inquiry. We further subdivided psychopathology according to its "object" of study: definition and distinction of individual phenomena, their diagnostic relevance, the empathic method to grasp subjective experiences and their meaningful connection, and the art of unfolding the underlying structure of subjectivity that makes possible the emergence of mental symptoms.

Fourth, we described the main tenets of some representative philosophers who are part of the European tradition generally called phenomenology, including existential and hermeneutic approaches. In doing so, we stressed similarities but also differences, acknowledging that such a tradition is a fruitful exchange of ideas in the discussion of such differences.

Fifth, we described the main methodological concepts that psychopathologists use in order to properly assess the qualitative specificities of mental phenomena and subjective structure: the distinction between form and content, that between explaining and understanding, the different forms of empathic understanding (static and genetic understanding), the phenomenological *epoché* and the resulting *eidos*, and the analysis of the way the human being projects (or encounters difficulties in doing it) his/her existence in the world with others.

Finally, a section was specifically dedicated to the hermeneutic approach in psychopathology, discussing the hermeneutic stance at three levels: the hermeneutics of mental symptoms, the hermeneutic circle in the relationship between symptoms and diagnosis, and finally the hermeneutics of the deep subjective structure on which the previous levels are grounded.

In conclusion, we argued for a philosophically informed approach in the clinical encounter in psychiatry, clinical psychology, and psychotherapy, especially for the task of exploring the patient's subjectivity. The main reason for this is that the assessment and the comprehension of a psychic state require a kind of analysis which largely exceeds the range of a naturalistic approach. Accordingly, a *personal level* of analysis is required to assess and confer meaning to psychopathological experiences. Indeed, it is within a personal history and a sociocultural context that their peculiar significance can emerge and be understood in their *peculiar feel, meaning, and value* for the subjects affected by them.

In endorsing the legacy of phenomenological psychopathology and its emphasis on the analysis of subjectivity, we have sketched a framework for the psychiatric and psychological encounter aimed to a wide-range, fine-grained assessment of the patient's morbid subjectivity, which can be useful not only in the clinical but also in the research setting (Stanghellini 2013).

In the clinic, this approach can provide the background for unfolding the phenomena of the life-world inhabited by the patient, moving toward the illumination of the structures of subjectivity that allegedly *generate and structure* the phenomenal world.

In research, the reconstruction of the complexities of the patients' subjectivity and life-worlds may prove helpful to rescue fringe abnormal phenomena that are not covered by standard assessment procedures. Thus, it provides the basis for exploratory studies, for the assessment of real-world, first-personal experiences of subpersonal impairments since this approach is concerned with bringing forth the typical feature(s) of personal experiences in a given individual to establish objective, transpersonal constructs helpful for empirical research (Stanghellini and Ballerini 2008).

Finally, reflection on the philosophical resources for the psychiatric interview may help to combat the hegemony of de-narratization in the mainstream psychiatric biomedical model with its emphasis on matters of fact rather than on intelligible relations. Hermeneutics looks for significance in our actions, experiences, and beliefs, aimed at a co-construction of meaning combining personal experiences into a coherent story related to the personal level of experience. In doing so, it can be an antidote to the dehumanization of psychiatry and of psychiatric patients.

References

American Psychiatric Association. (2013). *Diagnostic and statistical manual of mental disorders* (5th ed.). Washington, DC: American Psychiatric Association.

Andreasen, N. C. (1995). The validation of psychiatric diagnosis: new models and approaches. *American Journal of Psychiatry, 152*, 161–162.

Andreasen, N. C. (2007). DSM and the death of Phenomenology in America: An example of unintended consequences. *Schizophrenia Bulletin, 33*, 108–112.

Aragona, M. (2009a). The role of comorbidity in the crisis of the current psychiatric classification system. *Philosophy, Psychiatry and Psychology, 16*, 1–11.

Aragona, M. (2009b). About and beyond comorbidity: Does the crisis of the DSM bring on a radical rethinking of descriptive psychopathology? *Philosophy, Psychiatry and Psychology, 16*, 29–33.

Aragona, M. (2009c). *Il mito dei fatti. Una introduzione alla filosofia della psicopatologia*. Rome: Crossing Dialogues.

Aragona, M. (2012). The study of subjective experience as a scientific task for psychopathology. *Journal of Evaluation in Clinical Practice, 18*, 155–156.

Aragona, M. (2013). Neopositivism and the DSM psychiatric classification. An epistemological history. Part 2: Historical pathways, epistemological developments and present-day needs. *History of Psychiatry, 24*, 415–426.

Aragona, M. (2014a). Rethinking received views on the history of psychiatric nosology: Minor shifts, major continuities. In P. Zachar, D. S. Stoyanov, M. Aragona, & A. Jablensky (Eds.), *Alternative perspectives on psychiatric validation* (DSM, ICD, RDoC, and beyond, pp. 27–46). Oxford: Oxford University Press.

Aragona, M. (2014b). Epistemological reflections about the crisis of the DSM-5 and the revolutionary potential of the RDoC project. *Dialogues in Philosophy, Mental and Neuro Sciences, 7*, 11–20.

Aragona, M., & Marková, I. S. (2015). The hermeneutics of mental symptoms in the Cambridge School. *Revista Latinoamericana de Psicopatologia Fundamental, 18*, 599–618.

Ballerini, A. (2003). La psicopatologia tra «comprendere» e «spiegare». In A. Garofalo & L. Del Pistoia (Eds.), *Sul comprendere psicopatologico* (pp. 31–48). Pisa: Edizioni ETS.
Batson, C. D., Fultz, J., & Schoenrade, P. A. (1990). Adult's emotional reactions to the distress of others. In N. Eisenberg & J. Strayer (Eds.), *Empathy and its development* (pp. 163–184). Cambridge: Cambridge University Press.
Berrios, G. E. (1993). Phenomenology and psychopathology. Was there ever a relationship? *Comprehensive Psychiatry, 34*, 213–220.
Berrios, G. E. (2013a). Jaspers and the first edition of Allgemeine Psychopathologie. *The British Journal of Psychiatry, 202*, 433.
Berrios, G. E. (2013b). Formation and meaning of mental symptoms: history and epistemology. *Dialogues in Philosophy, Mental and Neuro Sciences, 6*, 39–48.
Berrios, G. E. (2013c). *Per una nuova epistemologia della psichiatria*. Rome: Fioriti Editore.
Binswanger, L. (1923). Über Phänomenologie. Referat, erstattet auf der 63. Versammlung des schweizerischen Vereins für Psychiatrie in Zürich am 25. November 1922. *Zeitschrift für die gesamte Neurologie und Psychiatrie, 82*, 10–45.
Cargnello, D. (2010). *Alterità e alienità, II edizione (1977)*. Rome: Fioriti Editore.
Cuthbert, B. N., & Insel, T. R. (2013). Toward the future of psychiatric diagnosis: The seven pillars of RDoC. *BMC Medicine, 11*, 126.
Dilthey, W. (1977). Ideas concerning a descriptive and analytic psychology (1894). In *Descriptive psychology and historical understanding* (pp. 21–120). The Hague: Martinus Nijhof.
Farina, G. (2014). Some reflections on the phenomenological method. *Dialogues in Philosophy, Mental and Neuro Sciences, 7*, 50–62.
First, M. B. (2012). The National Institute of Mental Health Research Domain Criteria (RDoC) project: Moving towards a neuroscience-based diagnostic classification in psychiatry. In K. S. Kendler & J. Parnas (Eds.), *Philosophical Issues in Psychiatry II: Nosology* (pp. 12–18). Oxford: Oxford University Press.
Fulford, K. W., Stanghellini, G., & Broome, M. (2004). What can philosophy do for psychiatry? *World Psychiatry, 3*, 130–135.
Fulford, K. W. M., & Stanghellini, G. (2008). The third revolution: Philosophy into practice in Twenty-First Century psychiatry. *Dialogues in Philosophy, Mental and Neuro Sciences, 1*, 5–14.
Gabbani, C., & Stanghellini, G. (2008). What kind of objectivity do we need for psychiatry? *Psychopathology, 41*, 203–204.
Gadamer, H. G. (1960). *Wahrheit und Methode: Grundzüge einer philosophischen Hermeneutik*. Tübingen: Mohr.
Heidegger, M. (1927). *Sein und Zeit*. Halle: Max Niemeyer.
Heidegger, M. (1982). *The basic problems of phenomenology (1927)*. Bloomington: Indiana University Press.
Hornsby, J. (2000). Personal and sub-personal: A defence of Dennett's early distinction. *Philosophical Explorations : An International Journal for the Philosophy of Mind and Action, 2*, 6–24.
Husserl, E. (2001). *Logical investigations* (Vol. 1, 1900). Abingdon and New York: Routledge
Insel, T., Cuthbert, B., Garvey, M., Heinssen, R., Pine, D. S., Quinn, K., Sanislow, C., & Wang, P. (2010). Research domain criteria (RDoC): Toward a new classification framework for research on mental disorders. *American Journal of Psychiatry, 167*, 748–751.
Janzarik, W. (1976). (Die Krise der Psychopathologie. *Nervenarzt, 47*, 73–80.
Jaspers, K. (1963). *General psychopathology (1947)*. Chicago, IL: University of Chicago Press.
Kraus, A. (2010). Existential a prioris and the phenomenology of schizophrenia. *Dialogues in Philosophy, Mental and Neuro Sciences, 3*, 1–7.
Kuhn, T. S. (1970). *The structure of scientific revolutions* (2nd ed.). Chicago and London: University of Chicago Press.
Kupfer, D. J., First, M. B., & Regier, D. A. (2002). Introduction. In D. J. Kupfer, M. B. First, & D. A. Regier (Eds.), *A research agenda for DSM-V* (pp. xv–xxiii). Washington, DC: American Psychiatric Association.

Maj, M. (2012). DSM-IV: Some critical remarks. In K. S. Kendler & J. Parnas (Eds.), *Philosophical issues in psychiatry II: Nosology* (pp. 161–164). Oxford: Oxford University Press.
Merleau-Ponty, M. (2013). *Phenomenology of perception (1945)*. London and New York: Routledge.
Miles, A., & Mezzich, J. E. (2011). The care of the patient and the soul of the clinic: Person centered medicine as an emergent model of modern clinical practice. *The International Journal of Person Centered Medicine, 1*, 207–222.
Murphy, D. (2006). *Psychiatry in the scientific image*. Cambridge, MA: MIT Press.
Needleman, J. (1963). Introduction. In L. Binswanger (Ed.), *Being in the world*. New York: Basic Books.
Othmer, E., & Othmer, S. C. (2002). *The clinical interview using the DSM-IV* (Fundamentals, Vol. 1). Washington, DC: American Psychiatric Publishing.
Oulis, P. (2014). The epistemological role of empathy in psychopathological diagnosis: a contemporary reassessment of Karl Jaspers' account. *Philosophy, Ethics, and Humanities in Medicine, 9*, 6.
Ricoeur, P. (1969). *Le conflit des interprétations*. Paris: Éditions du Seuil.
Rosini, E., Di Fabio, F., & Aragona, M. (2013). 1913-2013: One hundred years of General Psychopathology. *Dialogues in Philosophy, Mental and Neuro Sciences, 6*, 57–66.
Rossi Monti, M., & Stanghellini, G. (1996). Nosografia e psicopatologia: Un matrimonio impossibile? *ATQUE, 13*, 179–194.
Rossi-Monti, M. (2013). Jaspers' 'Critique of Psychoanalysis': Between past and future. In G. Stanghellini & T. Fuchs (Eds.), *One century of Karl Jaspers' general psychopathology* (pp. 27–41). Oxford: Oxford University Press.
Sartre, J.-P. (2004). *The imaginary: A phenomenological psychology of the imagination (1940)*. New York and London: Routledge.
Schneider, K. (1975). *Klinische psychopathologie* (10th ed.). Stuttgart: Thieme.
Sirgiovanni, E. (2009). The mechanistic approach to psychiatric classification. *Dialogues in Philosophy, Mental and Neuro Sciences, 2*, 45–49.
Stanghellini, G. (2007). The grammar of the psychiatric interview: A plea for the second-person mode of understanding. *Psychopathology, 40*, 69–74.
Stanghellini, G. (2010). A hermeneutic framework for psychopathology. *Psychopathology, 43*, 319–326.
Stanghellini, G. (2013). Philosophical resources for the psychiatric interview. In K. W. M. Fulford (Ed.), *The Oxford handbook of philosophy and psychiatry* (pp. 320–355). Oxford: Oxford University Press.
Stanghellini, G., & Ballerini, M. (2008). Qualitative analysis. Its use in psychopathological research. *Acta Psychiatrica Scandinavica, 117*, 161–163.
Stanghellini, G., & Broome, M. R. (2014). Psychopathology as the basic science of psychiatry. *British Journal of Psychiatry, 205*, 169–170.
Stanghellini, G., & Fuchs, T. (Eds.). (2013). *One century of Karl Jaspers' general psychopathology*. Oxford: Oxford University Press.
Stanghellini, G., Fulford, K. W. M., & Bolton, D. (2013). Person-centered psychopathology of schizophrenia. Building on Karl Jaspers' understanding of the patient's attitude towards his illness. *Schizophrenia Bulletin, 39*, 287–294.
Stanghellini, G., & Rossi, R. (2014). Pheno-phenotypes: A holistic approach to the psychopathology of schizophrenia. *Current Opinion in Psychiatry, 27*, 236–241.
Strauss, J. S. (1992). The person-key to understanding mental illness: Towards a new dynamic psychiatry-III. *British Journal of Psychiatry, 161*(suppl 18), 19–26.
Tatossian, A. (1997). *La phénoménologie des psychoses. L'art du comprendre, numéro double, Juillet*. Paris: Le Cercle Herméneutique.
Turner, S. M., & Hersen, M. (2003). The interviewing process. In M. Hersen & S. M. Turner (Eds.), *Diagnostic interviewing* (3rd ed., pp. 3–11). New York, NY: Spring Street.

Villareal, E., & Aragona, M. (2014). El concepto de "comprensión" (Verstehen) en Karl Jaspers. *Vertex, 116*, 262–265.

Walker, C. (2013). Form and content in Jaspers' psychopathology. In G. Stanghellini & T. Fuchs (Eds.), *One century of Karl Jaspers' general psychopathology* (pp. 76–94). Oxford: Oxford University Press.

Zachar, P., & Jablensky, A. (2014). Introduction: The concept of validation in psychiatry and psychology. In P. Zachar, D. S. Stoyanov, M. Aragona, & A. Jablensky (Eds.), *Alternative perspectives on psychiatric validation* (DSM, ICD, RDoC, and beyond, pp. 3–24). Oxford: Oxford University Press.

2 Phenomenological Investigation of Obsessive-Compulsive Disorder

Martin Bürgy

2.1 Phenomenological Methodology

It is not always immediately apparent what the term "phenomenological" actually means. There is no coherent methodology of phenomenology. Instead, each individual phenomenological method used must, depending on the subject under investigation, be redetermined and described anew (Blankenburg 1991; Kraus 2001; Schmidt-Degenhard 2011).

The etymological alignment with the concept of the phenomenon (Greek, *phainomenon*) refers to "that which appears" quite generally to whatever is perceived via the senses (Schischkoff 1991). The concept itself therefore already contains on outline of the polarity between the imagined object and the consciousness which envisions it which is common to all the phenomenological approaches in their heterogeneity. The first philosophical and systematic examination of *The Phenomenology of the Spirit* by Hegel in 1807 was intended to demonstrate that the spirit takes on a materialised form in history and, in the consciousness of humans, comes to awareness of itself (Hegel 1988). The history of philosophy in the second half of the nineteenth century was marked by a growing disillusionment about the opportunities of gaining knowledge by means of speculative idealism and a romantic metaphysics, which, together with the progress in the natural sciences, led to an orientation of philosophy towards the factual (Lembeck 1994). The immediate experience is the starting point for a phenomenological philosophy, which sets out to describe phenomena in way which surpasses those provided by all forms of science and reflection. Heidegger later described this development as a "return to the things themselves!" (Heidegger 1979, p. 27). His own thinking was also initially still oriented around the pole of the object only later, with the publication of *Being*

M. Bürgy (✉)
Center of Mental Health, Klinikum Stuttgart, Germany

University of Heidelberg, Heidelberg, Germany
e-mail: M.Buergy@klinikum-stuttgart.de

G. Stanghellini, M. Aragona (eds.), *An Experiential Approach to Psychopathology*,
DOI 10.1007/978-3-319-29945-7_2

and Time (*Sein und Zeit*) in 1927, to complete the change from phenomenology to a hermeneutics oriented on the existential basic structures of human being (Pöggeler 1983). Husserl is the actual founder of the first phenomenological philosophy, which he conceived of as being a theory of experience and which he claimed to be a fundamental science (Husserl 1901). "Getting to the thing" therefore means, for Husserl, undertaking as precise a description as possible of the objects of which a person is directly aware. Through this process concepts were led back to their "original sources in imagination" (Husserl 1984, p. 154). Description is a struggle for imagination and idea, as well as to bring these together in the experience of evidence. Husserl called this "descriptive psychology" or the "descriptive method". Jaspers transferred the descriptive method into psychopathology and thus brought the experiences of people with mental illness into focus (Langenbach 1995). The later developments of Husserl, moving away from the pole of the descriptively recorded object towards the pole of the constituting consciousness, i.e. to transcendental phenomenology, were not followed by Jaspers (Jaspers 1977). Throughout his life, he retained his adherence to descriptive proximity to the object under investigation and to the clarity of the method used. This subdivision into two poles, one oriented descriptively to the object and the other hermeneutically oriented to the consciousness of the person experiencing the object, has remained determinant of the phenomenological method until the present day (Schmidt-Degenhard 1997). Because Jaspers, and in clinical practice following him above all Kurt Schneider, placed the emphasis in methodology on descriptive phenomenology and on the investigation of the profile of experience altered by psychopathology, they have continued to have a decisive influence on psychiatric classification into the present day. The use of more hermeneutic approaches was ruled out in order to exclude speculative understanding and to secure the fundamental boundary between psychotic and nonpsychotic experiences for the purposes of psychiatric nosology (Bürgy 2008). At the same time, however, there are indeed approaches towards a broader conception of understanding in Jaspers which, however, did not find their way back into clinical theory and practice. In the "general psychopathology", we encounter three different ways of understanding which Jaspers continued to modify from the first edition of 1913 up to his final revision of the last edition of 1959 (Jaspers 1913, 1959). Here understanding always means "the conception of the psychological which is gained from within" (1959, p. 24), which has an impressive immediacy and which is developed in a methodical sequence of stages. The first stage is that of "static understanding", which focuses on the direct experience of the patient in the here and now and which is classed as being descriptive phenomenology. The second stage is that of "genetic understanding" in which an attempt is made to put oneself in the patient's view in order to investigate how psychological phenomena arise from one another. The "empathetic understanding" was initially presented by Jaspers as a stand-alone method, but it was later logically subsumed under the genetic understanding. Jaspers initially still called his third stage "understanding and interpreting" but he later renamed this as "seizing the totality". By this he meant that research which has as its subject the individual and the specific cannot succeed without an orientation to the whole. The movement from the individual to the whole, for example, from individual phenomenon to the total experience of the person or from the individual symptom to the prototypical unity of the mental disorder, is completed in the hermeneutic circle (Spitzer 1985). In the rest of this article, I will therefore refer to this third level of understanding as "hermeneutic understanding". These three ways of understanding described here are built on one another and are intertwined. The further understanding is removed from the direct object of experience by the choice of the method used, and the more it brings into focus the genesis or the entirety of the person and the illness, or the general points underlying it, the more interpretive and speculative, but also the more complete the findings made will be. These methodological procedures have either not yet explicitly or only in part been realised in relation to mental illnesses. Even the two major case studies by Tellenbach on Melancholy (Tellenbach 1971) and by Blankenburg on Schizophrenia (Blankenburg 1971) lack this methodological order. In his later work on *Phenomenology as the Foundation Discipline of Psychiatry* (*Phänomenologie als Grundlagendisziplin der Psychiatrie*) of 1991, Blankenburg correctly wrote: "For the future, it will remain an important task to bring descriptive and genetic or hermeneutical phenomenology into a close relationship with one another" (Blankenburg 1991, p. 99).

Phenomenological investigation of obsessive-compulsive disorder should follow the specified sequence of stages from the static understanding, via the genetic understanding, to the hermeneutic understanding. We have therefore selected historical and clinical findings accordingly and ordered them in accordance with the specified stages of understanding. The clinical examples here are intended above all to illustrate the static understanding and its transition into the genetic understanding.

2.2 The Static Understanding

The first description of a patient with obsessive-compulsive disorder in the sense of a fear of touching is found in Esquirol in 1839. He emphasises the two characteristics of the constant fight against the obsessive thoughts whilst at the same time maintaining the insight into their ridiculousness (Esquirol 1839). In the German-speaking countries, it was von Krafft-Ebing who introduced the term of obsessive ideas in 1867. However, he used this term to describe an obsession which the melancholy state of mind exercises on imagination (v. Krafft-Ebing 1867). In an 1868 lecture to the Berlin Medical-Psychological Society, Griesinger described three patients who had obsessive ideas which were not supported by affect (Griesinger 1868). Westphal was, in 1877, the first person to provide a definition of obsessive-compulsive syndrome, and this definition, though it has since been modified, remains valid to this day. "By obsessive ideas I mean those ideas which, with otherwise normal intelligence and without being determined by an emotional or affect-like state appear in the mind of the person affected by them, against and contrary to their will and which they cannot remove, such that these ideas prevent and intersect with the person's normal course of ideas. These ideas are always experienced by the person as being abnormal and alien to him and as being ones which he would oppose were he in full control of his consciousness" (Westphal 1877, p. 669). In his work *Conceptual Investigation into Obsession* (*Begriffliche Untersuchung über den Zwang*) in 1939, Kurt Schneider explicitly disputes the work of Westphal and arrives at a "core definition" which is linguistically simpler and extremely sharp and which later found its way into his clinical pathology. "We speak of obsession when a person is unable to displace contents of his consciousness even though he finds these to be nonsensical or experiences them to be dominating his thoughts without good reason to do so" (Schneider 1939, pp. 23–24). With this formulation Schneider not only created the preconditions for making a differential diagnostic delimitation between delusional and affective disorder but he also created an orientation for the diagnostic classification of obsessive-compulsive disorder which has remained valid until the present day. His definition was accepted into the psychiatric classification systems even though it has since undergone further modifications.

Whilst ICD-10 places obsessions (obsessive thoughts) and compulsions (compulsive actions) in a relationship to one another in which they are both of equal value and equivalent to one another, DSM-IV (APA 1994) allocates the obsessive-compulsive disorder to the category of the anxiety disorder which means that a dynamic relationship is implied between the primary obsession (usually obsessive thoughts, which create anxiety) and the secondary compulsion (usually compulsive actions which serve to control the anxiety) (Kapfhammer 2008). DSM-5 (APA 2013) does indeed set aside the subordination of the obsessive-compulsive disorder to the category of anxiety disorder, and it introduces degrees of insight into the foolishness of the compulsions, but it retains the structure of conditions in relation to obsessions and compulsions (Ehret and Berking 2013). Kurt Schneider had already preformulated this relationship between primary and secondary compulsions in his work cited of 1939: An item of the contents of consciousness intrudes to which the "I" then adopts a position. Schneider maintained his descriptive position, and this is presumably why he never made any reference to the works of Binder who, a few years previously, had characterised the primary compulsion as being the actual "disturbing psychism" which is followed by the "defence psychism" (Binder 1936). In a publication on obsession in the strict sense, I pointed especially to the importance for differential diagnostic purposes of the distinction between primary obsessions and secondary compulsions (Bürgy 2007). Using three case reports, I was able to demonstrate that on the behavioural level, it is only unspecific symptoms, above all compulsive washing and compulsive checking, which impress us. On examination of the primary phenomena which underlie the actions, however, it becomes clear that we are dealing here with delusional and primarily paranoid thoughts rather than obsessive thoughts.

The organisation of the obsessive-compulsive phenomena described found its way into the further attempts at differentiating between obsessive-compulsive disorders because, despite their great formal similarity, obsessive-compulsive symptoms vary very widely in their extent and their phenomenological embodiment. One advance in this field is provided especially by the factor-analytical determination of subtypes (Bloch et al. 2008; Leckman et al. 2010). Concentrating on the four most important groups, the behavioural therapists Hoffmann and Hofmann have in an exemplary manner presented in detailed phenomenological terms the aspects of threat and defence inherent in the obsessive-compulsive disorder which means that the original significance of the anxiety affect for the initiation of secondary compulsions has been further relativised (Hoffmann and Hofmann 2004).

1. *Compulsive checking:* The perceived threat to the individual which is at the root of compulsive checking is that feeling of incompleteness which Janet was the first to describe in relation to obsessive-compulsive disorder (Ecker and Gönner 2006). In an act of defence, this primary feeling is externalised and symbolically fought against. There is therefore, for example, no end to the checking of electrical appliances and plug sockets because neither the person's affect nor his insight arrives at the conclusion that the action has been completed. The patient suffers from the conviction that there is a permanent threat emanating from him, which always seeks and finds new contents.

Case Report

A 40-year-old patient worked as a laboratory technician. In his own words, he derived all of his feelings of self-worth from his career and from the fact that he was able to handle carcinogenic and radioactive substances in a responsible manner. He had been having a relationship with his girlfriend for many years during which time he had only seen her at weekends. His girlfriend had, however, recently moved in with him and, combined with the pressures of his job, this had become too much for him to handle. He had adapted himself too much to meeting her needs and to doing everything to please her. This became an ever-increasing strain on him and he felt anger and a fear of loss at the same time. He finally developed feelings of disgust and felt increasingly exhausted. Because of this inner confusion and tension, he became less and less able to concentrate on his work. What had previously seemed obvious to him was now suddenly no longer obvious. Suddenly he no longer knew whether he had closed the containers containing the poisonous substances properly or not. He began to check the lids of all the containers and this took him longer and longer to do. He could not stop performing these checks, and he could no longer say at what time he had closed the containers. The things which he perceived became alien to him—in the sense of derealisation/depersonalisation—and he became obsessed only with his checking the lids of the containers. Finally he attempted to institute only a very exact number of checks and to follow a very particular procedure for them. This, however, no longer gave him any feeling of certainty or security, and he finally even began to remove any supposed impurities from the

(continued)

laboratory. He began to clean the laboratory, to wash his hands and to disinfect them. Once again he was less and less able to stop doing these things but started doing them more and more, even outside the laboratory.

We can see the transition to the genetic understanding in the very accounts which the patient gives us of his experiences as he himself tried to understand what the consequences of all his checking the lids of the containers might be. He reported that during his childhood, he had suffered severe physical abuse at the hands of his father which had left him with scars on his back. He also reported that his mother had been powerless and had only felt able to stand up to his father by threatening to commit suicide. By doing this, however, she had also frightened the patient who feared losing his mother. The patient had always cared for his mother and he still made sure she was alright today. At the time the patient was, however, only able to understand that because of his childhood experiences of human relationships, he felt that he was at his girlfriend's mercy and experienced inner tension and confusion. He was, however, not able to understand why his actions got out of control and why he was no longer able to set proper limits for completing his actions.

2. *Compulsive repetition, compulsive orderliness and obsessive thoughts:* These are all related to the threat posed to a person by his thoughts about blasphemy, his own serious misdeeds, illness, dirtiness, contamination as well as of shame in relation to his own person or body. Compulsive repetition and compulsive orderliness are attempts to neutralise this threat. The psychological disturbance at the root of this behaviour is not, for example, the fear that a fire could break out or that a close relative could be harmed in an accident, but rather it is the fear that one could have caused the fire or the accident oneself and without anybody else noticing this. This kind of thinking is magical thinking and indicates the person has deficiencies in his self-perception. His consciousness and awareness are not reliable.

Case Report

A clinical example concerning a female patient can help us to understand obsessive thoughts and their relationship to compulsive actions. A 29-year-old woman reported that her grandmother whom she adored had been living in an old people's home for some years. Her grandmother's health had recently been continuously deteriorating. During the patient's last visit to her grandmother, her grandmother had suffered from particularly severe pain which really upset the patient. Her grandmother's doctor happened to be present and he suggested that since the grandmother's pain relief medication had so far proved to be ineffective, he would give her pregabalin. The patient wanted her grandmother's pain to be reduced and so she strongly supported

(continued)

the doctor's suggestion. Because, however, the patient's grandmother became very tired after being given the medication, the patient became convinced that she had killed her grandmother. She therefore felt that she had to visit her grandmother more often so that she could make sure that her grandmother was still alive and that she had not killed her. In addition to her feelings of guilt, during her visits to her grandmother, the patient also experienced a fear that she had either thought or imagined something bad which could also have harmed her grandmother. For example, she imagined that there was a knife sticking into her grandmother and there was blood everywhere. She tried to think of other things to counteract these thoughts and kept checking to see if there was any blood anywhere and whether or not her grandmother was still alive. She finally became trapped by her feelings of guilt and could no longer even visit her grandmother. Instead she sent her parents and her boyfriend to check whether her grandmother was still alive.

3. *Washing, polishing and cleaning compulsions:* A thorough examination of the roots of these phenomena shows that they are not based on a fear of the threat of contamination but that central to them is a disgust at the thought of potentially touching or having touched the objects in question. A closer examination of the fear of contamination and disease shows that this is merely a secondary rationalisation of a primary, overpowering sensitivity to disgust. As a representative of the German phenomenological-anthropological school, von Gebsattel had in 1954 already described the "disgust-phobia of the obsessive-compulsive patient" and stated this to be the original cause of compulsive washing (v. Gebsattel 1954).

Case Report

A 26-year-old patient developed a significant washing compulsion over the course of her pregnancy. Quite a long time previously, she had stopped having sexual intercourse with her husband because she feared that this would cause bleeding. This had actually happened during her pregnancy. As towards the end of her pregnancy her baby descended lower into the birth canal, she began to experience feelings which she could no longer differentiate from one another with any certainty: She did not know whether these were her unborn baby's movements, labour pains or whether they were caused by sexual excitement. She was afraid that she would lose her baby and sad about her feelings whilst at the same time feeling ashamed about talking about them. She felt disgusted by dirt and her head was so full of thoughts and she felt so confused that she began to wash herself frequently. She knew that this was mad but she was trying to wash away her thoughts and her inner confusion. She washed her entire body but "it" was also hiding in her

(continued)

clothing. After being visited by her gynaecologist, who had manipulated parts of her body and who had therefore also triggered the feelings described, she threw away the clothes which she had been wearing during the doctor's visit. She felt a very deep sense of disgust at having to touch these clothes. She said that towards the end of her pregnancy, she was only able to sit for many hours each day in the bath whilst her husband had to rub cream into her skin which had become macerated by all the constant washing.

4. *Collecting and hoarding:* Compulsive collecting and hoarding relate to objects of relatively low value, which over the course of time fill living spaces, making them unusable for the purposes of actually living. Secondary rationalisations for this type of behaviour are thriftiness or providing against times of emergency. The patient feels an intimate connection with the objects for which the patient is responsible and to which he in part ascribes mental or spiritual emotions. The function of these behaviours is to create a sense of security against the threat posed by dissolution and emptiness by indulging in this hoarding behaviour. Authors such as Lang, Quint and Bürgy have therefore attributed the origins of this phenomenon to a "disorder of the self" or to a "weakness in the integration of the I" (Lang 1986; Quint 1988; Bürgy 2001).

Case Report
A 61-year-old patient became preoccupied with recording conversations which he had overheard. This first happened after he had once overheard a brief conversation that two people were having as he walked past them. Later on, this scene came into his mind again and he felt an urge to reconstruct the conversation he had overheard word for word. He was indeed able to reconstruct most of it but even whilst he was doing this, he did not know why he was doing it. Perhaps it was because he did not want to surrender a little piece of his own experience, a little piece of his own life story, into oblivion and thus into final dissolution. On another occasion he had been able to remember everything about a conversation which he had overheard in the neighbouring town except for one single phrase. He really taxed his brain but he could not remember this phrase. The next morning everything became clearer and he had narrowed it down to a choice between two possible phrases. Each of these would, however, have given an entirely different meaning to the conversation, depending on which one of them he selected. Because he was unable to choose between these two phrases, he got into such a state of anxiety and tension that he travelled to the neighbouring town and stood at the spot where he had overheard the conversation. He stood there waiting until one of the protagonists came along so that he could ask him about the exact words which had been used in the conversation he had overheard. In the same way that this

(continued)

patient wanted to hold on to conversations he had overheard, he also hoarded everyday items such as newspapers, tin cans, exercise books and so on. He was unable to part from these things because each of these things was experienced as being a part of himself. In his own words, separation from any of these things would cause him a sense of inner emptiness which he would not be able to bear (Hoffmann and Hofmann 2004, S. 223–224).

This search for this experience of obsessions and compulsions and its dynamics in the patient and establishing a connection to personality and its development, to cognition and emotions, takes from the static to the genetic understanding of obsessive-compulsive disorder.

2.3 The Genetic Understanding

Up until the nineteen eighties, the view had stubbornly persisted that an obsessive-compulsive character has formed the personality basis for the development of obsessive-compulsive disorder (Bürgy 2005a). Kretschmer, Jaspers and Schneider had, however, already pointed out that sensitive personality features were a prerequisite of obsessive-compulsive disorder. Kretschmer wrote in his last revision of his book *Physique and Character* of 1931: "The sensitive person is sentimental, impressionable but restrained and processes experiences retrospectively. He has a long lasting hidden affective tension, is ethically sensitive and ambitious, feeling unsure of himself he tends to feelings of guilt and hides behind an asthenic façade a pronounced, if also inhibited wish to assert his own will" (Kretschmer 1977, p. 183). In 1986 Lang extended the dimension of inner conflict psychic around the social view of the obsessive-compulsive neurotic person by terming him an "inhibited rebel" (Lang 1986). These findings are supported by the results of comorbidity studies which show that in 51–75 % of cases of obsessive-compulsive disorder, there is also a personality disorder from Cluster C of the DSM classification system which is described as follows: a tendency to be easily offended by criticism and rejection, the exaggeration of potential problems, continuous tension and anxiety, a feeling of helplessness and dependency, enormous separation anxieties, excessive conscientiousness, a lack of flexibility and passive aggression (Csef 2001; Zaudig 2011).

The question remains, however, as to how obsessions and compulsions develop on the basis of this personality configuration. In the classical psychiatric literature, there are two basic approaches to the explanation of obsessions and compulsions. On the one hand, in authors like von Kraepelin, Aschaffenburg, Störing and von Gebsattel, the focus is on the genesis of affect. In the other approach, obsessions and compulsions are seen as being a disorder of thought content and are therefore moved closer to delusion. This approach is found in the works of authors like von Westphal, Binder and Schneider (Bürgy 2005b, 2007). Freud was one of the first researchers who attempted to combine these two positions. In his work *Notes on a Case of Obsessional Neurosis* (*Bemerkungen über einen Fall von Zwangsneurose*) of 1909, he described the primary battle between two strongly contradicting feelings, especially between love and hate, which leads to strong feelings of insecurity, ambivalence, weakness of will and the creation of neurotic symptoms in the form of symbolic compulsive actions. As a secondary effect, the obsession becomes isolated from the affect so that in the case of obsessive-compulsive disorder, virtually no affect is present. Binder felt that the cause of the start of obsessions resulted from a failure of integration and von Gebsattel traced it back to the disintegration of affect (Binder 1936; v. Gebsattel 1968). Von Gebsattel describes in subtle casuistry the case of man with a washing compulsion. He, however, fails "to integrate the feeling of disgust in an ordered way into the structure of the person" (p. 193). Affect and cognition are always closely associated with one another. Hoffmann and Hofmann also stress the importance of the intensity of feelings and the confusion between them at the start of the illness. The person will above all experience affects such as pain, grief, loneliness, anxiety, disgust and rage (Hoffmann and Hofmann 2004). In some of my works, I have described on a casuistic basis the situation which triggers the obsessive-compulsive condition as follows: At the root of obsession, the person feels a deeply anchored sense of insecurity and anxiety and the associated inner tension and also has inadequately differentiated affects. By this, I merely mean that the person has a poorly developed ability to identify, express and communicate affects. On this basis, the person feels, in a situation where he is emotionally overwhelmed, a confusion between contradictory affects which take control in turn and are intensified in a vicious circle of powerlessness, helplessness and isolation. The obsessional thought which appears suddenly attaches itself to a biographically charged, external object in order to subdue the inner chaos, whilst compulsive actions are, in addition, attempts to re-establish the control which has been lost. The strengthening of defences against these, however, does not bring calm to the person but instead serves to further build up the obsessive-compulsive symptoms so that these are appreciably extended.

Case Report

A case study of the start of an illness can help us to understand how the symptoms develop, via confusion of affect, from a biographically relevant event: A patient who was at the time 26 years old reported on the background events in her life story. She said that her father had been especially egotistic and self-opinionated. He had been dissatisfied with his life and indifferent towards his family. Her mother had, on the other hand, been strict but fair and had gone back to work immediately after the patient's birth because they needed the money. She said that working and bringing up her children had been too much for her mother which is why she overwhelmingly reacted to

(continued)

her daughter with impatience and irritation. The patient had gone to great lengths to get on with her parents, especially her mother, but without success. She remained uncertain and anxious during her interactions with her mother. In kindergarten she had felt excluded and in school she had felt as though her opinions did not go down well with the other children. They often teased her until she exploded. When she was 16, the boys had made her really afraid that they were going to attack her in the school magazine. She said that she had then run all the way home, afraid, furious and in despair. She had wanted to talk to her mother about it in order to calm herself down but her mother had just carried on doing the ironing and had, as always, reacted to her dismissively and with irritation. She said that at this point she had experienced a tremendous rage against her mother and had imagined strangling and stabbing her. She also said that she had imagined the iron exploding. Her mother had then, in the confusion which she had created, actually forgotten to switch off the iron which nearly caused a fire in their apartment. The patient had blamed herself for this and had developed a fear of losing her mother. She had also subsequently not been able to switch off her thoughts that the electrical appliances in her apartment might catch fire and explode. She had therefore started to check everything. She reported that she had become visibly less certain and threatened that her compulsions could be transferred to other situations and objects. She said she had thought that someone might break into her house and that she herself might carry harmful bacteria into the home on her hands and infect the other members of the family. She said that this was why she had begun to constantly check doors and windows and to wash her hands. She said that she had doubted the success of these actions which she was, however, not able to stop performing. She said she had known that her thoughts made no sense but that she had made no further progress in combating her anxiety and insecurity. (Bürgy 2005b, S. 223).

In the context of the behaviour therapy treatment involving exposure to the traumatic stimuli and prevention of a reaction to them, the original affects and thoughts associated with the trigger situation and their associated biographical memories are brought to the surface time and time again. The original confusion is then followed by the therapeutic differentiation of the emotions, the establishment of a sense of reality and the activation of the self-system which includes all the person's previous experiences, feelings, convictions and values as well as the constitution of an active I subject (Hoffmann and Hofmann 2010).

2.4 The Hermeneutic Understanding

The primary threatening aspect in obsessions and compulsions is characterised by an inner state, which can be described as a confusion of affect including the danger of disintegration, a sense of incompleteness and depersonalisation. Von Gebsattel attempted to summarise all the different ways of experiencing threat and specified them above all as "immobility", "a tendency to remain in the same state", "relative lack of emotion", "severe isolation" and a "directionless, free-floating character" (v. Gebsattel 1954). As a consequence of the defensive aspects of this condition, the person therefore develops an inability to complete actions. Von Gebsattel therefore describes the anthropological dimension of obsessive-compulsive disorder as a discontinuation of a person's personal development in time. Time and life at stand still and future is switched off. In von Gebsattel's *Prolegomena to a Medical Anthropology*, which has already been mentioned, he describes the consequences of this disruption to personal development as follows: "For the obsessive-compulsive person, what has happened in the past does not take the form of a completed action, it assails him as something uncompleted and overwhelms him with symbols of impurity, dirtiness and death" (p. 144). The standing still of time with the associated loss of the future leads over into the theme of death in obsessive-compulsive disorder.

In 1938 Erwin Straus published the autobiographical account of a female patient whose compulsive washing developed from an original fear of death which is only secondarily displaced, and always in external respects, into the experience of disgust (Straus 1938). In 1965 Skoog found unsettling death motifs in more than 70 % of obsessive-compulsive patients who were specifically asked about this by him (Skoog 1965), and in 1972 Schwidder found that the fear of a death which could occur at any time was the central fear of people with obsessive-compulsive disorder (Schwidder 1972). The topic of death is still even important in current publications for people with obsessive-compulsive disorder (Hoffmann and Hofmann 2013). Conventional symbols of death, such as crosses, people in mourning clothes, hearses and cemeteries, etc., create a strong feeling of unease in people with obsessive-compulsive disorder as well as the magical expectation that a disaster will happen. The fear of decay, illness and death, mixed with disgust, is regularly hidden behind compulsive washing.

Probably the most intensive and the most differentiated treatment of the death motif is that of the Göttingen psychiatrist J. E. Meyer. In Meyer's opinion the phobic element which already manifests itself in the initial phase of obsessive-compulsive neurosis points to the avoidance of death which is always immanent in life and thus at the same to a life which is unlived (Meyer 1973, 1975). Meyer included obsessive-compulsive disorder amongst the thanatophobic neuroses (Meyer 1982) and thus provided an interpretation, which is also found in the structural-anthropological approach of Hermann Lang (Lang 1998). Lang takes up Freud's idea of the special importance of the death wish in obsessive-compulsive disorder. Using the example of Shakespeare's dramatic character Lady Macbeth, he develops the significance of compulsive washing as a defence against guilt and death.

The fear of death and dying is to be found in the many of the fears of an obsessive-compulsive patient: the fear of dead creatures, of corruptible matter, of dirt and of dust; and the fear of anything which is definitive, unrepeatable or unpredictable in life. And this fear of death is hidden behind hopeless and exhausting battles, extreme caution, care and vigilance. These security systems are used to fend off a more primal experience, which cannot be fully relinquished in the present moment with all its dangers and possibilities.

2.5 Conclusions

At the beginning of the paper, I presented a methodological classification system, which has indeed already been defined as being "phenomenological", but for which no single model has yet been worked out and transferred into clinical practice. In the present study, this was illustrated using selected material in relation to obsessive-compulsive disorder as an example of this method. Under the heading of the static understanding of this topic, there was an initial description of the development of obsessive-compulsive disorder and its subtypes. The disruptive and the threatening aspects with the basic confusion of affects, depersonalisation and feeling of incompleteness were brought into focus, and it is on these that the defensive aspects of the condition are based. There is an inner tension which is deeply rooted in the personality, and the biographical development of the obsessive-compulsive person who finds it very difficult to accept reassurance is at the same time inhibited. This can most clearly be seen in the situation which triggers the onset of the condition. Both in the experience of the person with obsessive-compulsive disorder and in the hermeneutic interpretation of the disorder, the fear of death and defence against it and thus the anthropological dimension of obsessive-compulsive disorder can be recognised. The thanatophobic obsessive-compulsive person attempts to stop time and impermanence and thus rapidly falls victim to the pressure of his passing and unlived life. The disruptive and threatening aspects of the obsessions and compulsions therefore permeate all levels of his understanding as far as his fear of death which becomes ever more apparent and which is not ameliorated by living a meaningful life.

Static, genetic and hermeneutic dimensions of understanding must be repeatedly associated with and related to one another in the hermeneutic circle. This will lead us to both the analytical classification of previous findings and to their synthetic combination in the wholeness of the patient which, to follow Jaspers on this point, must always remain open and incommensurable.

References

American Psychiatric Association. (1994). *Diagnostic and statistical manual of mental disorders: DSM-IV*. Washington, DC: American Psychiatric Association.
American Psychiatric Association. (2013). *Diagnostic and statistical manual of mental disorders: DSM-5*. Washington, DC: American Psychiatric Association.
Binder, H. (1936). Zur Psychologie der Zwangsvorgänge. In: Ausgewählte Arbeiten (Selected Works) (1971). Band 1. Huber, Bern, S. 221–317.
Blankenburg, W. (1971). *Der Verlust der natürlichen Selbstverständlichkeit. Ein Beitrag zur Psychopathologie symptomarmer Schizophrenien*. Stuttgart: Enke.
Blankenburg, W. (1991). Phänomenologie als Grundlagendisziplin der Psychiatrie. *Fundamenta Psychiatrica, 5*, 92–101.
Bloch, M. H., Landeros-Weisenberger, A., Rosario, M. C., Pittenger, C., & Leckman, J. F. (2008). Meta-analysis of the symptom structure of obsessive-compulsive disorder. *American Journal of Psychiatry, 165*, 1532–1542.
Bürgy, M. (2001). The narcissistic function in obsessive-compulsive neurosis. *American Journal of Psychotherapy, 55*, 65–73.
Bürgy, M. (2005a). Psychopathology of obsessive-compulsive disorder. A phenomenological approach. *Psychopathology, 38*, 291–300.
Bürgy, M. (2005b). Zur Psychopathologie des Zwangs. Zeitschrift für klinische Psychologie. *Psychiatrie und Psychotherapie, 53*, 213–229.
Bürgy, M. (2007). Obsession in the strict sense. A helpful psychopathological phenomenon in differential diagnosis between obsessive-compulsive disorder and schizophrenia. *Psychopathology, 40*, 102–110.
Bürgy, M. (2008). The concept of psychosis: Historical and phenomenological aspects. *Schizophrenia Bulletin, 34*, 1200–1210.
Csef, H. (2001). Zwang und Persönlichkeit. *Persönlichkeitsstörungen, 5*, 81–90.
Ecker, W., & Gönner, S. (2006). Das Unvollständigkeitsgefühl. Neuentdeckung eines alten psychopathologischen Symptoms bei Zwangserkrankungen. *Nervenarzt, 77*, 1115–1122.
Ehret, A. M., & Berking, M. (2013). DSM-IV und DSM-V: Was hat sich tatsächlich verändert? *Verhaltenstherapie, 23*, 258–266.
Esquirol, E. (1839). *Des maladies mentales considérées sous les rapports medical, hygiénique et médico-legal*. Paris: Bailliére.
Freud S (1909) Bemerkungen über einen Fall von Zwangsneurose. In: Gesammelte Werke, Band 14. Fischer, Frankfurt, 1941, S. 379–463.
Griesinger, W. (1868). Über einen wenig bekannten psychopathischen Zustand. *Archiv für Psychiatrie und Nervenkrankheiten, 1*, 626–635.
Hegel, G. W. F. (1988). *Phänomenologie des Geistes (1807)*. Hamburg: Meiner.
Heidegger, M. (1979). *Sein und Zeit (1927)*. Tübingen: Niemeyer.
Hoffmann, N., & Hofmann, B. (2004). *Expositionen bei Ängsten und Zwängen*. Weinheim Basel Berlin: Beltz.
Hoffmann, N., & Hofmann, B. (2010). *Zwanghafte Persönlichkeitsstörung und Zwangserkrankungen*. Berlin Heidelberg: Springer.
Hoffmann, N., & Hofmann, B. (2013). *Wenn Zwänge das Leben einengen* (14th ed.). Berlin Heidelberg: Springer.
Husserl, E. (1901). *Logische Untersuchungen*. Halle: Niemeyer.
Husserl, E. (1984). Logische Untersuchungen II. Untersuchungen zur Phänomenologie und Theorie der Erkenntnis. Husserliana Band 19. Nijhoff, Den Haag.
Jaspers, K. (1913). *Allgemeine psychopathologie*. Berlin: Springer.
Jaspers, K. (1959). *Allgemeine psychopathologie* (7th ed.). Berlin: Springer.
Jaspers, K. (1977). *Philosophische autobiographie*. München: Piper.
Kapfhammer, H-P. (2008). Zwangsstörung. In: Möller H-J, Laux G, Kapfhammer H-P (Hrsg) Psychiatrie und Psychothrapie. Band 2. 3. Auflage. Springer, Heidelberg, S. 633–658.

Kraus, A. (2001). Phenomenological-anthropological psychiatry. In F. Henn, N. Satorius, H. Helmchen, & H. Lauter (Eds.), *Contemporary psychiatry* (Vol. 1, pp. 339–356). Berlin Heidelberg: Springer.

Kretschmer, E. (1977). Körperbau und Charakter. 26. Auflage. Springer, Berlin.

Lang, H. (1986). Zur Struktur und Therapie der Zwangsneurose. *Psyche, 11*, 953–970.

Lang, H. (1998). Ätiologie und Aufrechterhaltung der Zwangsstörungen aus psychodynamischer Sicht. In H. Ambühl (Ed.), *Psychotherapie der Zwangsstörungen* (pp. 23–30). Stuttgart, New York: Thieme.

Langenbach, M. (1995). Phenomenology, intentionality, and mental experiences: Edmund Husserl's Logische Untersuchungen and the first edition of Karl Jaspers's Allgemeine Psychopathologie. *History of Psychiatry, 6*, 209–224.

Leckman, J. F., Denys, D., Simpson, H. B., Mataix-Cols, D., Hollander, E., Saxena, S., Miguel, E. C., Rauch, S. L., Goodman, W. K., Philips, K. A., & Stein, D. J. (2010). Obsessive-compulsive disorder: A review of the diagnostical criteria and possible subtypes in dimensional specifiers for DSM-V. *Depression and Anxiety, 27*, 507–527.

Lembeck, K. H. (1994). *Einführung in die Phänomenologische Philosophie*. Darmstadt: Wissenschaftliche Buchgesellschaft.

Meyer, J. E. (1973). *Tod und Neurose*. Göttingen: Vandenhoeck & Ruprecht.

Meyer, J. E. (1975). Die Todesthematik in der Entstehung und im Verlauf von Zwangsneurosen. *Zeitschrift für Psychotherapie und medizinische Psychologie, 25*, 124–128.

Meyer, J. E. (1982). *Todesangst und das Todesbewußtsein der Gegenwart* (2nd ed.). Berlin Heidelberg New York: Springer.

Pöggeler, O. (1983). *Heidegger und die hermeneutische Philosophie*. Freiburg: Alber.

Quint, H. (1988). *Die Zwangsneurose aus psychoanalytischer Sicht*. Berlin Heidelberg: Springer.

Schischkoff, G. (1991). *Philosophisches Wörterbuch* (22nd ed.). Stuttgart: Kröner.

Schmidt-Degenhard, M. (1997). Zur Standortbestimmung einer anthropologischen Psychiatrie. *Fortschritte Neurologie und Psychiatrie, 65*, 473–480.

Schmidt-Degenhard, M. (2011). Anthropologische Aspekte psychischer Erkrankungen. In H.-J. Möller, G. Laux, & H.-P. Kapfhammer (Eds.), *Psychiatrie, Psychosomatik, Psychotherapie, Band 1* (4th ed., pp. 383–396). Berlin Heidelberg: Springer.

Schneider, K. (1939). Begriffliche Untersuchung über den Zwang. *Allgemeine Zeitschrift für Psychiatrie und ihre Grenzgebiete, 112*, 17–24.

Schwidder, W. (1972). Klinik der Neurosen. In K. P. Kisker, J. E. Mayer, C. Müller, & E. Strömgren (Eds.), *Psychiatrie der Gegenwart, Band II/1* (2nd ed., pp. 351–415). Berlin Heidelberg New York: Springer.

Skoog, G. (1965). Onset of anacastic conditions. A clinical study. *Acta Psychiatrica Scandinavica Supplement, 184*, 1–82.

Spitzer, M. (1985). *Allgemeine Subjektivität und Psychopathologie*. Frankfurt: Haag & Herchen.

Straus, E. (1938). Ein Beitrag zur Pathologie der Zwangserscheinungen. *Monatsschrift für Psychiatrie und Neurologie, 98*, 61–81.

Tellenbach, H. (1971). *Melancholie: Problemgeschichte, Endogenität, Typologie, Pathogenese, Klinik*. Berlin: Springer.

v. Gebsattel, V. E. (1954). Die Welt des Zwangskranken. In: Prolegomena einer medizinischen Anthropologie. Springer, Berlin, S. 74–128.

v. Gebsattel, V. E. (1968). Die anakastische Fehlhaltung. In: Imago Hominis. Müller, Salzburg, S. 173–199.

v. Krafft-Ebing, R. (1867). Beiträge zur Erkennung und richtigen forensischen Beurteilung krankhafter Gemützustände für Ärzte, Richter und Verteidiger. Enke, Erlangen.

Westphal, C. (1877). Über Zwangsvorstellungen. *Berliner Klinische Wochenschrift, 46*, 669–672.

Zaudig, M. (2011). Heterogenität und Komorbidität der Zwangsstörung. *Nervenarzt, 82*, 290–298.

The Window and the Wound: Dysphoria and Anger in Borderline Disorders 3

Mario Rossi Monti

3.1 Carla

Carla is a 25-year-old young woman with pensive and penetrating eyes. She looks dynamic and intelligent. She has come to see me unwillingly, pushed by her mother. Their relationship, she tells me, is (and always has been) a very conflictual one. Her mother "accuses" her of being constantly distracted, careless, and inefficient both in life and at work; she also reproaches her for being extremely oppositional and for making life impossible for everyone in the family with her constant outbursts. Carla, with a ferocious tone, claims that, on the contrary, it is her mother who makes life impossible for her. This is, she goes on, the source of the incessant clashes plaguing their family life. Her father seems to be a helpless witness to all this. He is described as a tiny, inconsistent man completely absorbed by his job.

Carla describes this situation with sadness. Hers, however, is a sadness full of impatience and dull anger. Such impatience and resentment emerge with particular harshness as soon as the subject shifts from a general description of her family situation to her own problems and her request for consultation. When I start inquiring about the reasons that lead her to me (for consultation), she immediately takes on an air of challenge:

C. "I thought *you* were supposed to tell me that. I had no reason to come here! I have really nothing to say!" (The tone is very provocative and grumpy. I sense a very bad mood.)

T. (Surprised) "If you have nothing to say, well... neither do I... But I guess if you came here, you must have done so for some reason."

C. "Of course! But I thought you were the one asking the questions... I don't feel like talking about all these things... I have nothing to say. Besides, it took me

M.R. Monti (✉)
'Carlo Bo' University, Urbino, Italy
e-mail: rossimonti53@gmail.com

G. Stanghellini, M. Aragona (eds.), *An Experiential Approach to Psychopathology*,
DOI 10.1007/978-3-319-29945-7_3

one hour to find parking! I also live on the other side of town... Plus, psychologists and psychiatrists do not understand a damn thing.... They are just 'shrinks' who don't really care about people!"

She goes on with the same tone, pouring innumerable insults on the whole professional category...When I ask her if she is often in such a bad mood, she replies that yes, it happens often, both when she is with her family and at work. Carla works for a pharmaceutical company and is responsible for quality control of the work of the other employees. "Not an easy situation," I remark, assuming that, having to evaluate the work of other people, she must often find herself in a difficult position due to recurring criticism and recriminations. Mine, I thought, was just a trivial observation. Carla did not think so. She reacts with an explosion of anger and discontent:

C. "Here we go again! You talk in clichés too! What you say is what everyone thinks. But it is absolutely false! What do people know? I'm not just another bitch!"—and so on.

After this verbal assault, which I witness in silence, she seems to calm down, at least momentarily:

C. "The truth is that in this world no one can understand anyone."
T: "I guess one must feel very sad and lonely in such a world."
Pause. Carla starts weeping. It is an intense, visceral crying. Slowly she curls up and slides down the chair, almost to the point of disappearing. I did not expect the crying, especially such a pain-filled one—at least not so early.
C. "My life is a mess, I feel broken, I don't understand anything, there's the big bang inside of me... I don't know who I am or what I want... Each time I feel different, according to the people I deal with. The fact is that I am not what I look like. I don't know who I really am."

She shows me a tattoo on her arm that nobody knows about (indeed, it is very difficult to spot: at a first glance it looks like a mole, but it is in fact a tattoo of a black dot). A black hole. It is the only image—she says—she identifies herself with.

> I feel like I am always riding a roller coaster. In one hour, I can turn from utmost joy to utmost sadness. Nothing simply brushes me by: things whether completely overwhelm me or leave me totally indifferent... Everyone tells me to take it easy... But how? When I go to bed at night I find it hard to fall asleep because I am assailed by a swarm of thoughts. I cannot stop them. Such thinking and rethinking just kills me.

As she would later explain, Carla is unable to connect with other people on an intimate level. She thinks all her relationships are inauthentic ("mine are all fake relationships") and—so to speak—doomed to evaporate. In fact, they quickly go into pieces without leaving any trace or deposit in her mind. All this, at times, gives her a terrible sense of emptiness and dizziness:

> Those who don't know about it believe that to feel empty inside is no big deal. It's just emptiness—they think—you cannot really feel it. None of them knows that it feels like compressed air... It is an emptiness that weighs more than a wall of lead, an emptiness in which you do not fly: you fall. I don't feel my bones, my organs. I only imagine a deep emptiness in which I fall endlessly, like a stone... And to fall in it and to be swallowed by it also hurts."

When this feeling becomes unbearable—Carla says—she must do something sudden and "violent" (at least with respect to the impulsive way in which it is enacted). She picks a fight with someone. She breaks some object in the house. She grabs the scissors and rips a dress to shreds. Or, more often, she takes a cutter and cuts herself. Carla regularly cuts her arms. Despite her awareness that this behavior is "crazy," she cannot restrain herself: "the cuts—she says—help me to black out, to stop. Within me, I feel the gray of a mushy and uniform clay. I must see something different, the red of blood." Other times, she stuffs herself with food until it hurts without inducing vomiting afterwards.

Often, in the course of our therapeutic work, Carla would initiate the session by saying "Here we go again, I did it again, I cut myself. Do not ask me why. It's because I'm a bitch." But also because "after I cut myself, my head is finally free from thoughts... and maybe I even start to listen to some music." The pain of the wound—she would tell me in a different session—helps her to "pad" another kind of "pain": "the tangle in my stomach." And again, "when I was cutting myself, it was as if my body was following me: a mental pain becomes a physical pain—namely, it is solved by being transformed into something physical, making me feel physically in a certain way."

At the end of the first year of psychotherapy, a significant episode occurs, one that opens another window on Carla's self-harming behavior. It is about 6 months that she has quit cutting herself. This seems to be due to the fact that she had the opportunity (first of all during the sessions) to put the content of her experiences into words. Carla has also begun to write down and describe her feelings by taking notes on her mobile phone. One day she arrives at the session in despair. Something terrible has happened. She has accidentally deleted all her notes. There were more than a hundred of them. It was a true emotional archive. She felt the usual feeling of ineptitude. At the height of the tension, she took a knife and began to cut into her forearm. It was not a deep cut, but it was a cut. Carla had not done this for a long time. She then threw the knife away and started to write down frantically on a piece of paper (which she brought to the session). The note reads:

> You are a disgusting bitch. I want to dismember you, kick you in the head and tear the skin off of you. Not even a finger must be spared. I will butcher your hands, then cut them with an ax. You won't be left with a single vein intact. I want to open you up to get to the anger, that most hard lump you have in the chest, but already I struggle and lose heart as I think about it and I slam that unbreakable lump on the ground. It is as hard as steel, but I want to pull it out and set it on fire as I would do with your body-parts. You make me sick, remove

yourself from me! I want to go all the way down with the knife and scratch you bones, and maybe then I will enjoy a moment of glory and stop for a while for having gone too far. The word is too narrow a window to allow this lump to get out.

3.2 From the Borderline Disorder to the Borderline World

In the case described above, it is easy to recognize many of the elements which, according to the current psychiatric nosography, constitute the borderline personality disorder (DSM 5): identity disturbance, affective instability due to marked mood reactivity, chronic feelings of emptiness, inappropriate and intense anger, impulsivity, and self-harming behavior. The identification and the description of these symptoms are sufficient to perform a diagnosis in DSM terms, namely, in accordance with a descriptively and categorically oriented psychiatry. However, even if it tells us something about her disorder, such diagnosis tells us nothing about Carla as a person, about her lived experiences and her way of dealing with (or taking a stand toward) those symptoms. It is, as always happens when one adopts the method of clinical psychiatry, a diagnosis made from a third, impersonal perspective, based on the supposedly impartial description provided by an "observer."

But what happens inside Carla's world, a world that in order to be seen needs to be observed through her own eyes and words? If a description in the first person is to be made accessible, one has first to pay attention to all of Carla's statements and focus on what she feels and expresses through her words, her behavior, and her ways of relating to the others (with particular attention to the therapeutic relationship). What is important, as Karl Jaspers taught us more than a century ago, is that we must not blot out the chaos of phenomena by applying some diagnostic label to them. For the purpose of psychopathological knowledge, a precarious and contradictory diagnosis works better than a synthetic and monolithic one.

Indeed, the discrepancies affecting each diagnosis—Jaspers (1913) insisted—play a fruitful role: instead of exhausting every desire for knowledge, the diagnosis must remain a torment for the psychopathologist. In this sense, in order to recover its specific meaning, each of the symptoms described by clinical psychiatry must be rethought and repositioned on the basis of Carla as a person, with her history and her experiences. Only from this point a therapeutic plan can be developed. In order to clarify the elements from which one such plan can be developed, I will follow the same path followed by Carla during our sessions and focus on these three aspects: (1) the anger; (2) the feeling of emptiness, loneliness, inconsistency, and inauthenticity; and (3) the self-harming behaviors.

3.3 Borderline Anger

The first element that emerges in the encounter with Carla is her anger. Such anger, which takes the form of impatience and resentment, points, on the one hand, to her relationship with her mother and, on the other, to her relationship with the therapist. In fact, Carla's impatience toward her mother seems to extend seamlessly into the atmosphere of anger and challenge pervading our sessions. This limitless propagation of anger is one of the distinctive features of the borderline world. Quite often, to deal with a borderline patient means to deal with an angry person who in turn elicits anger. Inevitably, a great deal of anger begins to circulate. In the case of Carla, anger works as a kind of "business card" that not only describes what Carla experiences in her relationships but also how she deals with a new interlocutor. The anger with which she reacts to the first questions triggers a circuit of anger which inevitably drags the therapist with it.

Many therapists, in reporting about their work experience, have described a similar pattern: borderline patients are able to elicit a high amount of aggression and anger, thereby triggering those mechanisms of stigmatization and marginalization to which they often fall victim in the context of psychiatric services. Nancy McWilliams (2014) writes that, at the beginning, strong emotional reactions both in the patients and in the therapists are to be expected; such reactions cannot be dealt with by simply trying to appear professional and well-meaning. At Menninger Hospital, Glenn Gabbard (1999) had a young psychiatrist under supervision who, one day, confessed that he had had enough of a patient he had in treatment. He said he hated her and felt like strangling her. He did not want to see the patient again and asked to be replaced by another therapist. The fact is—as Gabbard clarifies—that the "treater's emotional reactions to the patient sweep through the course of treatment like a tempest with the potential to create havoc for the patient and the therapist."

How is one supposed to control oneself in front of such angered reactions? In fact, these reactions do not match the (often idealized) picture of the standard therapeutic relationship. According to Nancy McWilliams (2014), treating one's countertransfert as an obstacle to overcome is not the best solution to this problem. Rather, what proves essential is the ability to maintain a reflective attitude, to live the moment instead of criticizing one's own *unacceptable* feelings, to ask oneself what can be learned about oneself through these intense reactions, and to contain these powerful and undesired feelings rather than trying to suppress them. It is important for the therapist who deals with borderline patients to know that this procedure of "initiation" must be gone through. Of course, this awareness will not neutralize the therapist's emotional response (which would not be useful anyway), but at least will mitigate it. Moreover, when the therapeutic relationship becomes volatile (as with Carla), this kind of attitude allows a central aspect of the borderline relational functioning to come into view. This newly discovered territory immediately becomes both a battleground and a meeting place.

What is often striking at the beginning of the therapeutic relationship is the tendency of borderline patients to behave negatively and aggressively: typically, these patients challenge, attack, and give the therapist a hard time, intruding into his or her emotional and personal life. For the borderline person, anger is, so to speak, a way to establish and maintain contact with the others and the world. This way, a traumatic event that probably belongs to the patient's past is reactivated. At the same time, however, such event finally finds in the therapist an interlocutor who is (or should be) willing to experience it—to a certain extent—with the patient, to share it in the common search for a meaning and a new and different solution. In the words of a psychiatric worker, the borderline patient "is like one who spits in your face, but does so because he is looking for someone who, like a human thermostat, can help him regulate his emotions... But it's not easy to play that part when it is your face being spit upon." It is hard to work at the incandescent temperature of anger; it becomes even impossible when one is unable to attribute some meaning to that anger, a meaning that has both a strictly personal side (as in Carla's existential troubles) and a more general sense related to the experience of the world typical of the borderline personality.

According to Otto F. Kernberg (1992, 1994), the main functions of anger, from the most primitive to the most evolved, are:

(a) To eliminate, by means of a violent reaction, a source of irritation or pain
(b) To remove an obstacle to gratification
(c) To restore—by an extreme and desperate attempt—a sense of autonomy in the face of a very frustrating situation, trying to recreate a state of narcissistic equilibrium

The first two functions gravitate around an object that acts as a "source" of pain or as an "obstacle" to gratification. In this sense, anger presupposes the identification and focalization of an object as a target for one's arrows. The third function identified by Kernberg, instead, concerns the self and the effect that anger has on its condition.

Overall, the anger unleashed by the therapist's attitude (as in the case of Carla) seems to respond to the need to immediately structure the relationship along the anger/resentment axis. The potential space opened by the clinical encounter closes around the element of anger/intolerance/challenge with the identification of a target for one's anger, which is deemed responsible for all the experienced pain. But to identify the therapist as a target for one's anger also allows one to give cohesion and consistency to a self otherwise experienced (as would emerge in the dialogue with Carla) as empty, inauthentic, and inconsistent.

In a certain sense, we could conceive of anger as one of the most common ways by which the borderline tries to "get acquainted" with someone. Through the intensification of his or her hypersensitivity—namely, the ability to identify what is lacking in any environment and in any relationship so to angrily lament its absence—the borderline offers to an interlocutor who is willing to stand it the drama of his or her emotional life on a silver platter. In such a life, the recurring outbursts of anger reveal, just as sporadic volcanic eruptions do, an underlying, chronic turbulence wearing down both oneself and the others.

Anger and impulsive behaviors of the hetero-aggressive or (more frequently) self-harming kind represent a kind of "barrage fire" which often appalls the therapist and force him or her to keep the distance or even to retreat. The increasingly widespread stigmatization and marginalization of borderline patients within the psychiatric services is the product of this barrage fire. Therefore, the relationships that the psychiatric workers end up establishing with borderline patients are charged with anger, flooded by acting-outs and corresponding counteracting-outs, or poisoned by moralistic judgments. As Chiesa et al. (2000) rightly emphasized, "staff misunderstand patients' behavior. Specifically, staff fail to appreciate the fears and vulnerabilities behind acting-out, aggressive behavior [...] which are approached in a moralistic and punitive fashion."

At this level of the relationship, it is not possible to deal with the patient correctly unless the connection between the outbursts of anger and the underlying dysphoric mood condition affecting the entire borderline existence is properly understood (Pazzagli and Rossi Monti 2000; Stanghellini 2000). This dysphoric condition is often the legacy of an early traumatic event which is not necessarily related to a history of physical or sexual abuse but can be also connected to severe neglect or unpredictability and elusiveness on the part of the key figures (caregivers). The dysphoric mood typical of the borderline existence is ultimately related to the constant perception of the unpredictability and inconsistency of both the other and oneself. How can one live in a state where everything is blurred, where it is impossible to focus and see clearly? In such a condition the perception of oneself and the other becomes fuzzy, blurry, uncertain, fluctuating, ambivalent, and ambiguous, while the atmosphere becomes saturated with unpredictability, alarm, anxiety, and incomprehensibility. In this context, everything can become (and does become) traumatic—even a seemingly trivial remark like the one that angered Carla.

If the frequent and intense outbursts of anger are the most severe sign of borderline emotional suffering, then the dysphoric mood that sustains them is the true companion of the borderline emotional existence. In turn, dysphoria, which spreads something like a mist or a toxic gas in the borderline's experience of oneself, the world, and the other, could be seen as a crust enveloping a lump of indistinct emotions that the borderline subject fails to experience clearly or even to name, as if trapped in a sort of emotional illiteracy. The borderline emotional instability described by current psychiatric nosology points precisely to this emotional lump.

While dysphoria seems to be the most stable and persistent component of this emotional instability, other emotions, such as fear and anger, are expressed in a more acute and violent fashion. This emotional kaleidoscope is what Carla very well describes as the feeling of "always riding a roller coaster." Such feeling is probably connected to environmental or relational micro-occurrences which Carla cannot even become aware of, since borderline emotional instability is highly dependent on the context and is associated with poor emotional awareness. In fact, every process of emotional self-regulation presupposes some form of emotional awareness. An impairment of this function severely interferes with the process of feedback regulation of the intensity of the emotions. This way, in the borderline personality, emotions are experienced as autonomous physical and mental states that cannot be easily modulated, mitigated, or oriented in one direction rather than another. In this condition, one easily loses the sense of being the agent and source of one's emotional states: the awareness that a particular emotion originates within the self, that it belongs to it and has much to do with it and with the vicissitudes of the inner and outer world, is lost. When the borderline patient is not able to see himself as an active agent, such emotional states start fluctuating like vague and menacing entities, in search of a place to settle. The main, persistent, and tormenting result of this indistinct emotional magma is the dysphoric mood. This is the underlying mood condition animating the emotional outbursts which give Carla the impression of riding a roller coaster. Every violent emotion represents, to some extent, an opportunity to escape the painful condition of dysphoria, which is an objectless, and therefore hopeless, form of discontent. The borderline person seems to be always looking for an opportunity to turn a (senseless) dysphoria into an emotion that has a cause and an (apparent and contingent) meaning. Anger provides such opportunity.

But what is dysphoria? From a *general* point of view, dysphoria is a mood condition experienced as unpleasant, uncomfortable, negative, and oppressive, which exhibits all the characteristics typical of other mood states (it is enduring, devoid of an intentional object, unmotivated, rigid, and difficult to articulate; it completely engulfs one's perception of and relationship with the world, the others, and oneself). In this sense, the term "dysphoria" indicates an emotional state hard to endure: while euphoria is comparable to the feeling of wearing a comfortable dress that fits the body like a glove, dysphoria points to the exact opposite feeling. In this case, the subject experiences a state that, literally, does not suit him or her. Dysphoria is a feeling of alarmed and unsociable discontent, of an unpleasant tension, and of chronic irritation and irritability (Berner et al. 1987; Gabriel 1987); it can be hardly modulated and shows a growing propensity to impulsive actions. Its main components are *tension*, *irritability*, and *urge* (Rossi Monti 2012). In short, the mood condition typical of dysphoria has to do with the perception of something that is askew—something that went wrong and hinders one's life. Indeed, in dysphoria, *everything* goes wrong. It is difficult for most of us to imagine a condition in which this emotional state is constantly endured instead of being simply confined to an isolated experience (whether temporary or transient).

In the borderline functioning, the subject, utterly incapable of recognizing his or her discomfort, to make sense of it and to find a way to modulate it, is overwhelmed by it and, desperate to find ways to reduce the tension, is dragged into the abyss of impulsive actions (outbursts of anger, aggressive behaviors, use of drugs, self-harming behavior, etc.). This pervasive mood condition is durable and devoid of an intentional object (in the sense that the subject cannot ascribe it to a specific situation). Such condition dominates the borderline existence, an existence in which dysphoria envelops the subject like a thick fog.

In this context, the anger directed to an interlocutor becomes an invaluable escape route from the unbearability of the dysphoric condition. Anger provides a way to fill such condition with meaning. Indeed, anger as an emotion has an object, is intentional, and is motivated. In a state of anger, the object becomes clearly visible and strongly delineated and stands out quite distinctively. Such object is definitely *not* vague, blurred, and confused, and its features are easy to recognize.

To get angry with someone (or with something) means to make the object present, to take it out of its ambiguity, and to delineate some of its features very clearly: these mostly negative features function as "handles" to which anger can cling to. In this sense, anger allows one to switch from a typically dysphoric state of dispersion and, so to speak, "centrifugal pull" (where the object's outlines and features are blurred, vague, and ambiguous), to a condition in which the boundaries and characteristics of the object stand out with great clarity. Anger exerts a "centripetal" pull and allows the emotional dispersion to coagulate. Moreover, the transition from dysphoria to anger contributes to the preservation or recovering of a precarious cohesion of the self. The chance to observe the effects of one's anger on another person can also contribute to the development of this sense of increased vitality and cohesion. To the extent that one is able to scare the others, one is and exists as an acting and powerful subject.

Dysphoria turns into anger each time a specific object has been identified as the source and cause of one's suffering. In this sense, dysphoria resembles a widespread and unsaturated magmatic state in search of an object to converge onto. Instead of losing its way inside the dysphoric cloud, anger hunts down the object; forces it out of its vagueness, inconsistency, and anonymity; and turns it into the target of a sniper rifle. This is also how therapists and health workers feel when they become the target of borderline anger: they feel loaded with an amount of responsibility that often exceeds their understanding and ability to endure. In the context of a temporality dominated by the "absorption into the immediacy," where only the moment counts (Bin Kimura 1992), the transformation of dysphoria into anger invariably provides the subject with the illusion that the emotional and relational tangle in which he or she has always been trapped has finally been unraveled.

At some level, the patient's outburst of anger signals the presence of hope. In other words, it implies the belief that under the blows of anger, the object, the environment, or reality itself can react and respond to the violence of the stimulus, thereby regaining the role they had never played or had lost. Anger, therefore, is not the same as resignation or annihilating despair; rather, it is a desperate, vital reaction that presupposes both an interlocutor to be held accountable and the possibility of a response. At the same time, anger plays a role in the management of the pain caused by the separation and the irreparability of the loss: somehow, a mind that engages in angry fantasies is still clinging to what it has lost.

3.4 Emptiness, Inconsistency, and Inauthenticity

This set of experiences shows the other side of the sequence dysphoria-anger. This particular sequence plays in fact an "organizing" function by allowing the dispersion characterizing the dysphoric mood to be transformed into a focused attention on a specific object which assumes a scapegoat function. Therefore, in the transformation of dysphoric mood into polarized anger toward an object, a fantasy for compensation is also fulfilled. On the contrary, the sequence leading to the experiences of emptiness exemplifies the "disorganizing" side of dysphoria. In this case, dysphoria does not have an interlocutor to deal with and cannot be objectified through the anger directed toward someone, thereby exhibiting all its "centrifugal" pull: as a result of such centrifugal force, the various aspects of the self are dispersed without reaching the critical mass necessary to aggregate in some form of recognizable identity. In a spiral difficult to stop, the indefiniteness of the self contributes to the indefiniteness of the other and vice versa. If anger gives meaning to dysphoria, emptiness, instead, brings meaning away from it. If anger expresses a resilient hope for compensation, emptiness is experienced as hopeless and exhibits their reparability of a traumatic existence. "While anger fulfills me, strengthens me, and gives me strength and power—a patient said—the sense of emptiness disembowels me and leaves me empty."

Otto Kernberg has identified "identity diffusion" as one of the core features of the borderline functioning. This condition is characterized by the absence of a stable and consistent image of oneself as a person, which involves fundamental uncertainties regarding the subject's lifestyle, life choices, friends, partners, sexual habits, and moral, religious, and political values. This is due to the subject's inability to integrate the contradictory aspects of the self and the object. The impossibility for these aspects to become integrated and cohesive condemns the borderline person to a state of perpetual suspension of identity. In this situation, identity ends to be nothing more than a momentary agglutination of dispersed and contradictory elements. To the identity diffusion that afflicts the subject in its relationship with the others as well as the external world corresponds, on the more private and inner level of the self (Meares et al. 2011), a series of agonizing experiences of emptiness, insubstantiality, and inauthenticity—the *lived side* of identity diffusion.

But what is this "emptiness" so often mentioned by borderline patients? Referring to his inability to evoke a mental picture of himself, Roberto, a patient described by Irene Ruggiero (2012), calls it the "syndrome of the empty mirror." When he tries to imagine himself, what Roberto "sees" is not his own face, but a terrifying black hole ready to swallow him up, which leads him to question the reality of his physical existence. This experience is not easy to describe, but Carla's terse words are illuminating. The emptiness—she says—is not absence. The experience is not rendered light, weightless, or "winged" by its very emptiness. This emptiness is not equivalent to loss or lack of something. While in the experience of lack the subject is completely absorbed by the suffering caused by the disappearance of the object and totally engaged in the attempt to regain it, in the experience of emptiness the subject suffers from a condition which is very difficult to name and objectify. It is a condition one wants to abandon as soon as possible because the feeling is that of having the rug pulled out from under one's feet. In fact, the experience of emptiness feeds on itself and is self-perpetuating: emptiness calls for more emptiness, and the subject finds itself imprisoned in an emptied, hemorrhagic identity. In such loneliness and emptiness, there is no hand hold to grip and no way out. For this emptiness is anything but light: it is heavy, and it crushes and oppresses those who experience it. It weighs like lead and drags one down, making one "fall" by sucking him or her into a black hole. The experience of emptiness seems to point to identity diffusion in the sense of lack of cohesion and continuity of the self: a painful incoherence that Wilkinson-Ryan and Westen (2000) have identified as the central element of the borderline identity diffusion.

Experiences of emptiness, however, are not all equal. There are many ways to live and express a sense of emptiness. In addition to the modality of painful incoherence (essentially linked to the impossibility of finding an intentional object), a sense of emptiness can also appear under different shapes. One example is the feeling of being inhabited by something dead. This feeling derives from the impression of having voided one's whole inner space, which generates an atmosphere of hopeless desolation. This kind of experience of emptiness easily turns into a physical state and is expressed with bodily metaphors. In the words of one patient: "I feel like an empty container. My skin, my skeleton are there, but inside of me there is nothing. There is nothing alive inside of me." This emptiness is less empty than the previous one because the subject has already come close to finding an intentional object through the identification of aspects of itself as deadly, lifeless, destructive, or unworthy. Fonagy et al. (2002) have described this condition as "the alien self."

In other cases, the borderline emptiness, which is always, so to speak, "relational" in nature, can be the result of a worn-out relationship, namely, of a continuous and consuming reciprocal intercourse: an emptiness caused by an exhausting proximity which blurs each other's boundaries. As Franco Lolli (2012) has written, "in the experience of emptiness the act of thinking disappears and the feeling of self dissolves [. . .] As if crippled by the weight of the feeling of emptiness, the borderline patient seems to have no thickness, reduced to a kind of film capable of assuming the shape and characteristics of the occasional partner." Something very similar to what Carla says when she tries to describe her situation: "I don't know who I am or what I want. . . Each time I feel different, according to the people I deal with. The fact is that I am not what I look like. I don't know who I really am."

This first outline of a phenomenology of borderline emptiness is based on a dialectical view of the experiences of emptiness: such experiences should be seen as the inevitable but momentary stages of a journey oscillating between the "organizing" dysphoria-anger sequence and the "disorganizing" dysphoria-emptiness sequence. As long as the experience of emptiness maintains its dynamic dialectical relationship with the sequence dysphoria-anger, the situation is relatively stable. However, if the journey ends with the experience of emptiness, the situation can turn dramatic: when the emptiness experienced in one's inner world is matched by a real emptiness in the outside world, when the subject has driven everyone away and there are no interlocutors with whom to "share" one's sufferings, the risk of suicide is particularly high. When a dysphoric irritability has become disconnected with the world, self-suppression often appears as the only solution available.

More frequently, however, a way out from the disorganizing dysphoria-emptiness sequence is found in impulsive actions. When the emptiness is caused by painful incoherence, impulsive actions increase one's sense of agency by giving greater cohesion and coherence to the self; when the emptiness is due to the inner presence of dead objects, such actions serve to restore a sense of vitality (in the context of what Stanghellini and Rosfort 2013 have called "desperate vitality") and to regain hope; finally, when the emptiness is caused by excessive proximity, impulsive actions can help to strongly reestablish the borders of the self.

3.5 Borderline and Self-Harming Behavior

The third and final element in the meeting with Carla which deserves attention is that of self-harming behaviors: this is one of the ways in which Carla tries to come to terms with her dysphoric mood and with her feelings of emptiness-inconsistency. Although Carla is perfectly aware of the abnormality of her behavior, the urge to cut herself is stronger than her will. In the words of another borderline patient, to cut oneself is like finding oneself in a blind alley: the idea and the urge to cut oneself seem to come directly from the skin. Self-cutting is performed because it works and because the alternatives are often worse; it helps to fight one's inner chaos, even if one does not know where it comes from (Kettlewell 1999). Self-cutting "works" for various reasons and in different ways: Carla claims that it helps her to "black out," to stop the uninterrupted flow of thoughts ("after I cut myself, my head is finally free from thoughts") or the sudden emotional changes.

Self-cutting, however, "works" also because it helps one to grasp something alive within instead of contemplating a "mushy and uniform clay." The red blood flowing out of the wound makes one feel the presence of something alive. The pain of the wound dispels other kinds of pain, such as the "tangle in the stomach," but also the tangle of thoughts and emotions in which the person feels trapped. To turn a mental pain into a physical one is a way to materialize and locate such pain, to make it visible first to oneself and then, if necessary, to the others. These, however, are just some of the ways in which self-harm is said to "work." Whenever a person cuts or burns herself—Potter writes (2003)—one should try interpreting the wound with as open a mind as possible in order to understand what that person can and cannot say (to the others as well as to herself). The greatest risk facing the therapist in such cases is that of remain enmeshed into monolithic, stereotyped, abstract, and absolutist interpretations, which supposedly would explain the self-harming behavior on the basis of a predetermined motive. If, however, the therapist is willing to "listen" to these wounds, especially through the patients' retrospective interpretation, he will discover that there is not just one meaning to the self-cutting but that, on the contrary, there is a whole range of experiences distributed along a continuum—and that in each cut multiple reasons are intertwined, in ways that also change over time. Within such continuum, it is then necessary to identify some possible "psychopathological organizers," understood as synthesizing schemes of comprehension aimed at connecting different pathological experiences into unitary cores of meaningfulness (Rossi Monti and Stanghellini 1996). We have identified at least six of them (Rossi Monti and D'Agostino 2009):

1. *Concretizing*: the wounds function as a means to transform a mental pain into a physical one, to control intolerable feelings through the body. It might be an attempt to give shape to an invisible, wandering, and boundless mental pain by localizing it in the body or to fill a distressing inner emptiness with a bodily sensation. Another patient said that when she cuts herself, she can look at the wounds and say: "this is my way of feeling bad... and it is real" (Leibenluft et al. 1987). One patient quoted by Straker (2006, 104) says: "it's as if the cut gives shape or form to what feels like boundless pain. At the moment of cutting time stops, and with the pain of the cut, always much less than the psychological pain, and with bleeding, everything becomes focused and concrete. Actually pain is not really the right word; it's more like suffering that feels endless, formless, nowhere and everywhere, like suffering without an object, suffering from emptiness, suffering from nothing. Your thoughts do not wander uselessly and aimlessly anymore suffering, but fix almost literally on the cut."
2. *Punishing-eradicating-purifying*: the wounds function as a means to punish/eradicate some inner "evil" in order to detoxify/purify oneself. It is a way to punish a bad self, to assail one's thoughts, feelings, and memories or even to unconsciously repeat an emotional sequence connected to a history of childhood abuse: repetition here replaces recollection, functioning as a shield against bad memories. Julia Pestalozzi (2003) has written that the metaphors employed to describe this experience show that cutting the skin creates an opening through which the inner tension can be released, and all the bad and the alien can gush out from the interior of the body. Jenny (another patient) says: "The deeper I cut and the more I bleed, the better it makes me feel inside because it feels like all the hurt inside of me is coming out. I can see it with blood. So the deeper I go, the better I feel" (McDonald et al. 2010 p. 95).
3. *Regulating dysphoria*: the wounds function as a tool to modulate the dysphoric mood typical of the borderline existence. The best example of this psychopathological organizer is provided by Carla's behavior toward the end of the first year of psychotherapy. For 6 months Carla did not cut herself. She started to express her discomfort with words and found an interlocutor in the psychotherapist. Outside of the sessions, Carla finds relief in putting her feelings into words. The dysphoric mood underlying her tormented existence has now turned into something different: an emotional state toward which Carla can take a stand.

   By writing down her feelings, Carla can objectify and visualize them without being overwhelmed by them. The place where Carla deposits all this material is her mobile phone. It is an unsafe place. One day, inadvertently, Carla erases all her notes. Once again, everything is lost. The object to which she had entrusted her personal thoughts has proven unreliable. Carla herself feels unreliable and unworthy. When the dysphoric mood mounts, the only way out for her is to resort to the "safe" mode of cutting herself so to release the tension. But after the first cut, she finds a way to regain her own perspective on her emotional upheaval. Carla takes a piece of paper and writes down her feelings with great ardor and vehemence. It is a kind of volcanic eruption in which the intense violence of the content is barely restrained by language: "The word is too narrow a window" to allow her to express what she feels. The window is too narrow, but strong enough to withstand the impact, so much so that these notes can be brought to therapy and become the focus of a joint interpretation. The therapeutic work begins to bear fruit. Until then, the wounds had been—as another patient said—the only possible "blow hole" for Carla's dysphoric suffering. Now, instead, she has finally started to mentalize her mental pain.

4. *Communicating without words*: the wounds function as a language to convey something inexpressible through words but also as a way to control the others' behavior and emotions by eliciting care giving responses from them. In this context, the word *manipulation* has been often employed. The term, however, is poorly chosen since manipulation is a mode of thought and behavior requiring complex and sophisticated mental functions which in most cases of severe borderline psychopathology are gravely compromised (Stanghellini 2014). Rather, what we have here is mostly, on the one hand, an inability—to use Winnicott's words (1969)—to freely treat the other as an autonomous and independent object and, on the other, the necessity to treat him or her as a "subjective object."
5. *Building a memory of oneself*: the wounds function as a way to secure a memory of oneself. The skin is a surface on which to carve and mark certain circumstances, events, and emotions that correspond to significant turning points. A patient calls her self-inflicted wounds "my notches." Self-cutting becomes a way to make sure that certain events have left a concrete and visible trace—a trace one can immediately locate on one's skin. Another patient speaks of her wounds as a way to mark on her skin the evil she felt inside of her. Another patient, who had long stopped cutting herself, considered having her scars removed through plastic surgery. But then she changed her mind out of "nostalgia" for the time when she used to cut herself: she is sure she would miss her scars.
6. *Turning active*: the wounds function as a way to transform passively endured or externally imposed experiences into active ones. This way, an intrinsically traumatic sense of helplessness is transformed into a more reassuringly self-inflicted "trauma." "The thing is—a patient says—if I can harm myself, then I believe I can bear the pain inflicted on me by the others, as if by cicatrizing I become immune to the rest of the world. I'd rather endure a self-inflicted pain than one received from the outside." However, self-cutting is also an attempt to *shed skin* instead of changing oneself. There is also a social dimension to the "wounds": they can take on the characteristics of a ritual through which one's need to feel in control of one's body is acted out (Lemma 2005); they can spread through a kind of social "contagion" due to their capacity to mark the identity of each individual (often by opposition to the others). The "wounds," in this sense, become brands to exhibit as truly distinguishing features.

Two concluding remarks: (a) these organizers are not mutually exclusive, but intertwined; they simply serve as points of reference for the interpretation of self-harming behaviors; (b) in their progression along the continuum, self-harming behaviors tend to acquire an increasingly social value while at the same time reducing their psychopathological characterization, thereby coming close to the so-called culturally approved self-harming conducts. Each self-harming behavior derives its structure from some of the experiences outlined above. Such experiences play a fundamental organizing function with respect to these behaviors, each time producing a synthesis in which one of the above elements prevails. Therapy provides the precious opportunity to identify these organizers and to follow their evolution over time.

Only toward the end of a long series of psychotherapeutic sessions a patient was finally able to accurately describe the lived experience and the function sustaining two different kinds of self-harming behavior, namely, cutting herself with a razor blade and burning her skin with a cigarette: "The cuts were made quickly, in order to see the blood... When two contradictory ideas made me confused and foggy, and I was unable to decide, the cuts helped me to wipe out everything." These were quick, furious, and superficial cuts, aimed at cleaning up a mess like a windshield wiper would do. Cigarette burns were a different thing:"I did not feel the pain. I would smoke a cigarette, burn myself with it, then smoke and burn myself again right on the same spot, namely, the back of my hand or my leg. [This happened] when I had a fixed idea incessantly pounding at my head, a single idea pounding and pounding.... Today, watching the cigarette burns makes me feel pleasure, tenderness—I don't want anybody to touch them! For me, to look at the cigarette burns is like looking at a tattoo." More generally, she says, "if I was struggling with some suffering, I would not allow myself the time to feel it. It had to go away immediately. For me, physical pain is a hundred times better [than mental suffering]! It was as if my body was following me: a sentimental suffering would turn into a physical pain."

Anger, emptiness, inconsistency, inauthenticity, and self-harming behavior are the main ways in which many borderline patients try to give shape to their inner chronic pain—"the pain of being borderline" (Zanarini et al. 1998; Zanarini, 2008). The success or failure of each therapeutic work depends on the common effort and willingness to find alternative ways to deal with this pain. Such therapeutic work begins by focusing not only on the symptoms but also on the quality of the experiences at stake.

References

Berner, P., Musalek, M., & Walter, H. (1987). Psychopathological concepts of dysphoria. *Psychopathology, 20*(93), 100.

Chiesa, M., Drahorad, C., & Longo, S. (2000). Early termination of treatment in personality disorder treated in a psychotherapy hospital. *British Journal of Psychiatry, 177*, 107–111.

Fonagy, P., Gergely, G., Jurist, E., & Target, M. (2002). *Affect regulation, mentalization and the development of the Self*. London: Other Press.

Gabbard, G. (1999). An overview of countertransference: theory and technique. In G. Gabbard (Ed.), *Countertransference issues in psychiatric treatment*. Washington, DC: American Psychiatric Press.
Gabriel, E. (1987). Dysphoric mood in paranoid psychoses. *Psychopathology, 20*, 101–106.
Jaspers, K. (1913). *Allgemeine Psychopathologie*. Berlin: Springer. English edition: Jaspers, K. (1997). *General Psychopathology. Volumes 1 & 2* (trans: Hoenig, J., Hamilton, M. W.). Baltimore: Johns Hopkins University Press.
Kernberg, O. F. (1992). *Aggression in personality disorders and perversion*. New Haven: Yale University Press.
Kernberg, O. F. (1994). Aggression, trauma and hatred in the treatment of borderline patients. *The Psychiatric Clinics of North America, 17*, 701–714.
Kettlewell, C. (1999). *Skin game: A cutter's memoir*. New York: St. Martin's Press.
Kimura, B. (1992). *Écrits de psychopathologie phénoménologique*. Paris: Presses Universitaires de France.
Leibenluft, E., Gardner, D. L., & Cowdry, R. W. (1987). The inner experience of the borderline self-mutilator. *Journal of Personality Disorders, 1*, 317–324.
Lemma, A. (2005). *Under the skin. A psychoanalytic study of body modification*. London: Routledge.
Lolli, F. (2012). *L'epoca dell'inconshow*. Milano: Mimesis.
McDonald, M., Pietsch, T., & Wilson, T. (2010). Ontological insecurity: A guiding framework for borderline personality disorder. *Journal of Phenomenological Psychology, 41*, 85–105.
McWilliams, N. (2014). La patologia borderline come livello di organizzazione della personalità. In M. Fontana & S. Zito (Eds.), *La patologia borderline in psicoanalisi. Modelli per l'intervento*. Milano: Franco Angeli.
Meares, R., Gerull, F., Stevenson, J., & Korner, A. (2011). Is self-disturbance the core of borderline personality disorder? An outcome study of borderline personality factors. *Australian and New Zealand Journal of Psychiatry, 45*, 214–222.
Pazzagli, A., & Rossi Monti, M. (2000). Dysphoria and aloneness in borderline personality disorder. *Psychopathology, 33*, 220–226.
Pestalozzi, J. (2003). The symbolic and concrete: Psychotic adolescents in psychoanalytic psychotherapy. *International Journal of Psychoanalysis, 84*, 733–753.
Potter, N. (2003). Commodity/body/sign: Borderline personality disorder and the signification of self-injurious behavior. *Philosophy, Psychiatry and Psychology, 10*, 1–16.
Rossi Monti, M. (2012). Borderline: Il dramma della disforia. In M. Rossi Monti (Ed.), *Psicopatologia del presente. Crisi della nosografia e nuove forme della clinica*. Milano: Franco Angeli.
Rossi Monti, M., & D'Agostino, A. (2009). *Autolesionismo*. Roma: Carocci.
Rossi Monti, M., & Stanghellini, G. (1996). Psychopathology: An edgeless razor? *Comprehensive Psychiatry, 37*, 196–204.
Ruggiero, I. (2012). The unreachable object? Difficulties and paradoxes in the analytical relationship with borderline patients. *International Journal of Psychoanalysis, 93*, 585–606.
Stanghellini, G. (2000). Dysphoria, vulnerability and identity. *Psychopathology, 33*, 198–220.
Stanghellini, G. (2014). De-stigmatising manipulation: an exercise in second-order empathic understanding. *South African Journal of Psychiatry, 20*, 11–14.
Stanghellini, G., & Rosfort, R. (2013). Borderline depression: A desperate vitality. *Journal of Consciousness Studies, 20*, 153–177.
Straker, G. (2006). Signing with a scar: Understanding self-harm. *Psychoanalytic Dialogues, 16*, 93–112.
Wilkinson-Ryan, T., & Westen, D. (2000). Identity disturbance in borderline personality disorder: An empirical investigation. *American Journal of Psychiatry, 157*, 528–541.
Winnicott, D. W. (1969). *The use of an object and relating through identifications. In: Playing and Reality*. London: Tavistock.

Zanarini, M. (2008). Reasons for change in borderline personality disorder (and other axis II disorders). *Psychiatry Clinics of North America, 31*, 505–515.

Zanarini, M., Frankenburg, F. R., DeLuca, C. J., Hennen, J., Khera, G. S., & Gunderson, J. (1998). The pain of being borderline: dysphoric states specific to borderline personality disorder. *Harvard Review of Psychiatry, 6*, 201–207.

Gender Dysphoria

4

Giovanni Castellini

4.1 A Case Study of Gender Dysphoria: Francesco

Francesco is a 23-year-old natal male. He was born in a small village close to Florence, Italy. He was referred to the CIADIG, the Gender Identity Disorder Service of the University of Florence at the age of 20 years. At the first visit, he said that he wished to continue his life as a girl. He had this dream since he can remember. When doctors asked him how he can be sure about this, he spoke about his *cross-gender* behaviors, beginning when he was 5 years old. Francesco reported that even before primary school, he had been secretly dressing up in his mother's clothes almost every day of his child life. He always spent time with Cecilia, his young neighborhood friend, instead of other guys in the village. With Cecilia, he liked playing with dolls and cuddly toys and spending time with "girls' games" such as "cooking," "preparing dresses," and "tidying up the house." Francesco reported marked cross-gender identification in role-playing, as he always acted as a mother or a bride. He told to the doctors that his recurrent dream was to wake up in the morning and to discover in the mirror that he had become a girl.

He had a good relationship with his family which consisted of his mother, his father, and his grandparents who lived close to their house. In general, his parents did not stigmatize neither encouraged his cross-gender behaviors. Francesco was used to speak a lot with his mother, and his mother reported that when he was 8 years old he had told her he wanted to be a woman when he grew up. However, the grandfather sometimes displayed intense negative reactions to wear dresses or other feminine attire.

His first feedback from the environment took place when Francesco went to primary school. At that time, for the first time he realized his own *gender identity for the others*. The way his classmates built up this representation of Francesco was

G. Castellini (✉)
Florence University, Florence, Italy
e-mail: giovannicastellini78@hotmail.com

G. Stanghellini, M. Aragona (eds.), *An Experiential Approach to Psychopathology*,
DOI 10.1007/978-3-319-29945-7_4

quite typical of this kind of stories. At school Francesco often wanted to play with girls and avoided rough-and-tumble play or other activities with boys. He was found to take a Barbie doll in his bag, and his mannerisms and style of walking were feminine. Since the second year of school, all the children in his class called him Francesca. The primary was a small school in the countryside, and for all the first 5 years of school, he did not particularly suffer for marginalization. The teachers did not encourage his feminine behavior, but they were supportive. The other children considered him a singular boy who resembled a girl, but nothing more. They always play together, given that teachers were very careful not to allow games exclusively feminine or masculine.

More problems came up with secondary school when he was 12 years old. Francesco managed not to change his behaviors. Indeed, girls and boys tried to hire a female/male role through clothing and behaviors resembling the first adolescent changes of their body. Therefore, Francesco emphasized his feminine behaviors to belong to the girls' world. In this phase he did not receive the same sympathy and comprehension of his first school experience. Teachers stigmatized his behaviors and often called his parents to ask them for more appropriate dressing. Francesco lacked confidence and was teased by other children, who called him "gay" and "drag queen." He spent most of the time alone, as he avoided playing with boys, and girls did not include him in their activities. At this time, he had the first problems with his father who tried to prevent Francesco's cross-gender behaviors. Francesco began to feel rejection by his father feeling that "he was wrong" and that "would have been better if he had not existed."

At this time, he suffered from symptoms of anxiety, including stomach upsets, dizziness, and headaches, and he lost many days of school, thus compromising his final evaluation. This was a relevant consequence for Francesco, because of his concern about school performances and his perfectionism. Therefore, the ordinary evaluation he received represented a great blow for his self-esteem.

The "real tragedy"—as Francesco reported—began with adolescence. When he was 13 years old, the development of secondary sex characteristics made Francesco realize that his body was incongruent with his perceived gender identity. His body changes were the mirror of his sense of "non-belonging" and of feeling of "being wrong." The discrepancy between the experienced gender and physical sex characteristics was accompanied by a desire to be rid of secondary sex characteristics and to acquire some secondary sex characteristics of the other gender. Indeed, Francesco was deeply concerned about imminent physical changes; he told Cecilia that he found his penis, testes, and hairs disgusting and that he wished them removed and to have a vagina. When visible signs of puberty developed clearly, he began shaving his legs. Erections were perceived with a profound sense of uneasiness and sometimes disgust. He reported that the penis was "a kind of alien, separate from my body and from my mind." He sometimes bound his genitals to make erections less visible. However, when he was at the beach, this kind of actions lost their significance.

During these years, when he was at high school, he brought increased sexual and aggressive drives almost for his own biological gender. The challenge of establishing his sense of sexual identity was really complex. While his heterosexual peers—as his friend Cecilia—took their sexual orientation for granted, he had a million of questions and doubts about the social acceptance of his desires. Especially when he got back to his small village, he must cope with feeling different, ostracism, and dilemmas about revealing his sexual identity that is discrepant from family and social expectations. His mother helped him with the "coming out": one day she spoke with Francesco telling him "I know you are different Francesco, I don't mind if you don't like girls." Francesco was uncertain about what this sentence implied for him. He realized he was a lucky person, as compared with a homosexual friend who received a very different feedback from his parents who told him "From this day you don't exist for us until you will accept that your homosexuality is an illness and you will treat it." However, the sentences "you are different..." or "you don't like girls..." pronounced by his mother—instead of "there is nothing bad in loving boys..."—confirmed his feeling that something went wrong with his birth and the only thing his parents could do was to tolerate him.

At high school, Francesco found a better environment as compared with secondary school. He sought friendships with girls and adopted a new name Giulia for his friends, consistent with his experienced gender. At the end of high school, he had his first involvement in a sexual relationship with a 2 years older bisexual boy. Sex was not perceived as a natural activity, as Francesco usually did show or allow his partner to touch his sexual organs.

Even though the school represented a good environment for Francesco, during this period he experienced first bullying episodes. One day when he was coming back to home, a group of peers surrounded him just close to his house and tried to threaten him. Francesco did not talk to anybody about this episode, but he suffered from a severe sense of humiliation. He always thought about how to "clean up" the shame of this harassment which he thought he could have avoided if he would be different. After this episode, when he started dieting: he had very rigid diet rules, with "danger" and "forbidden" foods. He usually ate alone, only foods of known calorie content, and after few months he had a dramatic weight loss, with body mass index reaching 15.6. For this reason he attended a cognitive behavioral program for eating disorder. It is remarkable that at the time of the first visit at CIADIG, Francesco was aware that his diet attempts were aimed at modifying his body as it resembled a feminine appearance. Therefore, it was clear that his "masked" eating disorder was not related to a typical body image distortion, rather it represented a dysfunctional way to change the body he hates. Thanks to psychological treatment he recovered weight; however, he never fully remitted from his pathological eating behaviors, and after a few years, he experienced sporadic loss of control binge eating episodes of small quantities of food. Every time he thought he failed dieting, he believed his failure was because of his weakness, rather than viewing his dietary rules as being too rigid and extreme. He always felt horrible about having broken his diet, and sometimes he forced himself to throw up what he had eaten.

When he started attending Literature Faculty at the University, he had good performances. However, his pathological eating behaviors worsened and he developed a serious depression, with severe anhedonia and suicidal thoughts.

Thanks to the psychotherapist he was referred to the Service for Gender Dysphoria of the University of Florence. At the Service clinicians confirmed that Francesco presented with the features of a very well-established gender dysphoria according to DSM 5 criteria. Francesco reported that he had a strong desire to be of a different gender and treated as such, and he may had an inner certainty to feel and respond as the experienced gender, seeking a medical treatment to alter body characteristics and after that taking into consideration an intervention of genital reassignment surgery. Francesco was determined to first resolve the incongruence between experienced and assigned gender by living in the desired feminine role. Given the difficulties encountered in his village and the reluctance of his parents to accept these changes, he accepted to temporarily adopt a gender role neither conventionally male nor conventionally female when he was in his house. However, after few months, his desire to live in a female role became very intense in all the context of his life, and the parents agreed to let him live as a girl also at their village, by dressing in female clothes and changing his name to Giulia.

In the months following the first contact with the Service, Francesco attended the psychoeducational program of the center, and he had regularly contacts with two mental health clinicians. The aims of the intervention were to clarify and explore gender identity and role, addressing the impact of stigma and minority stress on one's mental health and facilitating a coming out process, which includes changes in gender role expression. The psychiatrist helped Francesco to explore and anticipate the implications of changes in gender role and to pace the process of implementing these changes. He provided a space for Francesco to begin to express himself in congruent ways with his gender identity and to overcome fears about changes in gender expression. Mental health professionals' intervention contributed also to improve self-consciousness on dysfunctional behaviors such as those associated with dieting and purging.

Francesco engaged a continuous months of living in a female gender role, experiencing a range of different life experiences and events such as family events, holidays, and meeting with friends. To help Francesco in exploring his female life and having a desired gender role, cross-gender hormonal treatment with feminizing hormone therapy was applied. Physical changes in his body included breast growth, decreased spontaneous erections, decreased testicular size, and increased percentage of body fat compared to muscle mass, softening of skin, and decreased skin oiliness. Clinicians could notice that the hormonal treatment reduced Francesco's body uneasiness not just for the objective modification on his own body, rather for the subjective perception and representation of one's own body. Francesco had a self-representation of his body as a less masculine and closer to his perceived identity. This phenomenon made him more self-confident in his new gender role exploration.

After 2 years, Francesco obtained the sentence from an Italian court to undergo genital reassignment surgery. After the penectomy and orchiectomy, he underwent other interventions such as augmentation mammoplasty (implants/lipofilling), as well as facial feminization surgery, thyroid cartilage reduction, and other aesthetic procedures. After 1-year follow-up, he indicated he had no regrets about the whole treatment. He was functioning well psychologically, intellectually, and socially. There were no clinical signs of physical imbalance; metabolic and endocrine parameters were in the normal reference range, as was bone density. At the end of his clinical course, he could ask for new name in his ID card. Now she is Giulia, an Italian woman who is going to graduate at the University of Florence. Her dream now is to be a journalist and to get married.

4.2 Gender Dysphoria: *Status Quaestionis*

4.2.1 Identity and Gender Identity

Everybody qualified himself/herself by means of different features which he/she thinks provide a more comprehensive description of one's own identity. Whenever I write or I speak to someone about myself, the very first inception of my sentence begins with "I am..." and the following might be "... a doctor" or "... a smart guy." In general the way I characterize myself depends on values attributed to different personal qualifiers. For example, an anorexia nervosa patient—before saying "I am a doctor" or "I am a smart girl"—might define herself as "a thin girl." Indeed, for most of the persons, the membership to the male/female gender is taken for granted, when they meet somebody; therefore, nobody says "Nice to meet you; I am a man and a doctor," because our body and our appearance "speak" for us. However, when an Italian person needs to get a job, he has to declare his/her gender in his CV. For the majority of people, *gender identity* is established in toddlerhood, is consistent with biological sex, and remains fixed. However, children like Francesco experienced gender nonconformity and a discomfort with their biological sex, from the very beginning of their life. They derive comfort from being perceived as, or a wish to be, the other sex.

Gender identity represents a person's private sense, and subjective experience, of their own gender (Money 1971). It has the significance of acceptance or desire of membership into a category of people: male or female. Gender membership is a fundamental component of our general *identity* and provides a sense of continuity of the self. According with a modern definition, *identity* constitutes itself as sameness and continuity in the face of continuous discontinuity in an individual's life and in the life of groups (Pfäffl 2014). The first conceptualization of a system of absolute identity was formalized by the philosopher and romantic writer Friedrich Schelling (Schelling 1801). His work made *identity* to become a central epistemological concept of the modern history of philosophy. The psychoanalyses further developed this construct with Freud's conceptualization of *ego-identity* and Erikson's (1970) *ego-identity* defined as the conviction that the ego is learning effective steps toward a tangible collective future and that it is developing into a defined ego within a social reality. Erikson described a *socialization process* in which each person—through the acquisition and rejection of identifications with primary significant persons—develops a sense of himself as a unique individual (personal identity, self-likeness, and continuity of the person in time). At the same time the individual—as belonging to a particular social group (group identity, constancy of the symbols of a group despite fluctuations in group membership)—finally finds his place in this group and experiences acceptance.

Psychoanalyses also took into consideration *gender identity*. According to Freud's position, *gender identity* becomes stable with the resolution of the Oedipus complex, and a child acquires a stable gender identity when he identifies himself with the same sex parent (Freud 1962). However, this theory has been commonly criticized; for example, Golombok argued that gender identification occurs in children much earlier than the stage at which Freud postulated the resolution of the Oedipus complex to occur (Golombok et al. 1995, 2001).

According to the contemporary literature in this field (Giordano 2011, 2012), *identity* (equivalent to ego-identity) refers to one's abstract sense of self within a cultural and social matrix, and it usually consolidated in adolescence. On the contrary, *gender identity* refers to an individual's personal sense of self as male or female, and it usually develops by age three, remaining stable over the lifetime. For most of the people, it is congruent with *sex*, in the sense of being male or female, referring to a person's anatomical sex. *Gender identity* and *sexual identity* have only more recently been considered as a subcategory of *personal identity* (Pfäffl 2014). Indeed, *gender identity* has been firstly conceptualized in a bipolar, dichotomous manner with a male gender identity at one pole and a female gender identity at the other pole. However, there are individuals who have an uncertain or confused gender identity or who are transitioning from one gender to the other who do not fit into this dichotomous scheme. Gender identity provides a biographical continuity of an individual, which can be either male or female but probably it is possible to speak about also a third, fourth or fifth gender.

4.2.2 Identity and the Body

In our life, the sense of self, and the membership to a gender category, develops with the progressive awareness of one's own body. As extensively reported, awareness and experience of the body are the original anchors of our developing sense of self (Kinsbourne 2002). Body awareness is a dynamic process; it is not a matter of retrieving information from a specialized area or module of the selectively attending brain. It follows that the sense of self as body is not something that is present from birth or that suddenly becomes available during maturation. Rather, it emerges gradually out of the increasing ability to attend selectively to various body parts. Infants may first experience themselves as individuals when they begin to move body parts against a background of undifferentiated body sensation.

This is the reason why adolescence represents a crucial period as in Francesco's story. Indeed, the perception of his incongruent gender identity became clear when his body provided the strong signs of gender-specific features. As for other persons, Francesco's gender identity remained indefinite until adolescent. When adolescence came, persons with gender dysphoria live in a cognitive state where their physical body is in contrast with their self-perceived identity (Gooren 2006), and this experience is a source of deep and chronic suffering (Gooren 2011). For persons like Francesco, the primary source of suffering is the sense of non-pertinence to the assigned gender based on anatomical sexual characteristics. *Gender dysphoria* is defined as the distress that may accompany the incongruence between one's experienced or expressed gender and one's assigned gender (American Psychiatric Association 2013).

The available literature reported that the body is the primary source of suffering gender dysphoria persons (Bandini et al. 2013; Fisher et al. 2014; Johansson et al. 2010). However, the uneasiness is not limited to sexual parts of the body, rather some studies reported GD persons are more dissatisfied with their body than subjects without GD, even with regard to nonsexual body parts and aspects (Vocks et al. 2009). However, as demonstrated by Francesco's story, the source of body uneasiness in gender dysphoria is generally not associated with a primary body image disorder such as the one we can find in eating disorder patients (Fairburn 2008). Indeed, it has been reported that successful treatments focused on relieving of gender dysphoria such as hormonal and surgical interventions are capable of reducing suffering related to the body (Bandini et al. 2013; Fisher et al. 2014; Johansson et al. 2010). Especially genital reassignment surgery showed a positive effect on body dissatisfaction, due to a reduction in the discrepancy between biological and desired sex (Kraemer et al. 2008).

From a phenomenological perspective, we can interpret gender dysphoria as the incongruence between the body people keep in their mind and by which they represent themselves and the body they have (anatomical body). In the light of phenomenology, we should distinguish between lived body (*Leib*) and physical body (*Koerper*) or body-subject and body-object. The first is the body experienced from within, the own direct experience of one's own body in the first-person perspective, oneself as a spatiotemporal embodied agent in the world; the second is the body thematically investigated from without, as, for example, by natural sciences as anatomy and physiology, a third-person perspective (Husserl 1912–1915; Merleau-Ponty 1996). One's own body can be apprehended by a person in the first-person perspective as the body-I-am. As previously reported, the perception of one's own body is a crucial phase for development of a primitive experience of oneself, the basic form of self-awareness. The cenesthetic apprehension of one's own body is the unmediated experience of one's own "facticity" including oneself as "this" body, its form, height, weight, and color, as well as one's past and what is actually happening. First and foremost, we have an implicit acquaintance with our own body from the first-person perspective (Stanghellini et al. 2012). The lived body turns into a physical, objective body whenever we become aware of it in a disturbing way. Whenever our movement is somehow impeded or disrupted, then the lived body is thrown back on itself, materialized or *corporealized*, and it becomes an object for me. This happened in Francesco's story during adolescence.

When he was a child, he only had an indefinite idea of his gender, as his physical body lacked of a "sexual shape." However, when adolescence came, he experienced the forced change of his body object and, as the psychoanalysts Di Ceglie and Freedman (1998) said, his lived gender identity became a *stranger* in his anatomical body. At that time he realized that he had a material sexually shaped body. In addition to these two dimensions of corporeality, Sartre emphasized that one can apprehend one's own body also from another vantage point, as one's own body when it is looked at by another person. When I become aware that I or better that my own body is looked at by another person, I realize that my body can be an object for that person. Sartre calls this the "lived body-for-others" (1943). "With the appearance of the Other's look," writes Sartre, "I experience the revelation of my being-as-object." Thus, one's identity becomes reified by the gaze of the other and reduced to the external appearance of one's own body (Stanghellini et al. 2012). Our behaviors, including clothing and gestures, are necessary to express our pertinence to once own gender identity. This is what concerns to the so-called *gender role* referring to activities, interests, use of symbols, styles, or other personal and social attributes that are recognized as masculine or feminine. In general, the lived body is not always present in our consciousness, rather the self remains abstracted from the body and it is intellectualized as the self-conscious mind. The lived body turns into a physical, objective body whenever we become aware of it in a disturbing way. Accordingly, in gender dysphoria persons, the perception of the incongruence between the lived and the physical body makes the body as a central feature in the uneasiness related with the self-representation. Therefore, gender dysphoria persons often live a sort of alienation from one's own body and from one's own emotions, disgust for it, shame, and an exaggerated concern to take responsibility for the way one appears to the others. This generally determines severe consequences in social life, sexual relationship, and personality development.

4.2.3 Psychopathology and Gender Dysphoria

During adolescence, Francesco experienced social isolation and severe depressive symptoms. As a matter of fact, gender dysphoria and related body uneasiness determine a pervasive impairment in self-esteem, depression sometimes with suicidal thoughts, as well as eating disorder symptoms (Vocks et al. 2009). Some studies reported a relatively high prevalence of psychiatric disorders among gender dysphoria patients (De Cuypere et al. 1995). However, almost all the data in this field confirm that gender dysphoria subjects lack severe primary psychopathology (Hoshiai et al. 2010; Haraldsen and Dahl 2000). Furthermore, it has been suggested that psychopathology may be the consequence of difficulties in coping with GD (Gómez-Gil et al. 2009), social stigma (Nuttbrock et al. 2010; Matsumoto et al. 2009), or rejection by family and friends (Factor and Rothblum 2007) rather than from a primary psychiatric condition. Indeed, hormonal and surgical sex reassignments have been reported to improve quality of life and psychological well-being (Wierckx et al. 2011).

The current term *gender dysphoria* is more descriptive and less stigmatizing than the previous DSM-IV term *gender identity disorder*, and it focuses on dysphoria as the clinical problem, not identity per se (American Psychiatric Association 2013). In contrast with a dichotomous approach, gender identity should be considered as a dimension, and it should be measured as a continuous non-dichotomous variable.

Indeed, even though persons requiring a genital reassignment surgery represent a very low percentage of the population (American Psychiatric Association 2013), some studies reported that there has been a recent increase in the number of individuals who identify as *transgender* (Feldman and Bockting 2003). Experienced gender may include alternative gender identities beyond binary stereotypes. *Transgender* refers to the broad spectrum of individuals who transiently or persistently identify with a gender different from their natal gender, while transsexuals are persons who seek a social transition from male to female or female to male, which eventually involves a somatic transition by cross-sex hormone treatment and genital surgery (sex reassignment surgery). According to De Cuypere et al., review of the literature (2007), the prevalence figures reported in these ten studies range from 1:11,900 to 1:45,000 for male-to-female individuals (MtF) and 1:30,400 to 1:200,000 for female-to-male (FtM) individuals. Therefore the commonly used term *transsexual* refers only to a tip of an iceberg of nonconforming gender identities. Accordingly there are a lot of intermediate conditions up to the subthreshold clinical gender dysphoria. For example, the so-called tranny boys who are frequent among young lesbian women (McCarthy 2003; Rochman 2006), frequently desire a "partial" sex reassignment such as mastectomy, but not masculinizing hormone treatment or vice versa. Moreover, it has been noted that female-to-male transsexual women and self-identified "butch" lesbians shared a common feeling of "anatomic dysphoria" (Lee 2001). Another example is represented by intersex conditions which often show variation in long-term gender identity outcome, both within and across syndromes (Zucker 1999). For example, persons with congenital adrenal hyperplasia often appear to differentiate a gender identity consistent with their gender assignment and rearing (Dessens et al. 2005), but only few of them develop full-blown gender dysphoria (Meyer-Bahlburg et al. 1996). In other conditions, such as 5-alpha-reductase 2 deficiency (Cohen-Kettenis 2005) or in genetic males with cloacal exstrophy (Meyer-Bahlburg 2005), gender dysphoria and gender change are much more common.

According to the new definition proposed by the DSM 5 to the fluidity of the real world of gender identity in the population, new instruments have been recently developed for gender dysphoria, such as the Gender Identity/Gender Dysphoria Questionnaire for adolescents and adults (GIDYQ-AA), which were designed to assess gender identity (gender dysphoria) dimensionally. This measure conceptualized gender identity/gender dysphoria as a bipolar continuum with a male pole and a female pole and varying degrees of gender dysphoria, gender uncertainty, or gender identity transitions between the poles.

Moreover, gender nonconforming individuals are not inherently disordered. Rather, the distress of gender dysphoria, when present, is the concern that might be diagnosable and for which various treatment options are available. The existence of a diagnosis for such dysphoria often facilitates access to health care and can guide further research into effective treatments.

4.2.4 Why Gender Dysphoria? Nurture and Nature

A still unresolved question regards why some persons develop a disease of such entity to ask for long-lasting hormonal treatment as well as for complex surgical interventions. How can one explain a felt incongruence between gender identity and sex of birth?

A first interpretation was provided by Freud. According to his theory on gender identity development, the resolution of Oedipus conflict leads the child to identify with the same sex parent and thus to acquire a stable sex and gender identity. If this process is inhibited by traumatic experiences, sex and gender identifications are likely to be hindered, and people can have problems in sex and gender identification. Even though the Freudian theory of gender identity development has been criticized, there are still authors supporting the idea that transgenderism results from situations of family conflicts that the child elaborates through rejection of their gender.

The dichotomy between *nature* and *nurture*—between what is biologically determined and the effect of the environment—is now considered outdated. Therefore, the biopsychosocial perspective appears to be adequate also for gender identity and gender dysphoria. Historically, the various authors that conceptualized their theories on gender identity development often adopted a biological, a psychological, or a social view.

Various theories have incorporated the importance of social factors for gender identity development. A strong support for an *exclusive nurture* theory on gender identity development was postulated by Money et al. (1955), who proposed the idea that core gender identity was malleable and could be formed by raising a child as male or female during a critical period in early childhood. Even though this extreme position was later considered wrong, further studies demonstrated the importance of social factors in gender identity development. For example, Kohlberg (1966), proposed that children develop gender identity only when they are cognitively able to understand that gender differences exist and understand the meaning of gender identity. Early social learning theory stressed the importance of gender role behavior and how it is shaped by reward (Maccoby and Jacklin 1987), and Bandura argued for the importance of gender role modeling (Bussey and Bandura 1999).

From a biological perspective, the *nature* "side of the coin" was supported by studies showing the structural differences between males and females in size and distribution of white and gray matter and that these differences are correlated with differences in cognitive functioning (Gur et al. 1999). Moreover, transsexuals showed a specific brain area similar in size to that of the identified sex instead of the assigned biological sex (Zhou et al. 1995). In particular, there is evidence that the central bed nucleus of the stria terminalis (BSTc), a hypothalamic structure implicated in sexual behavior, is small in male-to-female transsexuals, similar to most females. Furthermore, individuals with gender discordance may differ in central nervous system lateralization from the general population (Bradley and Zucker 1997). Indeed, they are more likely to be non-right-handed, to have abnormal EEG findings, and to have lateral otoacoustic processing consistent with their gender identity compared to a non-gender discordant population.

As far as hormonal theories are concerned, it has been noted that variations in prenatal sex hormones may influence later gender identity but do not appear to fully determine it (Meyer-Bahlburg 2005).

Finally, genetic factors have been implicated, as genetic males with gender discordance tend to have a later birth order and lower birth weight, suggesting an influence of prenatal events (Bradley and Zucker 1997).

In conclusion, there is no evidence that transgenderism is monocausal and upbringing has a large role in its development (Gaffney and Reyes 2009).

4.3 Diagnosis and Treatment

4.3.1 Diagnosis

In our clinical practice with gender dysphoria, we often have to face the common ignorance spread in the general population regarding gender identity/dysphoria. It is quite common that persons confuse gender dysphoria with homosexuality. Even though these two concepts are mutually correlated, gender identity and sexual orientation do not represent the same construct. *Sexual orientation* refers to the sex of the person to whom an individual is erotically attracted. It comprises several components, including sexual fantasy, patterns of physiological arousal, sexual behavior, sexual identity, and social role. Scientific studies demonstrating the healthy, adaptive functioning of the great majority of gay and lesbian adults paved the way toward removal of homosexuality as an illness from the DSM in 1973 (Bayer 1981). Therefore, homosexuality is now recognized as a non-pathological variant of human sexuality.

Moreover, clinicians should be aware that gender atypical does not always underlie a pathological condition, rather it refers to somatic features or behaviors that are not typical (in a statistical sense) of individuals with the same assigned gender in a given society and historical era. For behavior, gender nonconforming is an alternative descriptive term. As for all the other clinical conditions included in the DSM, mental health professionals should consider to take care of persons with gender atypical features only when they identify an individual's affective/cognitive discontent with the assigned gender, the so-called dysphoria.

Many times, gender dysphoria persons are not aware about the significance of their disease. Unrecognized conditions are occasionally diagnosed when patients are seen with anxiety, depression, conduct disorder, substance abuse, dissociative identity disorders, borderline personality disorder, sexual disorders, and disorders of sex development (Cole et al. 1997a, b).

On the contrary, inexperienced clinicians may mistake indications of gender dysphoria for other psychiatric conditions, and the diagnosis is not meant to merely describe nonconformity to stereotypical gender role behavior (e.g., "tomboyism" in girls, "girly boy" behavior in boys, occasional cross-dressing in adult men). Indeed, gender dysphoria should be distinguished from simple nonconformity to stereotypical gender role behavior by the strong desire to be of another gender than the assigned one and by the extent and pervasiveness of gender-variant activities and interests (American Psychiatric Association 2013). A distinction should be made with transvestic disorder, which occurs in heterosexual persons for whom cross-dressing behavior generates sexual excitement and causes distress and/or impairment without drawing their primary gender into question. Body uneasiness is a core psychopathological feature for gender dysphoria as well as for other psychiatric disorder such as eating and body dysmorphic disorders. However, an individual with body dysmorphic disorder focuses on the alteration of a specific body part which he perceived as abnormally formed, not because it represents a repudiated assigned gender. Finally, among schizophrenic patients, there may rarely be delusions of belonging to some other gender. However, phenomenologically, there is a qualitative difference between the presentation of gender dysphoria and the presentation of delusions or other psychotic symptoms. Moreover, the vast majority of children and adolescents with gender dysphoria are not suffering from underlying severe psychiatric illness such as psychotic disorders (Steensma et al. 2011).

A relevant issue is represented by the diagnosis among children and young adolescent. The diagnosis of gender dysphoria in children is controversial (Meyer-Bahlburg 2010). Several different categories of gender discordance, each characterized by a unique developmental trajectory, have been described (Steensma and Cohen-Kettenis 2011). They differ in regard to whether gender discordance emerges in childhood, adolescence, or adulthood; whether the gender discordance is persistent or transient; and whether there is a post-transition homosexual or heterosexual orientation. In follow-up studies of prepubertal boys with gender discordance—including many without any mental health treatment—the cross-gender wishes usually fade over time and do not persist into adulthood, with only 2.2 % (Green 1987) to 11.9 % (Zucker and Bradley 1995) continuing to experience gender discordance. Rather, 75 % become homosexual or bisexual in fantasy and 80 % in behavior by age 19; some gender-variant behavior may persist (Zucker and Bradley 1995). The desistence of gender discordance may reflect the resolution of a "cognitive confusion factor," (Zucker et al. 1993) with increasing flexibility as children mature in thinking about gender identity and realize that one can be a boy or girl despite variation from conventional gender roles and norms.

4.3.2 Therapy

In the last years treatment for patients with gender identity concerns has shifted considerably. “Sex change” operations are freely available in many centers around the globe. While once patients and doctors had to fight for the legitimization of such operations, the discourse has now changed radically. In the last 50 years, health professionals began to provide assistance to alleviate gender dysphoria by supporting changes in primary and secondary sex characteristics through hormone therapy and surgery, along with a change in gender role. Treatment options include hormone therapy to feminize or masculinize the body and surgery to change primary and/or secondary sex characteristics (e.g., breasts/chest, external and/or internal genitalia, facial features, body contouring). Both hormone therapy and surgery have been found to be medically necessary to alleviate gender dysphoria in most of the people (American Medical Association 2008; Brown 2009, The World Professional Association for Transgender Health, 2008), including the severe body uneasiness often reported (Bandini et al. 2013; Fisher et al. 2014). Satisfaction of genital reassignment surgery rates across studies ranged from 87 % of MtF patients to 97 % of FtM patients (Green and Fleming 1990), and regrets were extremely rare (1–1.5 % of MtF patients and <1 % of FtM patients; Pfäfflin 1992).

However, a variety of therapeutic options should be considered, as the number and type of interventions applied and the order in which these take place may differ from person to person (Rachlin et al. 2010). For example, while many individuals need both hormone therapy and surgery to alleviate their gender dysphoria, others need only one of these treatment options and some need neither (Bockting and Goldberg 2006). Often with the help of psychotherapy, some individuals integrate their trans- or cross-gender feelings into the gender role they were assigned at birth and do not feel the need to feminize or masculinize their body. Sometimes, changes in gender expression and role (which may involve living part time or full time in another gender role, consistent with one’s gender identity) represent the best and unique therapeutic option. Psychotherapy includes individual, couple, family, or group interventions. It is aimed at exploring gender identity, role, and expression, addressing the negative impact of gender dysphoria and stigma on mental health, alleviating internalized transphobia, enhancing social and peer support, improving body image, or promoting resilience.

For children and adolescents, a combined approach includes administration of medical therapies as well as psychotherapy, social intervention, and family work (Di Ceglie and Thümmel 2006; Cohen-Kettenis et al. 2008). The main aim of this approach is to alleviate distress and improve the child’s quality of life and not to reduce cross-gender behavior or realign the child’s perceived gender with the gender of assignment.

References

American Medical Association. (2008). Resolution 122 (A-08). Retrieved from http://www.ama-assn.org/ama1/pub/upload/mm/471/122.doc

American Psychiatric Association (2013) Diagnostic and Statistical Manual of Mental Disorders, Fifth edition. Washington, DC London, England.

Bandini, E., Fisher, A. D., Castellini, G., Lo Sauro, C., Lelli, L., Meriggiola, M. C., et al. (2013). Gender identity disorder and eating disorders: Similarities and differences in terms of body uneasiness. *The Journal of Sexual Medicine, 10*(4), 1012–23.

Bayer, R. (1981). *Homosexuality and American psychiatry: The politics of diagnosis*. New York: Basic Books.

Bockting, W. O., & Goldberg, J. M. (2006). Guidelines for transgender care (special issue). International Journal of Transgenderism, 9(3/4).

Bradley, S. J., & Zucker, K. J. (1997). Gender identity disorder: A review of the past 10 years. *Journal of the American Academy of Child and Adolescent Psychiatry, 36*, 872–880.

Brown, G. R. (2009). Recommended revisions to The World Professional Association for Transgender Health's Standards of Care section on medical care for incarcerated persons with gender identity disorder. *International Journal of Transgenderism, 11*(2), 133–139.

Bussey, K., & Bandura, A. (1999). Social cognitive theory of gender development and differentiation. *Psychological Review, 106*, 676–713.

Cohen-Kettenis, P. T. (2005). Gender change in 46, XY persons with 58-reductase-2 deficiency and 179-hydroxysteroid dehydrogenase-3 deficiency. *Archives of Sexual Behavior, 34*, 399–410.

Cohen-Kettenis, P. T., Delemarre-van de Waal, H., & Gooren, L. J. G. (2008). The treatment of adolescent transsexuals: Changing insights. *Journal of Sexual Medicine, 5*(8), 1892–1897.

Cole, C. M., O'Boyle, M., Emory, L. E., & Meyer, W. J., III. (1997a). Comorbidity of GID and other major psychiatric diagnoses. *Archives of Sexual Behavior, 26*, 13–26.

Cole, C. M., O'Boyle, M., Emory, L. E., & Meyer, W. J., III. (1997b). Comorbidity of gender dysphoria and other major psychiatric diagnoses. *Archives of Sexual Behavior, 26*(1), 13–26.

De Cuypere, G., Janes, C., & Rubens, R. (1995). Psychosocial functioning of transsexuals in Belgium. *Acta Psychiatr Scand, 91*, 180–184.

De Cuypere, G., Van Hemelrijck, M., Michel, A., Carael, B., Heylens, G., Rubens, R., Hoebeke, P., & Monstrey, S. (2007). Prevalence and demography of transsexualism in Belgium. *European Psychiatry, 22*(3), 137–41.

Dessens, A. B., Slijper, F. M. E., & Drop, S. L. S. (2005). Gender dysphoria and gender change in chromosomal females with congenital adrenal hyperplasia. *Archives of Sexual Behavior, 34*, 389–397.

Di Ceglie, D., & Freedman, D. (1998). *A stranger in my own body: Atypical gender identity development and mental health. Front Cover*. London: Karnac Books.

Di Ceglie, D., & Thümmel, E. C. (2006). An experience of group work with parents of children and adolescents with gender identity disorder. *Clinical Child Psychology and Psychiatry, 11* (3), 387–396.

Erikson, E. H. (1970). *Identität und Lebenszyklus*. Frankfurt am Main: Suhrkamp.

Factor, R. J., & Rothblum, E. D. (2007). A study of transgender adults and their non-transgender siblings on demographic characteristics, social support, and experiences of violence. *Journal of LGBT Health Research, 3*, 11–30.

Fairburn, C. G. (2008). Eating disorders: The transdiagnostic view and the cognitive behavioural theory. In *Cognitive behavior therapy and eating disorders* (pp. 7–22). New York: Guilford Press.

Feldman, J., & Bockting, W. (2003). Transgender health. *Minnesota Medicine, 86*(7), 25–32.

Fisher, A. D., Castellini, G., Bandini, E., Casale, H., Fanni, E., Benni, L., Ferruccio, N., Meriggiola, M. C., Manieri, C., Gualerzi, A., Jannini, E., Oppo, A., Ricca, V., Maggi, M., & Rellini, A. H. (2014). Cross-sex hormonal treatment and body uneasiness in individuals with gender dysphoria. *The Journal of Sexual Medicine, 11*(3), 709–19.

Freud, S. (1962). *Three essays on the theory of sexuality*. New York, NY: Avon. Original work published in 1903.

Gaffney, B., & Reyes, P. (2009). Gender identity dysphoria. In M. Lanyado & A. Horne (Eds.), *The handbook of child and adolescent psychotherapy: Psychoanalytic approaches*. New York, NY: Routledge.

Giordano, S. (2011). Sex and gender: Issues of public health and justice. In M. Boylan (Ed.), *The morality and global justice*. Colorado: Perseus Academics. Chapter 18.

Giordano, S. (2012). *Children with gender identity disorder, a clinical, ethical and legal analysis*. London and New York: Routledge.

Golombok, S., Cook, R., Bish, A., & Murray, C. (1995). Families created by the new reproductive technologies: Quality of parenting and social and emotional development of the children. *Child Development, 66*, 285–289.

Golombok, S., MacCallum, F., & Goodman, E. (2001). The 'test-tube' generation: Parent–child relationships and the psychological well-being of in vitro fertilization children at adolescence. *Child Development, 72*, 599–608.

Gómez-Gil, E., Trilla, A., Salamero, M., Godás, T., & Valdés, M. (2009). Sociodemographic, clinical, and psychiatric characteristics of transsexuals from Spain. *Archives of Sexual Behavior, 38*, 378–92.

Gooren, L. (2006). The biology of human psychosexual differentiation. *Hormones and Behavior, 50*, 589–601.

Gooren, L. (2011). Clinical practice. Care of transsexual persons. *The New England Journal of Medicine, 364*, 1251–7.

Green, R. (1987). *The "sissy-boy syndrome" and the development of homosexuality*. New Haven: Yale University Press.

Green, R., & Fleming, D. T. (1990). Transsexual surgery follow-up: Status in the 1990s. *Annual Review of Sex, 1*, 163–174.

Gur, R. C., Turetsky, B. I., Matsui, M., Yan, M., Bilker, W., Hughett, P., et al. (1999). Sex differences in brain gray and white matter in healthy young adults: Correlations with cognitive performance. *The Journal of Neuroscience: The Official Journal of the Society for Neuroscience, 19*, 4065–4072.

Haraldsen, I. R., & Dahl, A. A. (2000). Symptom profiles of GID patients of transsexual type compared to patients with personality disorders and healthy adults. *Acta Psychiatrica Scandinavica, 102*, 276–81.

Hoshiai, M., Matsumoto, Y., Sato, T., Ohnishi, M., Okabe, N., Kishimoto, Y., Terada, S., & Kuroda, S. (2010). Psychiatric comorbidity among patients with gender identity disorder. *Psychiatry and Clinical Neurosciences, 64*, 514–9.

Husserl, E. (1912–1915). Ideen zu einer reinen Phaenomenologie und phaenomenologische Philosophie. II. Phaenomenologische Untersuchungen zur Konstitution. Den Haag: Nijhoff.

Johansson, A., Sundbom, E., Höjerback, T., & Bodlund, O. (2010). A five year follow-up study of Swedish adults with gender identity disorder. *Archives of Sexual Behavior, 39*, 1429–379.

Kinsbourne, M. (2002). Brain and body awareness. In T. F. Cash & T. Pruzinsky (Eds.), *Body image: A handbook of theory, research, and clinical practice*. New York: Guilford Press.

Kohlberg, L. A. (1966). A cognitive-developmental analysis of children's sex role concepts and attitudes. In E. E. Maccoby (Ed.), *The development of sex differences* (pp. 82–173). Stanford, CA: Stanford University Press.

Kraemer, B., Delsignore, A., Schnyder, U., & Hepp, U. (2008). Body image and transsexualism. *Psychopathology, 41*, 96–10027.

Lee, T. (2001). Trans(re)lations: Lesbian and female to male transsexual accounts of identity. *Women's Studies International Forum, 24*, 347–357.
Maccoby, E. E., & Jacklin, C. N. (1987). Gender segregation in childhood. *Advances in Child Development and Behavior, 20*, 239–287.
Matsumoto, Y., Sato, T., Ohnishi, M., Kishimoto, Y., Terada, S., & Kuroda, S. (2009). Stress coping strategies of patients with gender identity disorder. *Psychiatry and Clinical Neurosciences, 63*, 715–20.
McCarthy, L. (2003). Off that spectrum entirely: A study of female bodied transgender-identified individuals. Unpublished doctoral dissertation, University of Massachusetts, Amherst.
Merleau-Ponty, M. (1996). Phenomenology of perception. Engl. Transl. by Colin Smith. New York: Humanities Press.
Meyer-Bahlburg, H. F. (2005). Gender identity outcome in female-raised 46, XY persons with penile agenesis, cloacal exstrophy of the bladder, or penile ablation. *Archives of Sexual Behavior, 34*, 423–438.
Meyer-Bahlburg, H. F. L. (2010). From mental disorder to iatrogenic hypogonadism: Dilemmas in conceptualizing gender identity variants as psychiatric conditions. *Archives of Sexual Behavior, 39*, 461–476.
Meyer-Bahlburg, H. F. L., Gruen, R. S., New, M. I., Bell, J. J., Morishima, A., Shimshi, M., et al. (1996). Gender change from female to male in classical congenital adrenal hyperplasia. *Hormones and Behavior, 30*, 319–332.
Money, J. (1971). Transsexualism and the philosophy of healing. *The Journal of the American Society of Psychosomatic Dentistry and Medicine, 18*, 25–26.
Money, J., Hampson, J. G., & Hampson, J. L. (1955). Hermaphroditism: Recommendations concerning assignment of sex, change of sex and psychologic management. *Bulletin of the Johns Hopkins Hospital, 97*, 284–300.
Nuttbrock, L., Hwahng, S., Bockting, W., Rosenblum, A., Mason, M., Macri, M., & Becker, J. (2010). Psychiatric impact of gender-related abuse across the life course of male-to-female transgender persons. *Journal of Sex Research, 47*, 12–23.
Pfäffl, F. (2014). Identity: A historical and political reflection. In P. C. K. Baudewijntje, T. D. Steensma, & A. L. C. de Vries (Eds.) *Gender dysphoria and disorders of sex development progress in care and knowledge*. Springer.
Pfäfflin, F. (1992). Regrets after sex reassignment surgery. *Journal of Psychology and Human Sexuality, 5*, 69–85.
Rachlin, K., Hansbury, G., & Pardo, S. T. (2010). Hysterectomy and oophorectomy experiences of female-to-male transgender individuals. *International Journal of Transgenderism, 12*(3), 155–166.
Rochman, S. (2006, April 11). Life in the T zone. The Advocate. Retrieved August 24, 2006, from http://www.advocate.com/print_article_ektid28281.asp
Schelling, F.W.J. (1801). *Darstellung meines Systems der Philosophie*. (cp. First outline of the philosophy of nature [2004]. New York: State University of New York).
Stanghellini, G., Castellini, G., Brogna, P., Faravelli, C., & Ricca, V. (2012). Identity and eating disorders (IDEA): A questionnaire evaluating identity and embodiment in eating disorder patients. *Psychopathology, 45*(3), 147–58.
Steensma, T. D., Biemond, R., de Boer, F., & Cohen-Kettenis, P. T. (2011). Desisting and persisting gender dysphoria after childhood: A qualitative follow-up study. Clinical Child Psychology and Psychiatry. Advance online publication.
Steensma, T. D., & Cohen-Kettenis, P. T. (2011). Gender transitioning before puberty? *Archives of Sexual Behavior, 40*(4), 649–650. doi:10.1007/s10508-011-9752-2.
Vocks, S., Stahn, C., Loenser, K., & Legenbauer, T. (2009). Eating and body image disturbances in male-to-female and female-to-male transsexuals. *Archives of Sexual Behavior, 38*, 364–77.
Wierckx, K., Van Caenegem, E., Elaut, E., Dedecker, D., Van de Peer, F., Toye, K., et al. (2011). Quality of life and sexual health after sex reassignment surgery in transsexual men. *The Journal of Sexual Medicine, 8*(12), 3379–88.

Zhou, J. N., Hofman, M. A., Gooren, L. J., & Swaab, D. F. (1995). A sex difference in the human brain and its relation to transsexuality. *Nature, 378*, 68–70.
Zucker, K. J. (1999). Intersexuality and gender identity differentiation. *Annual Review of Sex Research, 10*, 1–69.
Zucker, K. J., & Bradley, S. J. (1995). *Gender identity disorder and psychosexual problems in children and adolescents*. New York: Guilford Press.
Zucker, K. J., Bradley, S. J., Sullivan, C. B., Kuksis, M., Birkenfeld-Adams, A., & Mitchell, J. N. (1993). A gender identity interview for children. *Journal of Personality Assessment, 61*, 443–456.

5 An Experiential Approach to Dissociative Phenomena

Luis Madeira and Maria Luisa Figueira

5.1 A Clinical Vignette

Eduard is a 22-year-old Portuguese male, single, Caucasian, with no children, born in Lisbon, and living in Lisbon. He performed outstandingly during high school in a science-based curriculum where he had "enjoyed my life as a student being an extroverted, warmhearted, enjoying and fostering a strong group of friends." At the age of 18, after a problematic breakup (a 2-year relationship), he became help-seeking for the complaints that are described next and started psychotherapeutic and psychiatric treatment. During the following 2 years, he underwent treatment with antidepressants (SSRI and SNRI) and benzodiazepines as well as completed a year of weekly psychoanalytical psychotherapy and a year of weekly cognitive behavioral therapy. He had no past medical diagnosis and no substance abuse or forensic history. There were no formal psychiatric diagnoses in any of his family members though he referred that his father had been diagnosed with psychotic episodes (with paranoid and persecutory delusions) but did not entertain any psychiatric assistance other than acute prescription at emergency department and his mother showed anxious and an anankastic personality traits.

Our initial contact with Eduard occurred 2 years after his original complaints through a visit to our emergency department in North Lisbon Hospital Centre. His main complaint was "I have lost contact with reality. The best way to translate it is in recognizing my face as familiar in the mirror or, in case of not having that notion of reality, I just do not recognize myself. I need to recover the notion of reality and myself." In his first psychopathological assessment, he showed restless behavior and general distress, syntonic contact, clear reference in time and space and also an auto-psychically, euthymic mood slightly unhinged, physical and psychic anxiety,

L. Madeira (✉) • M.L. Figueira
Psychiatry Department, Hospital Santa Maria, Lisbon, Portugal

Faculdade de Medicina, University of Lisbon, Lisbon, Portugal
e-mail: luismadeiramd@gmail.com; unknownplace@gmail.com

G. Stanghellini, M. Aragona (eds.), *An Experiential Approach to Psychopathology*,
DOI 10.1007/978-3-319-29945-7_5

severe depersonalization and derealization (d&d), no apparent thought disturbances other than pressure of speech and rumination about his d&d experiences (no formal thought disorders), and no eating or sleeping disturbances. After an initial psychiatric follow-up, he commenced weekly client-centered psychotherapy treatment, which lasted for a year, and 3 years of psychiatric treatment. We attempted most psychopharmacological drugs from antipsychotics (including clozapine), antidepressants (including clomipramine), and mood stabilizers (including carbamazepine) with no consistent improvement. Despite enduring continuous symptoms and experiencing them as severe, restricting and disabling his performance fluctuated dramatically irrespective of the symptom burden ranging from (1) periods of loss of contact with reality, severe social isolation, and being restricted to home care (once he admitted to an in-patient unit and he spent 1 month at a day-hospital) to (2) average to good functioning with good social life and being esteemed worker and good student. Extensive neuropsychiatric tests were performed twice and suggested normal executive functions and no other disruption.

Eduard sent emails spontaneously, almost as a log of his daily activities referring mostly to anxious and d&d phenomena. The phenomena listed here (providing a glimpse into Eduards subjective world) and in Sect. 5.3 refer to those presented in (1) psychotherapeutic sessions (client-centered psychotherapy) which were taped for supervision purposes (tutoring) and (2) over a thousand detailed emails in the past 3 years.

> "I'm getting crazy, for times this is just anxiety but then I start being saturated and destroyed, losing pleasure in the things that I do"…"I don't feel time passing by, I can feel space, I can't feel my body. There are so many everyday life things that I cannot feel. I'm not available to reality. And this state is progressive a fact which always brings me down. Sometimes I feel that someone should open my chest with a machine-gun. I just can't "let it be", the lack of pain and feeling is not a good thing of course"…"I do not allow myself to become close to others, I've lost my inner center, I even fear of being homosexual, it is really as if I'm living a parallel history of my life, and the worse is that in this story I'm a bystander—I don't feel anything. You've led to try and see "how I feel" but that's just too vague and I don't feel much anything besides emotional distance and apathy"…"Sometimes I think this represents my lack of mental health while many other moments I feel I just lack disposition to do whatever"… "I'm worried with my emotional apathy. I see my girlfriend crying and I cannot cry, not even sadness, not guilt nor anything. I'm very worried because I'm becoming rigid. This rigidity is very worrying because it takes away my power"…"I think this is the lack of mental well-being and it is because I have suffered too much. I feel like I always have a cloud in my head"… "I feel as if I had suffered so much that I cannot believe that such amount of suffering could exist and it was more plausible that reality didn't exist" "I cannot stand this anguish, I can't stand this. This is sick. I can find a solution and I spend all days in my room. I can't feel this anymore. I already finished with her why am I left in this state, why? Enough. I'm not suicidal. But I cannot stand this suffering anymore"…"I can't feel sorry or shame. I can't feel anything. I have no identity, I feel no connection to others, everyone is a stranger to me, I feel no shame, I have no self concept"…"my head is going berserk, everything is just a mess, I'm all mixed up inside, fantasy gets mixture with reality. Yes I did get to some conclusions but today I got worse for staying home. My thoughts have become diffused and I can no longer separate things, I don't know why I keep making these associations"…"Everyone says I'm

obsessive-compulsive, as I don't show a critical appraisal the contents of my thoughts. But that critical stance exists thought only projected because I'm restless, it is an appraisal that reminds me that before it wasn't like this and the tendency is to vanish as I'm reinforcing my state and each time less my healthy readings of reality"..."I'm becoming paranoid, I feel that my friends talk to my girlfriend behind my back"..."My previous therapist just destroyed the rest always asking questions like "do you ever feel that persons in the newspaper are spying you?" For 3 months I felt that everyone was a spy by always testing myself. Convincing myself otherwise was almost impossible, made tests to myself lose the test I always lose the test and feel that I do feel that."

5.1.1 Appraising His Clinical Record

Despite a 5-year follow-up, Eduard has been challenging from the standpoints of diagnosis and treatment. At symptom level he displayed trait features of psychical and physical anxiety, derealization, and depersonalization experiences and states of psychomotor agitation and retardation, dysphoric, euphoric, and depressed moods with times of mood instability. His thought disturbances included experienced and observed thought pressure as well as overvalued, obsessive, and quasi-delusional ideation. A disturbing feature of his emails was the perseverance of ideas, as they seemed, from time to time, to recapitulate themselves on examples (he had little insight for such persistence). Along the 5 years there were no disturbances in appetite, sleep-wake rhythm, or suicidal ideation. According to ICD-10 classification system, there were periods where criteria were present for the diagnosis of general anxiety disorder, obsessive-compulsive disorder, dissociative fugue, psychotic episode, bipolar disorder, major depressive disorder, substance abuse, and several traits of borderline and anxious personality disorders.

His psychopharmacological treatment was decided largely to address anxiety and also, at times where diagnoses (nosology) were implied, for direct treatment of each diagnostic impression. Large arrangements of prescriptions were attempted along the years comprising most antipsychotics (including clozapine), antidepressants (including most tricyclic antidepressants), mood stabilizers (including lithium), and benzodiazepines. No improvement was acknowledged with exception of the reduction of anxiety through diazepam and other benzodiazepines. Indeed his enduring and severe symptomatic presentation seemed to improve and worsen across his life events. These comprised (1) a breakup form a long-standing relationship, (2) a rehousing process (left for a period from his parents' house), (3) voluntary and involuntary unemployment, and (4) permanent change of his friendships.

Eduard presently considers psychopharmacological treatment noneffective and psychiatric follow-up as negative to his recovery, and yet he accepts them both. He takes that psychodynamic and cognitive behavioral therapies were both prejudicial to his recovery by increasing or adding more elements to the intricateness of his chain of thoughts and increasing his cognitive strain. Along the 2 years where he decided just for sole psychiatric treatment, he described that the year of weekly client-centered therapy "was fruitful in decision-making and clarifying difficult moments in his life" moreover it allowed him to focus and explore his experiential features. . .there were times in the sessions where he felt he was "in contact with reality and himself." Recently he decided to resume his weekly therapy sessions. An interesting take on his experiences arising from the last therapy sessions includes "I think it is my creativity and my intelligence that makes me this way, they took hold and I came to be in this state of everlasting diffidence, there is no proof for the things I doubt, the things I lack we all take for granted, but there are moments, there are always moments, I take it as happiness but they are also ecstatic where I can get a peek into experiencing reality—this state of well-being is really rare this time. This is what I want to achieve."

Therapist and psychiatrist agree with Eduard that his symptom constellation was unaffected by most treatments and that the patient remained help-seeking for the last 5 years. Despite the extreme suffering experiences and important fractures in his performance, the features of his personal contact, including his empathy, warmheartedness, and care, countered the possibility of the diagnosis of schizophrenia and to some point suggested to us that his restlessness might be hypomanic. Also his most relevant subjective distress was permanent depersonalization and derealization, features that were expressed in rich metaphorical language and some of which are described along the discussion of this chapter.

5.2 A Conceptual History of Dissociation

Eduard's main complaint is of suffering from dissociative phenomena (DP) particularly depersonalization and derealization (DD). By its nature, the distress of depersonalization experiences refers to the subject of complexity of human subjective experience suggesting the possibility of suffering not only through the presence of a feeling but also by the lack of feelings. Derealization implies that the meaning of experiences is not immediate but a process of inner attribution of meaning (and conceptualization) in which if disturbed can lead to different amounts of perplexity (or even loss of natural evidence). Most of Eduard's descriptions are made by metaphors adding to the overall idea that these changes in engagement with the world, enactment of meanings, and periods of loss of awareness are not easily transmittable. As a group, DP are complex as they involve (1) a large range of phenomena and (2) they occur in a large number of psychiatric and neurologic disorders as well as in healthy persons. The idea of dissociation in psychiatry has had various inputs and such is expressed in symptomatology (conceptual halo) and nosology, as in the different stances about dissociative disorders expressed in DSM-5 and ICD-10 (APA 2013; World Health Organization 1992). As with other psychiatric symptoms, DP are in need of increased conceptual and phenomenological inquiry. Dissociative disorders as a broad category raise criticism on the "lack (of) a single, coherent referent . . . that all investigators in the field embrace" [chapter by Cardena in Lynn and Rhue (1994)], and yet some of its central categories have shown phenomenological consistency [as is the case of depersonalization (Sierra and Berrios 2001)]. Dissociative amnesia, depersonalization (and derealization), conversion symptoms (somatic symptoms), pseudo-hallucinations, trance, and self-disturbances are taken as classic dissociative phenomena.

Our up-to-date manuals including the ICD-10 (World Health Organization 1992) and the DSM-5 (APA 2013) use mainly an epistemology of changes of consciousness and the separation of "mental functions" (Hilgard 1973). The ICD-10 takes dissociative phenomena as a partial or total loss of (1) an integrated memory system, (2) a conscious awareness of identity or sensations, and (3) the control of bodily movements, and DSM-5 details it as a "separation of mental functions usually integrated and consciously accessible" comprising both/either memory, identity, perception, emotions, and/or will (Hilgard 1973). The DSM-IV was reorganized in the DSM-5 to increase the homogeneity of the categories—depersonalization/derealization disorder instead of depersonalization and accepting dissociative amnesia as encompassing dissociative fugue. Overall the clinical use of both classifications involves intense criticism as patients are frequently assigned with the diagnosis of "dissociative disorder not otherwise specified" (Saxe et al. 1993; Kihlstrom 1994).

An historical review of the conceptual models for dissociation is out of the scope of this chapter and can be found in a comprehensive review by Onno van der Hart and Martin Dorahy (Rosenthal 2009). From their analysis we retrieve some important ideas. First the conceptualization of dissociation is driven from the very start as (1) a detachment of parts of personality in Puysegur, Moreau de Tours, Gros Jean, and Taine or (2) the occurrence of double consciousness described in Charcot, Feinkeind, Janet, and Binet (see more in the previous reference). The former suggests a disorganization of the incorporation of personality elements. The latter proposes a behavioral override by an independent mental structure that the subject is unaware and that bursts directly as a response to a stimulus.

An important epistemological quarrel included dissociation being considered a phenomenon, a neurological explanation, or a psychological understanding. As an explanation dissociation is seen as the mechanism of the conversion symptoms in psychiatry and of functional symptoms in neurology. The latter has provided dissociation another delicate aura—functional symptoms stand for absence of an organic explanation that neurologists would claim real (dissociation = absence of a real cause). As a psychological explanation (e.g., psychoanalytical inputs), dissociation stands as the most relevant conceptualization of hysterical symptoms by the separation of psychological elements under the light of preceding stressors (traumatic experiences). Further studies have suggested a consistent psychological and biological correlation between trauma and dissociative phenomena [see seminal work by Ferenczi Putnam (1989)]. As a phenomenon, dissociation is also represented in the ideas of depersonalization, fugue state, and dissociative amnesia. Dissociative phenomena as a group are troubling as each phenomenon occurs in contrasting situations (e.g., depersonalization in anxiety disorders and dissociative amnesia arising in patients that do not express clear anxiety symptoms and can sometimes show "la belle indifference"). Linking the previous considerations leads to even more intricate possibilities as depersonalization is being considered as a dissociative phenomenon with an anxious explanation (Baker et al. 2003; Sierra et al. 2012) or as a mechanism (detachment) of dissociative phenomena (Holmes et al. 2005).

Dissociative phenomena must also be distinguished if they occur (1) as a lifelong trait as in patients with schizoid, borderline, and anxious personality disorders or (2) in particular states as in depressive episodes, panic attacks, or epilepsy (Krüger and Mace 2002). Trait dissociation also appears to be phenomenologically related to the idea of schizophrenic autism and other basic symptoms. This discussion renders some troubles in the conceptualization of other dissociative phenomena as, for instance, amnesia in its anterograde form (inability to encode while in the situation) appears as a state, while retrograde amnesia (inability to retrieve elements of past situations) might occur as trait.

Another input is that dissociative phenomena could also accept lighter deviations of consciousness (e.g., daydreaming) suggesting that it is dimensional with non-pathological states (e.g., meditation). This discussion is age-old and materialized in the seminal quarreling by (1) Pierre Janet who supported that true dissociation only occurred in mental patients, specifically in hysteric subjects (Janet 2012) and (2) William James (James 1950) and Morton Prince (Prince 2012) who suggested it was dimensional occurring in adaptive and useful experiences (e.g., during stressful events) or in pathological situations. Some empirical studies support that a class of dissociation is pathological (Waller et al. 1996) and yet still with no nosological bearing as it occurs indistinctively in diverse taxonomical categories such as dissociation, schizophrenia, or PTSD (Waller and Ross 1997).

5.3 Dissociative Phenomena Through the Prism of Subjective Experience of Self

The idea that changes in the self are linked with dissociative phenomena is not new in psychiatry, but recently the research on this topic has increased (Parnas et al. 2003; Fuchs and Schlimme 2009; Stanghellini et al. 2012; Sass et al. 2013). Of all the conceptualizations, the idea of three interdependent levels of subjective experience of self seems to us useful to grasp differences between dissociative phenomena. In standard subjective experience of the self, the levels are attuned leading to a coherent narrative, effortless cognitive introspection, and a readily accessible body. Disturbances of the subjective experience of oneself take place when any of these levels are disturbed or there is a disconnection between them. The latter represents the dissociative mechanism that in this model would prime classic dissociative phenomena. Yet this model also accepts various phenomenological mimics due of these phenomena (e.g., derealization occurring due to a cessation of pre-reflexive level or due to its disconnection).

5.3.1 The Minimal Self

This first level, portrayed in the idea of a minimal self (Cermolacce et al. 2007; Legrand 2007), encompasses pre-reflexive experiential involvement with oneself and the world (and its pre-reflexive meaning). It incorporates the (multifaceted) notions of "myness" (the feeling of oneness with experience), "ipseity" (a nonpropositional acquaintance with oneself), "agency" (and the experience of embodied intentionality), self-awareness (ecological awareness of being in the world and awareness of the environment), vital feelings [see more in Scheler (1992)], "self-affection" and affective resonance (possibility for interpersonal synchronization), and self-continuity (retentional-protentional unity of internal consciousness and temporal coherence). Important attributes of the experience of the minimal self include (1) its nature of being implicit and involuntary and the subject oblivious to its existence under ordinary circumstances and (2) bearing hierarchical importance to other levels and edifying their foundations (its disturbances leading to devastating consequences on other levels of self-experience). So when fully operational, the pre-reflexive level allows effortless relatedness to (and understanding of) reality leading to an intuitive and transparent activity in the world. Disturbances in this level make the subject aware of being separate from oneself or of a sense of unfamiliarity or unreality of the environment. Also such immediate understanding allows the subject to act upon his perceptual experiences without cognitive effort. So beyond the experiential feature (which is discussed in Sect. 5.4), the minimal self refers to an immediate, pre-reflexive, or experiential meaning that imbues experience before any cognitive enterprise.

A disturbance in the minimal self could be conceptualized in Eduard's complaints including having to think more on what occurred ("I cannot stop thinking about what is happening to me, thinking it's a necessity as I feel that I'm always at risk of becoming perplexed"), losing the understanding about the other's behaviors ("I freeze in front of others as if I cannot understand usual gestures"), or even loss of familiarity ("my house doesn't seem my house, I feel I had never been here"). In descriptive psychopathology, these experiences refer to derealization experiences and yet also might refer to different phenomena including the (1) loss of the ability for ordinary undertakings (labeled as enacting and affordances), (2) loss of common sense and the manifestation of perplexity and a permanent struggle by introspection and cognitive reasoning, (3) attendance of new and private meanings about life, and (4) loss of a sense of acquaintance to one's world. The possibility of the subject accessing an embodied meaning (and its disturbance) is key to understanding situations where patients feel derealized while, at the same time, keeping on performing fine in their everyday functions.

5.3.2 The Cognitive Self

A second level is conceived as cognitive and includes the voluntary and semi-voluntary effort to cognitively introspect on experiences. The phenomena involved in this level include (1) judgments and beliefs on oneself and the world (self-reflection); (2) body image, the reflexive concept of oneself; and (3) perspective taking—possibility to assess reality through different perspectives. As described, commotions in the previous level can lead to major disturbances in this level, and examples include (1) compensatory and primary forms of hyper-reflexivity, (2) delusional interpretation of reality, and (3) abstract idealization—"a kind of spiritual or intellectual utopian ideology, detached from concrete daily interpersonal life" (Stanghellini 2004).

Together with the derealization feeling, Edward complained that a part of his suffering was due to being restlessly thinking about experiences aiming to regain "contact with reality" through "thinking about reality," a straining cognitive effort in which, for times, he risked reaching farfetched conclusions against his actual objective and cultural milieu. This painful, frustrating and involuntary process of introspection had become out of control and was now imposed upon him—he felt that thoughts arose independently of his own will. In descriptive psychopathology symbols, these phenomena would be quoted as thought pressure, obsessive and compulsive ideas, and hyper-reflexivity. He also complained of losing the capacity to "think clearly" both by feeling that other person's ideas were saturating his way of seeing the world or as if he wasn't the author of his thoughts. Some of these disturbances that are well represented in other chapters of classical descriptive psychopathology (obsessive ideation, ruminations, passivity experiences) seem also to constitute d&d experiences by a felt sense of losing control of the frequency, proprietorship, and presentation of thoughts as well as a feeling of loss of control of the contents of thoughts. Such changes (together with insight) lead the patient to an overall strangeness and loss of harmony of his way of thinking. These disturbances have a close relation with other categories (discussed in Sect. 5.2 in the epistemology of subjective self-disturbances) as they are conceived as referring to a primary loss of other faculties (cognitive disturbance is the endpoint of other processes). Becoming derealized through changes in cognition could turn out to be (1) disturbances of the form of thoughts (see classical formal thought disorders), (2) hyper-reflexivity (as involuntary thinking processes), (3) disturbances of the cadence of thoughts (acceleration or slowing of thoughts), or an (4) altered hierarchical relation between thoughts and one's consciousness (the feeling that thoughts are not originated in oneself).

5.3.3 The Biographical Self

The third level of self-experience entails the cohesive judgment over one's own attitudes and memory arrangements that add up to the experience of having a biography and to the possibility of portraying oneself through a story (Gallagher and Shear 1999). The experience of oneself includes a coherent narrative for one's life that is different from all experiential, physical, or cognitive milieus. Such is portrayed in Proust "the corporeal envelope of our friend had been so well stuffed with all this (narrative details), as well as with a few memories relating to his parents, that this particular Swann had become a complete and living being, and I have the impression of leaving one person to go to another distinct from him, when in my memory, I pass from the Swann I knew later with accuracy to that first Swann whom I rediscover the charming mistakes of my youth and who in fact resembles less the other Swann than he resembles the other people I knew at the time, as though it were the same in life as in a museum where all the portraits from one period have a family look about them, one tonality." (in The Way by Swann's, Proust, 1913) The author alludes to the idea that narratives (both autobiographical and of others) are part of one's identity. Disturbances at this level entail the (a) incongruence between one's autobiographical narrative and one's experience (experiencing experiential features that no longer adapt to previous narrative) and (b) periods of life to which one has experienced but cannot find a narrative for. Dissociative fugue and borderline personality disorder could be taken as examples of a disturbance of the narrative level of self-experience (Gallagher 2013; Bennouna-Greene et al. 2012).

The loss of autobiographical coherence reports to a feeling of having become someone else—again seeing oneself from a subjective third-person perspective and feeling that something has changed." These ideas report to the "narrative dimension" of patients' self-concept and how one can endure the loss of this autobiographical sketch, including the memory of personal life and existential determinations. In the case of Edward, he felt that ever since the loss of "contact," he was no longer himself—"I'm no longer myself, I can't recognise myself as if my narrative was stolen from me, what I'm living now doesn't make any sense, and there is no meaning possible for his existence in the world, I don't have a sense of a present or a future"; "I'm no longer myself—I don't act the way I did before"; "I feel as I must follow the rules and I cannot escape society dictatorship", "sometimes I have empty blocks in my life, as if nothing was attributed to them nor I feel to have lived them." Such autobiographical dimension of self-experience covers different experiences including (1) having autobiographical distinctiveness (e.g., a specific role in the world), (2) the consistency of autobiographical memories (e.g., if subject feels that his past makes sense as a whole), (3) continuity (there are no gaps in one's history), (4) personal consideration on how the narrative account develops, and (5) social integration (relation with personal and social norms). The first category refers to the presence or absence of the feeling he has a role in the world whether it is in micro-sense with his family/friends or macro-sense—that he has world importance. The second category characterizes the insight to a loss of (or an increased) contact with past moments in life (e.g., struggling to remember recent or distant occurrences in life as in dissociative amnesia) and has to do with the feeling that when one is portraying his life, he struggles for the description or he feels that such description is strange. The third category refers to the patients "Present" and to the feeling that there appear to be gaps in it, parts which the patient cannot explain (e.g., being aborted to a point of losing contact to what he is doing just to feel lost a moment after that). The fourth and fifth categories include various idiomatic expressions which have been put forward previously in the EASE interview (Parnas et al. 2005) by Tellenbach (see the discussion by Giovanni Stanghellini (Stanghellini et al. 2006), which refer to how the person stands on his stance toward social norms (follows norms, even crushed by norms or has his own personal rules) and his overall existential inclination (stances toward reality). Having insight into changes of this dimension leads the subject to feel that he is autobiographically disengaged or desynchronized with himself or the world—which will fall under the ideas of dissociative fugue, depersonalization, or derealization.

Interestingly Edward's case illustrates that the relation between these levels of experience of the self might not be unidirectional (primacy of the pre-reflexive) as he considered that the disturbances of the minimal self started at the narrative level—through the breaking up with his girlfriend "I could not hold up to my ideas and through pain and suffering I had to depersonalize. . . I had to lose a part of me so that I could bear discussions with her but then, after the breakup, I didn't know how to turn-on the button to feel again. It was forever ruined."

5.4 Dissociation Through the Prism of Perceptual Experience

In this section we follow a parallel discussion of dissociative phenomena under the prism of anomalous perception of oneself and the world. Perception is here regarded as different from sensation as (1) being contingent to intentionality (e.g., humans attach relevance to items to which they are related to), (2) for times disregarding real objects (as in hallucinations) and (3) pre-reflexively meaningful and so not really a raw experience (Merleau-Ponty 1980). As in the case of the self, we consider human perception as having three moments that are weaved implicitly (which the subject is unaware). If these moments become disjointed, the subject experiences a disturbance of the perception of the world. Such disruptions we take here to be associated with dissociative forms of experiencing (loss of connection between different parts of experience). For understanding purposes, we discuss separately the disturbances of the perception of reality, of the lived body, and of the physical body.

5.4.1 Perception of Reality

Following the ideas of the previous section, for perception we consider that there is also an immediate meaning which allows the subject to live without experiencing the "effort to understand what he is living" (and only if that fails does the subject exerts a cognitive effort to value what he is experiencing). Cognitive understanding is only one of the facets of understanding experience, and the vast majority of the meaning of experience is readily available before the subject is able to cognitively portray it. Such "pre-theoretical realm meaning" appears to be as original as experience itself, and such primacy could mean either (1) that experience is already meaningful (meaning imbued in experience) or (2) that there is a previous translational effort which comprises an implicit pre-theoretical/precognitive understanding of the world. The first advocates that symbolization and thoughts are built over another type of meaning—a meaning that is immediate to experience (e.g., when understanding someone extending his hand to invite us to shake it, the meaning comes with us seeing the hand). The second reports to the fact that the acquisition of meaning of concepts is mainly practical (hands on appraisal). Indeed, most of the concepts we use for building cognitive judgments are founded in an applied knowledge (e.g., we know exactly what "time" means although it might be hard to define it). So not only the understanding of reality has little to do with "thinking about experiences," even when attending to such cognitive form of meaning we are bound to practical knowledge imbued in our concepts.

The experiential access to the world and to others can become disturbed referring to a disturbed perception of the world. In the case of Eduard, such had changed and he indicated that "the world is no longer as it was, I cannot feel the realness of reality—it all seems a part of my imagination", "I lost my ability to feel in contact with others", "sometimes I think that everything around me is menacing, as if I was the target of some evil plan", "I can't act according to my ideas as I am forced to act according to others", "It is not only as if I'm not present, but also that the world appears simulated or feigned", "I'm always in an introspective world, thinking about what is happening within me, trying to make sense of it, I cannot contact the world as if I was cut off from it." Such portrays (1) experiences of detachment or invasiveness of reality (saliency, loss of the feeling of realness), (2) becoming overwhelmed by its features (some which might constitute true hallucinations), and (3) disturbance of the interpersonal dimension of experience (the possibility of willing or unwilling synchronization for others).

We propose that it should be clarified if the person feels derealized as he feels that the world is distant and lacking authenticity [e.g., Truman symptoms (Fusar-Poli et al. 2008)] and or if he feels that the world is menacing or invading him [e.g., Conrad's trema phase of delusional atmosphere as in Mishara (2010)] or if there are new and fearful elements as true hallucinations.

5.4.2 Perception of the Lived Body

In perceiving one also finds a subjective awareness of the body (Leib) which is in nature different from the corporal dimension (Korper) and has been an extensive study of phenomenological authors of the last century [see more in Sartre (1993)]. It represents the cenesthetic indulgence of this-body-I-am—what one experiences while occupying the first-person perspective and being conscious of oneself. It is the prerequisite to the experience of belongingness and to the particular relation one has with the world. The presence of this dimension of perception of the body is greatest in intensity when fully involved in an activity and when devoid of any cognitive effort (meaning arising is pre-reflexive). This experience is not a physical occurrence and so when there are only phatic inputs to perception the body and reality feels immaterial.

In Eduard's case (along with the increased feeling that his body had become physical), the most prevalent experiential feature was the loss of the experiential features of his living body. He portrayed an unwilling detachment from the world, a "feeling of not being himself," "feeling he was not the one acting in the world," and "feeling total absence of pleasure or having become callous by a total lack of affection for other's experiences" (lack of first-person perspective empathy). These experiences are similar to depersonalization and derealization but also to other extensively described phenomena such as anedonia and blunting of affect. We present here that the experience of the lived body (leib) includes subjective awareness of oneself (ipseity, vitality, pleasure, agency, engagement), the changes in the structure of lived time and temporality and also some cenesthetic experiences. These concepts are complex and discussing them is not the aim of this chapter. They are idiomatically bound to ideas coming from phenomenological psychiatry such as (1) ipseity [descriptions in Gallagher et al. (2004)]; (2) changes in temporality including the ideas of intra-, ante-, and post-festum [see Stanghellini and Fuchs (2013) and Kimura (2003)]; (3) cenesthopathic changes and pain-like experiences [see Stanghellini et al. (2012)]; or (4) Tellenbach's despair and remanence (Stanghellini et al. 2006). In descriptive psychopathology, patients experiencing a disturbance of such lived body dimension would be classified as suffering from passivity experiences, depressive mood, or general derealization and depersonalization experiences.

5.4.3 Perception of the Physical Body

Lastly, perceiving the body is also experiencing it as materialized, objective, or physical (we take our body not as an experience but as reality due to the fact that perception involves a corporal/physical dimension). By "resisting" us, our body leaves the experiential dimension and appears to us as real—as when I hit a maple while moving in a house—or if my body cannot attend what is requested (as when I fall ill with the flu). In everyday routine, our awareness to such corporal dimension is a small part of its perception, and yet we can become hyperaware of their physical dimension (e.g., the flu or when experiencing shame). When falling ill as in the flu, our body cannot attend what is requested, and the corporal experience of self-world becomes manifest as a "resistance." In shame, the experience of external reification of oneself gives rise to objective apprehension of one being physical.

Many of Eduard's complaints focused on his body becoming "as flesh" when (1) his body became explicit, resisting movement, or estranged (increased awareness, materialized in flu-like syndromes), (2) his body became strange or changed in the mirror (here referred as mirror-related phenomena), and (3) the perceptualization of his thoughts which became similar to his own speech (here perceptual thoughts). This dimension has been present in seminal phenomenological (and philosophical) literature and psychiatric literature with respect to different psychiatric disorders from depression to schizophrenia (Fuchs and Schlimme 2009; Ratcliffe and Stephan 2014; Stanghellini et al. 2012). As pointed out previously, coining depersonalization and derealization can cloud rich phenomenological descriptions of (1) uncanny experiences of objectification or (2) immateriality of body or mind and disturbances of the experiential features of specific parts of the body or increased awareness of properties of movement. This section groups

15 different experiences and distributes them across 5 different categories: (1) intensity of body expressiveness, (2) change in the manifestation of mind, (2) change in the manifestation of the body, (4) change in the appearance of the body, and (5) changes in bodily movements. All seem to correspond to a feeling that the corporal dimension of experience is disturbed either by becoming ever-present (e.g., flu-like experiences) or by disappearing all-entirely (e.g., feeling of immateriality or passivity).

Lastly, the models we discussed here can interact, and there can be various assortments of disturbances of the experience of self and of perception leading to distinctive accounts of dissociative experiences. Therefore, we conceive mixed forms over a spectrum of two poles: (1) a full experience of selfhood that is disturbed due to the loss of relevant parts of perceptual experiences to (2) a disturbed experience of self while perception is preserved or amalgam disturbances both of self and perception.

The proposed models and the conceptual background presented for dissociative experiences stresses the complexity of their status as mental symptoms. Also, and irrespectively of these considerations finding or not further empirical validity, it should be added how artificial (and nonnatural/man-made) may turn to be their organization into classifications.

5.5 Discussion on Diagnostic and Therapeutic Implications

This essay was established on an unpretentious clinical issue—the feeling that writing "depersonalization" and "derealization" in Eduard's clinical file did not make justice to phenomenological detail we were achieving. Also, such detail appeared to us as relevant for clinical decision-making as all other symptomatic features revealed to be fluctuating and unreliable. Therefore our endeavors were to analyze these phenomena both from (1) their past and present epistemological understandings and (2) the phenomenological inputs that literature provided on the assortment of phenomena. In Sect. 5.2, we presented the theoretical ground of dissociation and the heterogeneity of inputs that fall under such topic. We found an assortment of inputs that seemed tomake dissociative experiences a complex field—even with some ideas being at odds—stressing that the inexistence of adequate diagnosis and consistent treatment plans could be due to conceptual and phenomenological impreciseness. Also we suggest that the tying bond of the whole group is not up-to-date with neuroscience research. Therefore we draw two present-day paradigms that are used for schizophrenia and depression to discuss them—disturbances of subjective self-experience and of the perception of reality, the lived, and corporal bodies. These are presented over Sects. 5.3 and 5.4.

Such parallel understanding can stimulate new research tracks that distance themselves from the age-old concepts on dissociation (e.g., separation of mental functions). Moreover, we suggest that exploring the presence or absence of singular experiences would help distinguish clusters that could account for depersonalization in specific psychiatric disorders (e.g., major depression, borderline personality disorder, depersonalization disorder, and schizophrenia). It is stated here that we can feel (and be considered) depersonalized because (1) we lack engagement in the world, (2) experience reduced vitality, (3) are absorbed in our minds, or even (4) that we are plighted to social rules and tasks and lost the ability to experience our present (post-festum). Indeed keeping with umbrella terms is not helpful to current translational efforts of dissociative disorders as brain mapping relies (1) on the clarity of the phenomena in study and its closeness to a natural category and (2) the possibility that these phenomena have meaning for charting a disorder. And reiterating it, the possibility of different classes of depersonalization phenomena is key to understand which of those occur in psychosis and schizophrenia and which are mainly happening in anxiety disorders. Our effort to depict the conceptual and phenomenological ground of dissociative experiences is nevertheless partial (incomplete or unsatisfactorily categorized) and in need of empirical substantiation.

We would like to emphasize two important intersecting premises raised in our appraisal, that subjective phenomena should be inquired and that phenomenologically based semi-structured interviews seem relevant for its psychopathological investigation. Many of the topics regarded in this chapter are subjective phenomena which have for long been absent in our diagnostic textbooks (Stanghellini et al. 2013). Also, there are increasing evidences that the validity of psychopathological inquiry is greatest when we use semi-structured interviews (Nordgaard et al. 2012) even for objective signs and symptoms. By the use of the phenomenological method, phenomena are untouched (provide the interviewer plain access to the persons way of experiencing), and there is space for a discussion of meaning being presented so that the interviewer clarifies the phenomena. Also here is stressed that person-centered phenomenologically based interviews share fundamental features with various schools of psychotherapy including person-centered and experiential schools adding the possibility that the inquiry itself might be therapeutic (Thorne and Lambers 1998). To Eduard such person-centered interview allowed him (1) "increased control about such experiences" as well as, for times, (2) even "reducing the occurrence of depersonalization and derealization phenomena."

All together, it seems to us that a more detailed inquiry about these experiences, allowing for phenomenological unpacking, including subjective phenomena, and keeping up with a semi-structured person-centered interview, might allow us to better clarify them. In the future we aim that dissociative phenomena have increasing diagnostic properties as well as suitable psychiatric and psychotherapeutic managements.

References

APA. (2013). *Diagnostic and statistical manual of mental disorders* (5th ed.), DSM-5. American Psychiatric Publishing.

Baker, D., Hunter, E., Lawrence, E., et al. (2003). Depersonalisation disorder: Clinical features of 204 cases. *The British Journal of Psychiatry, 182*, 428–433. doi:10.1192/bjp.182.5.428.

Bennouna-Greene, M., Berna, F., Conway, M. A., et al. (2012). Self-images and related autobiographical memories in schizophrenia. *Consciousness and Cognition, 21*, 247–257. doi:10.1016/j.concog.2011.10.006.

Cermolacce, M., Naudin, J., & Parnas, J. (2007). The "minimal self" in psychopathology: Re-examining the self-disorders in the schizophrenia spectrum. *Consciousness and Cognition, 16*, 703–714. doi:10.1016/j.concog.2007.05.013.

Fuchs, T., & Schlimme, J. E. (2009). Embodiment and psychopathology: A phenomenological perspective. *Current Opinion in Psychiatry, 22*, 570. doi:10.1097/YCO.0b013e3283318e5c.

Fusar-Poli, P., Howes, O., Valmaggia, L., & McGuire, P. (2008). "Truman" signs and vulnerability to psychosis. *The British Journal of Psychiatry, 193*, 168. doi:10.1192/bjp.193.2.168.

Gallagher, S. (2013). *The Oxford handbook of the self.* OUP Oxford.

Gallagher, S., & Shear, J. (1999). *Models of the self.* Thorverton: Imprint Academic.

Gallagher, S., Watson, S., Brun, P., & Romanski, P. (2004). *Ipseity and alterity*. Publication Universite Rouen Havre.

Hilgard, E. R. (1973). A neodissociation interpretation of pain reduction in hypnosis. *Psychological Review, 80*, 396–411.

Holmes, E. A., Brown, R. J., Mansell, W., et al. (2005). Are there two qualitatively distinct forms of dissociation? A review and some clinical implications. *Clinical Psychology Review, 25*, 1–23. doi:10.1016/j.cpr.2004.08.006.

James, W. (1950). *The principles of psychology* (Vol. 1). New York: Dover Publications.

Janet, P. (2012). *L'automatisme Psychologique 1889* (French ed.). Ulan Press.

Kihlstrom, J. F. (1994). *One hundred years of hysteria.* New York: Guilford Press.

Kimura, B. (2003). Disturbance of timing and selfhood in schizophrenia. *Seishin Shinkeigaku Zasshi, 105*, 729–732.

Krüger, C., & Mace, C. J. (2002). Psychometric validation of the State Scale of Dissociation (SSD). *Psychology and Psychotherapy: Theory, Research and Practice (formerly the British Journal of Medical Psychology), 75*(1), 33–51.

Legrand, D. (2007). Pre-reflective self-as-subject from experiential and empirical perspectives. *Consciousness and Cognition, 16*, 583–599. doi:10.1016/j.concog.2007.04.002.

Lynn, S. J., & Rhue, J. W. (1994). *Dissociation: Clinical and theoretical perspectives*. New York: Guilford Press.

Merleau-Ponty, M. (1980). The nature of perception. *Research in Phenomenology, 10*, 9–20.

Mishara, A. L. (2010). Klaus Conrad (1905-1961): Delusional mood, psychosis, and beginning schizophrenia. *Schizophrenia Bulletin, 36*, 9–13. doi:10.1093/schbul/sbp144.

Nordgaard, J., Revsbech, R., Saebye, D., & Parnas, J. (2012). Assessing the diagnostic validity of a structured psychiatric interview in a first-admission hospital sample. *World Psychiatry, 11*, 181–185.

Parnas, J., Handest, P., Saebye, D., & Jansson, L. (2003). Anomalies of subjective experience in schizophrenia and psychotic bipolar illness. *Acta Psychiatrica Scandinavica, 108*, 126–133. doi:10.1034/j.1600-0447.2003.00105.x.

Parnas, J., Møller, P., Kircher, T., et al. (2005). EASE: Examination of anomalous self-experience. *Psychopathology, 38*, 236–258. doi:10.1159/000088441

Prince, M. (2012). *The dissociation of a personality; a biographical study in abnormal psychology*. Hardpress Publishing.

Putnam, F. W. (1989). *Diagnosis and treatment of multiple personality disorder (Foundations of modern psychiatry)* (1st ed.). New York: The Guilford Press.

Ratcliffe, M., & Stephan, A. (2014). *Depression, emotion and the self.* Andrews UK Limited.

Rosenthal, H. (2009). *Dissociation and the dissociative disorders: DSM-V and beyond* (1st ed.). New York: Routledge.

Sartre, J-P. (1993). *Being and nothingness*, Reprint. New York: Washington Square Press.

Sass, L., Pienkos, E., Nelson, B., & Medford, N. (2013). Anomalous self-experience in depersonalization and schizophrenia: A comparative investigation. *Consciousness and Cognition, 22*, 430–441. doi:10.1016/j.concog.2013.01.009.

Saxe, G. N., Van der Kolk, B. A., & Berkowitz, R. (1993). Dissociative disorders in psychiatric inpatients. *The American Journal of Psychiatry, 150*(7), 1037–42.

Scheler, M. (1992). *On feeling, knowing, and valuing*. Chicago: University of Chicago Press.

Sierra, M., & Berrios, G. E. (2001). The phenomenological stability of depersonalization: Comparing the old with the new. *The Journal of Nervous and Mental Disease, 189*, 629–636.

Sierra, M., Medford, N., Wyatt, G., & David, A. S. (2012). Depersonalization disorder and anxiety: A special relationship? *Psychiatry Research, 197*, 123–127. doi:10.1016/j.psychres.2011.12.017.

Stanghellini, G. (2004). *Disembodied spirits and deanimated bodies: The psychopathology of common sense (international perspectives in philosophy and psychiatry)* (1st ed.). Oxford: Oxford University Press.

Stanghellini, G., Ballerini, M., Poli, P. F., & Cutting, J. (2012). Abnormal bodily experiences may be a marker of early schizophrenia? *Current Pharmaceutical Design, 18*, 392–398.

Stanghellini, G., Bertelli, M., & Raballo, A. (2006). Typus melancholicus: Personality structure and the characteristics of major unipolar depressive episode. *Journal of Affective Disorders, 93*, 159–167. doi:10.1016/j.jad.2006.03.005.

Stanghellini, G., Bolton, D., & Fulford, W. K. M. (2013). Person-centered psychopathology of schizophrenia: Building on Karl Jaspers' understanding of patient's attitude toward his illness. *Schizophrenia Bulletin, 39*, 287–294. doi:10.1093/schbul/sbs154.

Stanghellini, G., & Fuchs, T. (2013). *One Century of Karl Jaspers' General Psychopathology (International Perspectives in Philosophy and Psychiatry)* (1st ed.). Oxford: Oxford University Press.

Thorne, B., & Lambers, E. (1998). *Person-centred therapy: A European perspective*. London: Sage.

Waller, N. G., & Ross, C. A. (1997). The prevalence and biometric structure of pathological dissociation in the general population: Taxometric and behavior genetic findings. *Journal of Abnormal Psychology, 106*, 499–510.

Waller, N., Waller, N., Putnam, F. W., et al. (1996). Types of dissociation and dissociative types: A taxometric analysis of dissociative experiences. *Psychological Methods, 1*, 300–321. doi:10.1037/1082-989X.1.3.300.

World Health Organization. (1992). *The ICD-10 Classification of Mental and Behavioural Disorders*. Geneva: World Health Organization.

Varieties of Mind-Body Disunity

6

Robert D. Stolorow and George E. Atwood

A number of attempted solutions to the so-called mind-body problem have appeared in the philosophical literature—reductionism, parallelism, interactionism, etc. (Wallace 1988). In each of these, both the mind and the body are regarded as metaphysical entities subsisting independently of one another, a legacy of Descartes' metaphysical dualism. In this phenomenological study, by contrast, both mind and body are regarded as regions of lived experience—the mind of lived experience or the lived mental and the body of lived experience or the lived body (Merleau-Ponty 1945). We are concerned in particular with varied forms of lived mind-body disunity.

We envision two broad types of such disunity—those mediated by concrete bodily symbols and those that might be characterized as failures to symbolize. The first type includes hysterical conversion symptoms, hypochondriacal anxieties, and certain severe dissociative states, whereas instances of the second can be found in psychosomatic disturbances.

6.1 Disunities Mediated by Concrete Bodily Symbols

We have come to believe that the process we call *concrete symbolization*—the encapsulation of structures of experience by concrete, sensorimotor symbols—is a ubiquitous and fundamental process in human psychological life that serves to

R.D. Stolorow (✉)
Institute of Contemporary Psychoanalysis, Los Angeles, CA, USA

Institute for the Psychoanalytic Study of Subjectivity, New York, NY, USA
e-mail: robertdstolorow@gmail.com

G.E. Atwood, PhD
Institute for the Psychoanalytic Study of Subjectivity, New York, NY, USA

Rutgers University, Newark, NJ, USA

G. Stanghellini, M. Aragona (eds.), *An Experiential Approach to Psychopathology*,
DOI 10.1007/978-3-319-29945-7_6

maintain the organization of emotional experience, whether that be specific organizations of experience or organization as such (Atwood and Stolorow 2014). Concretization can assume a number of forms, depending on what pathways or modes of expression it favors, For example, when motor activity predominates in the mode of concretization, then behavioral enactments are relied upon to actualize required configurations of experience. When motor activity is curtailed, as in sleep, then perceptual imagery may become the preferred pathway of concretization, as in dreams. Here we are specifically concerned with concrete *bodily* symbols and how they mediate several forms of mind-body disunity.

6.2 Conversion

The early psychoanalytic discovery that hysterical conversion symptoms and other neurotic inhibitions could be resolved by unveiling their unconscious *meanings* (Breuer and Freud 1893–1895) was perhaps the first major demonstration of the role of concretization in the genesis of psychopathological constellations. However, in resorting to metapsychological notions of crypto-physiological energy transformations to explain this phenomenon, Freud and others obscured the important finding that the use of concrete, sensorimotor symbolism was central to the process of symptom formation. As this phenomenon is by now well known, one brief example will suffice.

Midway through the course of her 4-year analysis, a 33-year-old woman reported a new symptom—a tightening of or lump in her throat, with difficulty swallowing. During the session she indicated that she had recently experienced some competitive successes in relation to a number of other women and that she felt vaguely uneasy about this. Her associations around this theme eventually led to memories of how unbearably guilty she had felt as a child whenever she would present some personal triumph to her chronically depressed mother, who always seemed so pathetic, so emotionally crippled, and so painfully unfulfilled. "Whenever I brought home an 'A' from school," she said, "it was like *shoving my success down my mother's throat*." The analyst interpreted that in the new symptom she seemed to be doing to her own throat what she feared her successes might do to her mother's. This single interpretation of the symptom's unconscious meaning as a "symbol written in the sand of the flesh" (Lacan 1953, p. 69, emphasis added) was sufficient to remove it permanently. The concrete bodily symbolism of the throat encapsulated her sense of guilt over the injury her success might inflict on her mother, and the concretization served the purposes of atonement and self-punishment.

6.3 Hypochondria

Whereas conversion symptoms ordinarily entail alterations in bodily functions, such alterations are usually not present in hypochondriacal states.

In these, the concretization process results in the formation of anxiety-ridden fantasies about the body, in which its parts are pictured as diseased, deteriorating, or under severe threat. In the imagery of failing body parts, concrete bodily symbols are employed to dramatize an impending catastrophe—the threat of psychological annihilation. Through bodily symbols, a nameless psychological catastrophe is replaced with namable and tangible threats to life and limb.

A 28-year-old man sought analysis in order to restore some emotional spontaneity to his regimented life and to correct the sexual inhibitions from which he suffered. He explained to his therapist that he believed that he possessed a limited supply of energy and bodily fluids that he had to conserve and that he could permit himself to have sexual relations only during the weekends for fear that sexual activity on weekdays would so drain him of these substances that he would have insufficient amounts of them left over for the performance of his work. Further exploration of his fear of being drained revealed that in the sexual situation he experienced his wife, much as he had experienced his mother, as a "bottomless pit" of never-ending needs and demands that he, perforce, was required to satisfy. The bodily imagery of dwindling energies and fluids symbolically encapsulated his dread of dissipating himself in servitude to the appetites of a mother-surrogate, and the concretization served a self-protective function in providing him with a feeling of control—he believed that he could conserve his energies and fluids and thereby protect against loss of selfhood by constricting and regimenting his sexual behavior.

In this case, interpretations of the meaning of the concrete bodily symbols were not effective in alleviating the sexual inhibitions. Increasingly, as the analysis progressed, the patient's associations drifted to his father, who crystallized in his memories as an elusive, uninvolved, emotionally absent figure, absorbed in a Walter Mitty-like world of private fantasy and reverie, and offering little in the way of strength and protection to his son. It was only when in the transference the analyst became established as an emotionally present, involved paternal figure whom, unlike his father, the patient could experience as a powerful ally against the "insatiable" demands of a mother figure that the sexual inhibitions abated. As the patient felt the integrity of his individual selfhood sustained and protected by the bond with the analyst, the self-conserving concretizations became less necessary, thereby freeing his sexual life to become increasingly spontaneous and a source of pleasure for him.

6.4 Severe Dissociation

Concrete bodily symbols can mediate severe dissociative phenomena, such as division into multiple personalities and out-of-body experiences. The case of a young woman whose sense of self had become fragmented into a set of separate, quasi-autonomous personalities richly illustrates the central role of bodily symbols in such dissociative states, as well as in behavioral enactments and dreams.

The family environment in which the patient grew up was one of extreme physical and emotional abuse. Both parents treated her as an extension of themselves and as a scapegoat for their frustrations and disappointments in life. Violent physical beatings represented a frequent form of interaction with the parents, and throughout her early childhood she thought they wished her dead. A sense of profound personal disunity had haunted the patient all her life, appearing even in her earliest recollections. For example, she recalled from her fourth year an obsession with the issue of how it could be that her mind controlled the movements of her body. A disturbance in mind-body unity was also indicated by quasi-delusional journeys outside of her body, which began during that same year. These journeys commenced on the occasion when she was visited by the benevolent ghosts of two deceased grandparents. The ghosts taught her to leave her body and fly to a place she called "the field," a peaceful expanse of grass and trees somewhere far removed from human society. She felt safe in the field because she was alone there and no one could find her.

The psychological disunity shown in the patient's out-of-body journeys was embedded in a broader context of self-division resulting from the violent abuse and rejection she had received in her family. Beginning at the age of two and one-half, when her parents abruptly ceased all affectionate bodily contact with her and continuing through a series of pivotal traumatic episodes over the next several years, she was successively divided into a total of six fragments, each crystallizing as a distinct personality, possessing its own individual name and unique personal attributes.

When the patient was 7 years old, she developed a renal tumor, causing agonizing pain. The need to escape the suffering generated by her condition became an additional motive underlying the journeys outside of her body. It was more than 1 full year before her illness was correctly diagnosed and the tumor finally removed. The surgery itself was handled with brutal insensitivity by her parents and doctors, and she experienced it as an overwhelming trauma. The impact of all these circumstances on her precarious selfhood was symbolized in a set of recurring nightmares that began during her recuperation from surgery and continued throughout her life thereafter. In these dreams she stood alone in the small train station of her town as flames sprang up all around her. Soon the whole building was engulfed in fire. After the station had burned to the ground, two eyeballs lay quietly in the smoking ashes and then began to quiver and roll about, conversing with each other by means of movements and glances. This dream of burning down to small fragments concretely depicted the disintegrating impact of a world persecuting her both from without and from within.

What psychological function can be ascribed to the patient's recurring dream of being burned down to isolated fragments? The repeated transformation of the experience of self-disintegration into an image of the physical incineration of her body enabled her to maintain the state of her sense of self in focal awareness and encapsulated her effort to retain psychological integrity in the face of the threat of total self-dissolution. By utilizing concrete bodily imagery, she was giving her disintegrating existence tangible form, replacing a precarious and vanishing sense of selfhood with the permanence and substantiality of physical matter. The image of the interaction and communication between the eyeballs at the end of the dream symbolized a further restitutive effort to reconnect the broken fragments and restore a measure of coherence to her splintered self-experience. The specific symbol of the eyeballs captured an essential feature of what became her principal mode of relating to her social milieu. She assumed the role of an ever-watchful, often disembodied spectator, perpetually scanning her environment for desirable qualities in others that she hoped to appropriate and assemble into a rebuilt sense of self. Thus, both her self-restorative efforts and what remained of her vanishing selfhood became crystallized in her waking life in the act of looking and in her recurring dreams in the bodily imagery of the eyes.

The central salience in the patient's emotional world of the need to maintain selfhood and recover a sense of personal unity was also indicated by an array of dramatic enactments that appeared concurrently with the onset of the recurring dream of being burned. These enactments included the self-administration of severe whippings with a leather belt, delicate cutting and puncturing of the surface of the skin on her wrists and arms, gazing tirelessly at the reflected image of her face in pools of water, fondling and staring into translucent pieces of glass, scratching and rubbing at cracks and crevices in hard physical surfaces such as walls and sidewalks, and stitching the skin of her separate fingers together with needle and thread.

The self-whipping ritual arose initially as an identification with the punishing treatment the patient had received during her earlier childhood. She tended at first to whip herself in response to acts that previously would have evoked her parents' wrath—e.g., acts of asserting her needs, seeking attention, or expressing unhappiness. The function of the self-punishments at this stage was primarily to master a sense of helplessness and counteract the dreaded feeling of being vulnerable to attack from the outside world. The ritual also came to include a wish-fulfilling and restitutive element in the form of a sequel to the actual whipping. After first violently beating herself on the back and buttocks, she would adopt the role of loving parent and say to herself in a soft voice, "It's all right honey, now there will be no more pain." Then assuming the role of comforted child, she would fall blissfully asleep. This hard-won feeling of peacefulness, however, was rudely shattered when she later awoke and found herself still entirely alone.

In addition to helping her master persecution anxiety and maintain needed images of herself being cared for by others, the whipping ritual also began to serve a more fundamental purpose in the patient's emotional life. One of the consequences of her profound and enduring emotional isolation was a feeling of being unreal, unalive, and insubstantial. This feeling was magnified by the continuing out-of-body journeys to the field. The increasing frequency of these journeys came to pose a new and even more menacing danger to her safety—namely, the severing of all connection to physical reality and the final obliteration of her embodied selfhood. The terror that she might permanently lose her physical form and somehow evaporate into thin air led her to return to the whipping ritual with redoubled intensity. The strong sensations of pain distributed on the surface of her skin were used to provide reassurance of her continuing embodiment and survival in the real physical world.

Essentially parallel functions were served by the patient's ritualistic cutting and puncturing of the skin on her wrists and arms. These behaviors seemed to originate as a restaging of the traumatically impinging medical procedures associated with her renal surgery. In addition to the operation itself, the procedures included a spinal tap, numerous injections, catheterization, intravenous administration of medications and fluids, etc. By cutting and puncturing her skin, she actively relived a passively endured trauma and sought mastery over her feelings of unbearable helplessness. Like the ritualized whipping, the cutting and puncturing activity also began to serve the function of strengthening the patient's conviction that she was substantial and real. By violating the physical boundary of her body with a needle or a knife, she dramatized the very existence of that boundary and reestablished a sense of her own embodiment. In addition, the stinging sensations and the droplets of blood produced by the delicate cutting provided her with concrete sensory evidence of her continuing aliveness.

The enactments involving water and glass were more complex, but also related to struggles with a precarious sense of self and a deep feeling of helpless vulnerability. The water ritual began when she gazed at her reflection in ponds and pools of rainwater. She recalled becoming fascinated by how the image of her face would disappear and then magically reappear when she disturbed the water's reflecting surface. One meaning of this activity pertained again to her need for mastery over passively experienced traumata—by actively being the cause of the disappearance of her image she was seeking to overcome the shattering impact on her sense of selfhood of her whole earlier history of victimization and abuse. In addition, in eliminating her reflected image she thought of herself as actually ceasing to exist and becoming nothing, which provided a feeling of safety because what does not exist cannot be made a target by a persecuting world. The water also seemed to function as a transitional object, giving reassurance that while her sense of self (concretized in a visual reflection) might be made to vanish on a temporary basis, it could not be annihilated permanently. A sense of self-continuity was thus tenuously achieved. A final significance of water to the patient was associated with its paradoxical quality of being both *transparent* and *reflecting*. There was something in the conjoining of these two properties with which she wishfully identified, and this identification was even more pronounced in her involvement with objects of glass.

The patient began to collect small glass objects during her early adolescence. The reflecting and refracting properties of crystal prisms and spheres particularly fascinated her. Acts of fondling and staring into such objects developed into a ritual behavior pattern duplicating and sometimes blending into her relationship with water. On occasion she would fill a crystal container with water and place it in a window where she could observe its interaction with the sun's rays. This ritual was enacted several times during the psychotherapeutic sessions. As she studied the interplay between the light, the water, and the glass, she would softly chant, "water . . . glass . . . water . . . glass." Her consciousness could become wholly absorbed in this preoccupation, which she seemed to experience as a refuge from the social environment. The psychological sources of the patient's attraction to glass were bound up with her difficulties in maintaining a feeling of her own personal selfhood. She was excessively vulnerable to the expectations and perceptions of others and tended to feel that she became whomever she was seen as being. For instance, when a grandfather told her wistfully how much she reminded him of his long-dead beloved wife, the patient felt the departed soul of the wife invading and assuming command over her body. Such episodes drastically affected her sense of being in possession of her own identity, and she responded to them by cultivating secret realms of herself protected from the annihilating potential of others' perceptions and definitions. Included in the elaboration of these hidden sectors of her emotional life was the development of her alternative personalities, each christened with its own secret name. The fact that no one knew her secret names made her feel safe from the engulfing potential of others' experiences of her. A consequence of the patient's defensive secrecy, however, was a further intensification of her feelings of estrangement. She was driven into isolation in order to protect herself from self-loss in relationships, but the isolation itself presented the danger of self-extinction through unendurable loneliness. Her preoccupation with glass sprang directly from the conflict between her need to retreat from others into a world of secrecy and her need to break out of isolation and reestablish bonds to the social environment. The glass concretized a wishful solution to this conflict by embodying the twin properties of translucency on the one hand and reflectivity on the other. The translucency of the glass meant that it was open to the passage of light from the outside, which served to lessen the patient's fear of isolation and entombment within her own secret world. The reflectivity of the glass objects, their solidity, and their firm boundaries, by contrast, meant that they were real and substantial, which made her feel safe from the dangers posed by involvement with her social milieu. A fusion of these properties also appeared in a recurring fantasy concerning a house she wished to build in the field she had been visiting in the out-of-the-body projections. She pictured this house as a beautiful construction of one-way glass, so that from the outside it would be a mirror, but from the inside transparent.

The remaining enactments to be considered were those in which the patient scratched and rubbed at cracks in solid surfaces and stitched her fingers together with thread. These enactments pertained to the patient's experience of being an assembly of disjointed parts. With regard to the scratching pattern, she explained that crevices and cracks in the external environment "itched" unbearably and compelled her to scratch them. The locating of the subjective sensation of itching in physical objects represented a transposition onto the plane of material reality of her feeling of her own fragmentation. She described herself as being like a jar filled with small spheres or cubes with concave surfaces and as a checkerboard filled with round checkers; even though the constituent elements might be packed together very tightly, they still would not form an integrated and smoothly continuous whole. The itching cracks and crevices in the external environment corresponded to the subjective interstices between the various fragmentary entities comprising her self-experience, and the scratching represented her effort to find relief from her distressing lack of a sense of cohesion.

Closely similar was the function of her pattern of sewing her fingers together with needle and thread. This ritual began with holding her hand up to the light and gazing at the spaces between her separate fingers. Then she would push a needle and thread just under the skin of her little finger, then under the skin of the next one, then the next, etc., and then back and forth several times until they were all tightly interconnected and pressed together. The act of weaving the fingers together was one in which separate parts of her bodily being were literally joined and made to appear whole and continuous, concretizing her effort to fashion an internally integrated identity out of the collection of parts into which she had divided during the course of her traumatic early history.

The enactments in which the patient engaged are functionally parallel to her recurring dreams of being burned to fragments. The essential feature the two sets of phenomena share in common is the reparative use of concrete bodily symbols to give an experience of self-disintegration a material and substantial form. In the dreams the emphasis appears on the concrete symbolization of the experience of self-dissolution, and the additional reparative trend of reassembling the broken pieces is hinted at in the image of the communication that develops between the eyeballs. In the enactments one finds analogous symbolizations and also the vivid expression of the patient's need to mend her brokenness by reconnecting the separate fragments into which she had disintegrated.

Each of the patterns of behavior discussed here was repeatedly enacted during the psychotherapeutic sessions. Some of these performances were extremely difficult for the therapist to witness, especially those in which she slapped, whipped, and cut herself. For the first year and a half of treatment, she brought knives, needles, pieces of broken glass, and a leather belt to the sessions on a regular basis and frequently used one or more of these objects against herself. When the therapist attempted to prevent this behavior by taking her objects away, she would scratch, slap, and beat herself with her hands and fingernails. The only means of ensuring that the patient would not engage in self-abuse was to physically restrain her until the self-destructive urges had passed. This physical restraining occupied a significant portion of many sessions during the early phases of the psychotherapeutic work and proved to be critically important in solidifying the therapeutic bond. In addition to the restraint required to prevent the patient from harming herself, there were a number of times when she approached her therapist and grasped him tightly, pressing her face against his body. After the first occasion of such an approach, she explained she had needed the physical contact to prove he was not an unreal apparition or hallucination she had conjured up. She reported having been shocked and surprised when her arms met the solid resistance of his flesh, for she had expected them to pass right through him as though he were made of mist. Contact with her therapist's bodily being served to differentiate him from the ghosts and other imaginary entities on whom she had previously depended. This contact also provided an anchoring point for the beginning stabilization of her own physical embodiment. It emerged in discussions of the meaning and significance of holding and being held that the patient had not experienced affectionate bodily contact with another human being since the age of two and one-half, when her parents ended all such interaction with her.

The first year and a half of the patient's therapy were devoted primarily to establishing a therapeutic relationship that would give her some relief from her estrangement and loneliness while at the same time strengthening her sense of individuality and separateness as a person. She oscillated during this period between expressions of suicidal despair and a merger-like closeness in which she seemed to want nothing but physical proximity to the therapist. The actual physical contact, together with the symbolic holding (Winnicott 1965) implicit in the therapist's consistent provision of acceptance, concern, and understanding, established a nexus of archaic relatedness in which the patient's aborted psychological development could move forward once again. Very gradually the functions inhering in the enactments we have described passed over to the bond that was becoming established. The nature of the patient's evolving reliance on her analyst at the beginning of this process was shown by her reactions to his periodic failures to comprehend or appropriately respond to what she tried to communicate. Such misunderstandings tended to be followed by a resurgence of one or more of the enactments, which then continued until the disrupted bond could be reestablished. As she increasingly came to rely on the therapist for the maintenance of her psychological organization, the ritualized enactments (and the out-of-body projections), which she had formerly needed for this purpose, lessened and finally disappeared. The repeating nightmares of being burned to fragments came to an end simultaneously.

The function of bodily symbols in dreams in maintaining the organization of a person's emotional world is to be seen not only in situations wherein structures are breaking down, as was the case with the patient at the time of the onset of her nightmares; dreams' symbols may also play an important role in consolidating and stabilizing new structures of experience that are in the process of coming into being. Let us turn now to a consideration of another dream of the patient we have been discussing, this one having occurred midway through the long course of her psychotherapy. The context of this dream in the treatment was one of intense conflict and struggle over the issue of self-unification. Two of the initial six self-fragments had at this point been assimilated into the remaining four, but the next steps of integration were being approached by the patient with trepidation and reluctance. Specifically, she feared that becoming one would render her vulnerable to being destroyed, either by attack from the outside world or by unendurable loneliness. At the same time, however, she had come to abhor the prospect of a life spent in continuing disunity.

In her dream she walked into the living room of her house and saw on the mantle above the fireplace four cement boxes resting side by side. There seemed to be bodies inside the boxes. The scene terrified her and she awoke but then fell back asleep and the dream continued. Now the four boxes were replaced by just one box, with four bodies arranged inside with their backs against the cement walls and facing inward toward a central point. The box seemed to be a coffin. In discussing this dream with the therapist, the patient spontaneously associated the four boxes with the four remaining self-fragments still requiring integration. A great deal of progress toward this goal had already been achieved, principally through the four parts growing less and less distinct from each other in the facilitating medium of the therapeutic relationship. The patient was oscillating, however, between experiencing herself as a single person with multiple facets on the one hand and as a collection of separate persons who happened to resemble each other and share the same body on the other.

The dream imagery concretizes one phase of this oscillation by replacing the image of four separate boxes with the image of just one that contains four bodies. The patient spontaneously offered the interpretation that the shift from four to one could be understood as a prelude to the integration of her personality, with the exterior boundaries of the final box representing the developing structure of a unitary person. The danger felt to be associated with her impending integration is also concretely symbolized in the dream, by the identification of the box as a coffin. The patient frequently expressed deep anxiety that becoming one would end her life, and she once even suggested that she was coming together as something dead.

The image of the box containing four bodies may also be understood as a symbol of her experience of the therapeutic relationship. The therapeutic bond, which by this time had become well established, was exercising a holding, containing, and integrating function in the patient's efforts to achieve psychological wholeness. Her ambivalence regarding this task emerged quite clearly in the transference, wherein she alternated between embracing her therapist's unifying comprehension and rejecting it as a deadly threat to the survival of the self-fragments. These alternations arose most fundamentally from the patient's deep conviction that she could never fully trust another human being, a conviction that was gradually overcome in stages closely paralleling the integration of her personality.

The dream of the transformation of four boxes into one box buttressed the patient's evolving self-integration by giving her developing unity a concrete physical form. In the same way that the earlier dream of being burned encapsulated her need to maintain her self-experience as she underwent psychological dissolution, this second dream expressed her need to maintain and consolidate the new but still unsteady structure of integrated self-experience that was gradually crystallizing. An enactment sharing this latter function appeared some 9 months after the dream of the boxes. During the interim the patient had continued to wrestle with the problem of unifying herself, with each of the residual fragmentary personalities making a common commitment to a shared future as one individual.

In the subsequent context of such statements as "We are me!" and "I am one now—we voted last night and we all agree," the patient began a therapy session by bringing out 12 small pieces of paper. On six of the slips were written the six names of the self-fragments and on the other six were short phrases designating the pivotal trauma she considered responsible for each of the self-divisions. After asking the therapist whether he thought he could match the self-fragments with their appropriate traumas, she cleared off his desk and assembled out of the 12 pieces of paper 2 closely juxtaposed columns displaying the temporal sequence of her shattering psychological history. The act of arranging the names and experiences into a single ordered structure clearly concretized the patient's increasingly successful efforts to synthesize an internally integrated, temporally continuous sense of self. By giving her newborn selfhood a tangible form and proudly demonstrating its unity and historical continuity to the therapist, she consolidated the structure of her experience more firmly than had been possible heretofore. Following the integrating enactment involving the 12 pieces of paper, the patient came to feel her own subjective integrity on a consistent basis, and the focus of the therapeutic work shifted to issues other than that of mending her self-fragmentation. The unity that had been achieved was completely lasting, as the patient went on in the ensuing years to finish her college studies, earn multiple graduate degrees, and eventually marry.

6.5 Disunities Deriving from Failures to Symbolize: Psychosomatic States

One can distinguish two closely interrelated developmental lines for affective experience (Jones 1995; Krystal 1974): (1) affect differentiation which is the gradual development of an array of distinctive emotions from the infant's diffuse ur-affect states of pleasure and unpleasure and (2) the symbolic integration of affect which is the gradual evolution of affect states from their earliest form as exclusively bodily states into emotional experiences that can be verbally articulated. Symbolic processes play a pivotal role in both of these developmental progressions. The capacity for symbolic thought comes on line maturationally at the age of 10–12 months, eventually making language possible for the child. At that point, the earlier, exclusively bodily forms of emotional experience can begin to become articulated in symbols—at first in imagistic symbols and then in words. Consequently, the child's emotional experiences increasingly can be characterized as *somatic-symbolic* or, eventually, *somatic-linguistic unities*.

We have long contended (e.g., Socarides and Stolorow 1984/85; Stolorow 2007) that these developmental progressions always take place within a relational medium or context. It is the caregiver's attuned responsiveness, phase-appropriately conveyed through words, that facilitates the gradual integration of the child's bodily emotional experience with symbolic thought, leading to the crystallization of distinctive emotions that can be named. In the absence of such verbally expressed attunement, or in the face of traumatically malattuned responses that make symbolic articulation of affect extremely dangerous, derailments of this developmental process can occur, whereby emotional experience remains inchoate, diffuse, and largely bodily. The persistence of psychosomatic states and disturbances in adults may be understood as remnants of such developmental derailments, failures to integrate bodily affective experience with images or words.

A striking example of such psychosomatic states and the therapeutic approach to them can be found in the following clinical vignette (a fictionalized composite). A young woman who had been repeatedly sexually abused by her father when she was a child began an analysis with a female analyst-in-training whom one of us was supervising. Early in the analysis, whenever the patient began to remember and describe the sexual abuse or to recount analogously invasive experiences in her current life, she would display emotional reactions that consisted of two distinctive parts, both of which seemed entirely bodily. One was a trembling in her arms and upper torso, which sometimes escalated into violent shaking. The other was an intense flushing of her face. On these occasions, the analyst was quite alarmed by her patient's shaking and was concerned to find some way to calm her.

The supervisor had a hunch that the shaking was a bodily manifestation of a traumatized state and that the flushing was a somatic form of the patient's shame about exposing this state to her analyst, and he suggested to his supervisee that she focus her inquiries on the flushing rather than the shaking. As a result of this shift in focus, the patient began to speak about how she believed her analyst viewed her when she was trembling or shaking: surely her analyst must be regarding her with disdain, seeing her as a damaged mess of a human being. As this belief was repeatedly disconfirmed by her analyst's responding with attunement and understanding rather than contempt, both the flushing and the shaking diminished in intensity. The traumatized states actually underwent a process of transformation from being exclusively bodily states into ones in which the bodily sensations came to be united with words. Instead of only shaking, the patient began to *speak* about her terror of annihilating intrusion.

The one and only time the patient had attempted to speak to her mother about the sexual abuse, her mother shamed her severely, declaring her to be a wicked little girl for making up such lies about her father. Thereafter, the patient did not tell any other human being about her trauma until she revealed it to her analyst, and both the flushing of her face and the restriction of her experience of terror to its nameless bodily component were heir to her mother's shaming. Only with a shift in her perception of her analyst from one in which her analyst was potentially or secretly shaming to one in which she was accepting and understanding could the patient's emotional experience of her traumatized states shift from an exclusively bodily form to an experience that could be felt and *named* as terror.

6.6 Concluding Remarks

This chapter presents a phenomenological study of varied forms of lived mind-body disunity. Two broad types of such disunity are envisioned—those mediated by concrete bodily symbols and those that might be characterized as failures to symbolize. The first type includes hysterical conversion symptoms, hypochondriacal anxieties, and certain severe dissociative states, whereas instances of the second can be found in psychosomatic disturbances.

As seen in our clinical examples, the therapeutic implications of this phenomenological distinction are profound. In the treatment of mind-body disunities mediated by concrete bodily symbols, an interpretive understanding of these bodily symbolizations, and of the emotional truths that they encode, is crucial for the therapeutic process. Such interpretive understanding, by contrast, is not relevant in the treatment of psychosomatic states, because there is no symbolism to be interpreted. Instead, as shown in our illustrative vignette, the therapist must investigate the dangers that oppose the symbolic/linguistic articulation of bodily affect.

References

Atwood, G. E., & Stolorow, R. D. (2014). *Structures of subjectivity: Explorations in psychoanalytic phenomenology and contextualism* (2nd ed.). London & New York: Routledge.

Breuer, J., & Freud, S. (1893–1895). Studies on hysteria. *Standard edition of the complete psychological works of sigmund freud* (2nd ed. & trans. J. Strachey). London: Hogarth Press, 1955.

Jones, J. M. (1995). *Affects as process: An inquiry into the centrality of affect in psychological life*. Hillsdale, NJ: The Analytic Press.

Krystal, H. (1974). Genetic view of affects. In *Integration and self-healing: Affect, trauma, alexithymia*. Hillsdale, NJ: The Analytic Press, pp. 38–62.

Lacan, J. (1953). The function and field of speech and language in Psychoanalysis. In B. Fink (ed.), *Ecrits: A selection* (pp. 31–106). New York: Norton, 2002.

Merleau-Ponty, M. (1945). *Phenomenology of perception*, trans. C. Smith. London & New York: Routledge & Kegan Paul, 1962.

Socarides, D. D., & Stolorow, R. D. (1984/85). Affects and selfobjects. *Annual of Psychoanalysis*, 12/13, 105–119.

Stolorow, R. D. (2007). *Trauma and human existence: Autobiographical, psychoanalytic, and philosophical reflections*. New York: Routledge.

Wallace, E. (1988). Mind-body. *The Journal of Nervous and Mental Disease, 176*, 4–20.

Winnicott, D. (1965). *The maturational processes and the facilitating environment*. New York: International Universities Press.

Anorexia Nervosa: Historical, Clinical, Biographical, and Phenomenological Considerations

7

Otto Doerr-Zegers and Héctor Pelegrina-Cetrán

7.1 Historical Considerations

We owe the first description of this syndrome we know today as anorexia nervosa (AN) to the English William Gull (1816–1890), who in 1868, at a meeting of the British Academy of Medicine, mentions the existence in young women of a "hysterical apepsy" leading to emaciation, "absent tuberculosis or some other somatic illness." In 1873, Gull publishes in *The Lancet* journal the clinical description of four patients between 14 and 18 years old, who suffered from a disease characterized by "anorexia, cachexia, bradycardia, diminished respiratory rhythm, amenorrhea, constipation, and paradoxical hyperactivity." In parallel form, the French author Lasègue (1816–1883) describes that same year, 1873, a similar picture, to which he gives the name "hysterical anorexia." But before continuing with Lasègue's work, we would like to mention the fact that Gull continued publishing on the subject. Thus, for example, in 1874, he recognizes that the disease does not start in the stomach, as he supposed at the beginning ("a failure in the powers of the gastric branches of the pneumogastric nerves"), but in a "psychic trauma," and he suggests calling it "anorexia nervosa." In 1888, in a new publication in *The Lancet*, accompanied by xilographies of patients before and after a successful treatment, he hypothesizes that this disease is due to a "perversion of the Ego, that being the cause and determining the course of the malady." This second

O. Doerr-Zegers (✉)
University of Chile, Santiago, Chile

Diego Portales University, Santiago, Chile

Centre of Studies on Phenomenology and Psychiatry, Diego Portales University, Santiago, Chile
e-mail: odoerrz@gmail.com

H. Pelegrina-Cetrán
Autonomous University of Madrid, Madrid, Spain

G. Stanghellini, M. Aragona (eds.), *An Experiential Approach to Psychopathology*,
DOI 10.1007/978-3-319-29945-7_7

publication had a great impact, and in the same year, an editorial article appeared in that journal, enthusiastically celebrating the discovery of a new disease (Schadewaldt 1965).

Lasègue's publication in France occurs the same year as that by Gull (1873): the disease affects young women between 15 and 20 years old, beginning with epigastric discomforts, progressive diminution of food ingestion, starvation, mutism, amenorrhea, and constipation. He calls it "hysterical anorexia," and he also refers to the paradox involving hyperactivity described by Gull, adding that it is also noteworthy that until the disease is very advanced, they insist that they feel very well. This author also makes an observation of the greatest clinical importance, which will constitute a key element for the differential diagnosis between anorexia nervosa and other cases of extreme emaciation. In 1871 Franco-Prussian War, he had had the opportunity of observing seriously malnourished persons, who, unlike anorectic patients, reported that their limbs were not under their control. Lasègue was also of the opinion that mental anorexia did not have its origin in a gastric disease, but rather what Charcot had called "perversion of the central nervous system" ("perversion du système central nerveux").

After Lasègue, other authors also showed interest in this subject. Thus, the German pediatrician Otto Soltmann (1844–1902) calls this disease "anorexia cerebralis" and attributes the cause to a disturbance of the central nervous system (Soltmann 1894). The same Charcot, who observed four fatal cases, had problems classifying this new illness and recognized it was not identical to hysteria. Thus, he wrote, referring to one of the deceased patients: "It was one of those cases on the borderline with hysteria, but fundamentally not belonging to it" (1886). Freud also makes references to the syndrome when in 1918 he states: "It is known that there exists in far later years of childhood in girls during puberty or immediately after, a neurosis in which the rejection to sexuality is manifested as anorexia. One could relate this syndrome with the oral phase of the development of sexual life." However, the picture is practically going to disappear as a result of the description of the Danish physician living in Hamburg, Morris Simmonds (1855–1925) of a cachexia, bearing his name, and caused by a lesion of the hypophysis (1914, 1916). From that moment until 1938, when the authors Farquharson and Hyland doubted that the diseases were in fact one and the same, all interest and research in these cases focused on the endocrinological aspects of this illness. Shehan's work about postpartum necrosis of the anterior lobe of the hypophysis was the final blow to the theory that Simmonds cachexia was the same as anorexia nervosa (1939).

But we owe to Jürg Zutt (1948) the clinical description that in a certain way sealed anorexia nervosa syndrome as an independent entity. This author analyzed six cases treated by him, carrying out at the same time an accurate differential diagnosis with respect to Simmonds' cachexia, to other forms of emaciation of organic origin, and to schizophrenia. Zutt finds an endogenous origin for AN, given the global form in which it affects people and the fact that it can be explained neither by somatic nor psychological mechanisms. He also disputes Leibbrand's interpretation (1939), in the sense that the essential characteristic of these patients is a profound fear of maturing, of becoming adults, finding it too vague and unspecific. Now the most complete description of this disease was given by the Swiss-German author Ludwig Binswanger (1881–1966), because it also includes a psychodynamic and an analytical-existential interpretation. He, however, apparently not knowing the existence of this disease, diagnosed the case as schizophrenia (Binswanger 1957).

Another question to be posed when analyzing the history of this disease is if there are mentions or elements of it in previous centuries. From Hippocrates on, there are some references to certain forms of emaciation in the woman, but with the exception of an isolated case described by the English author Richard Morton (1637–1968), none of them could be fully identified with the syndrome we know through the descriptions of Gull and Lasègue. In Corpus Hippocraticum, for example, there is no reference to this syndrome. However, in the treatise about Young Women's Diseases, anorexia here is no mention, but it is stated that when young women present amenorrhea, they can develop serious physical illness. The term "anorexia" appears only with Galeno, but as a symptom of gastric diseases, and interpreted according to the theory of the humors of the time. In the following centuries, the term went on being employed in the same sense. The first change occurs with the famous physician of the city of Hamburg, Johannes Schenck von Grafenberg (1530–1598), who uses this term to describe different ways of fasting, be it for religious, occult, or show business reasons. Regarding occult reasons, we have to remember that witches were always very thin women. Nobody could imagine a plump witch. However, this thinness almost necessarily accompanying these transgressor women who practiced magic has nothing to do with the "anorectic ideology," of which we will talk later and which practically appears as one of the three criteria of AN in DSM V (2013). In the sixteenth century, there existed several cases of famous practitioners of fasting like Margarete Ulmer, for example, who was reputed to have fasted for 4 years and was visited by hundreds of people until it was discovered that she ate at night (see Schadewaldt, p. 7). Already at the end of the sixteenth century, these cases were disqualified as "mere misleading attention-getting maneuvers of young girls" (Fabry von Hilden, 1560–1634). A separate case is constituted by the abovementioned English physician Richard Morton (1637–1698), as he described two cases which approach, considerably more than the previous one, the description of Gull and he called this syndrome "phthisis nervosa," and it was characterized by amenorrhea, lack of appetite, extreme emaciation, constipation, and conservation of work capacity, in spite of cachexia.

The big question, when it deals with the problem of the history of anorexia nervosa, is if some saints who were thin, as it is the case of Saint Catherine of Siena and Saint Rose of Lima, could have suffered from this illness. In our opinion, in these cases, it is not a matter of an anorexia nervosa as such, but of extreme cases of asceticism in women who had mystical experiences. Asceticism was present as a frequent religious practice throughout the first few centuries of Christianity and remained until well into the Middle Ages. The most important difference between these ascetic behaviors and of anorexia nervosa as such lies in the fact that fasting for these saints was a way to approach God, the absolute You, while our patients, as we will see later in detail, are entirely self-centered in control and manipulation of their body. Unlike what occurred with the fasting saints, there is no transcendence in their strange relationship with food and with their body. The historian Caroline Walker Bynum (1987), in her book "Holy Feast and Holy Fast," illuminates enough the relation of religious women with food and body in the Middle Ages. According to her, the medieval woman had little control over property, money, and power, and on the contrary, they had control over food. This was their territory, and if suffering was a way of imitating Christ, the most natural way they had to do it was by refusing it. And later she states: "The redemption of all humanity lay in the fact that Christ was flesh and food... God, like woman, fed his children from his own body (the Eucharist symbolizing Christ's broken body)... Thus, women found it very easy to identify themselves with a deity whose flesh, like theirs, was food" (p. 275). Here, we see clearly how the fastening of the medieval saints had a transcendent sense, unlike the absolute immanence of anorectic behavior.

What Conclusions Can We Draw from the History of This Illness?

1. That AN as such just appears in the second half of the nineteenth century, that is to say, in full modernity. Previous descriptions point to some elements of the syndrome, but not to the disease described by Gull and Lasègue.
2. That what we understand today as AN coincides up to the details with the descriptions of the nineteenth century, for example, furtive eating, hyperactivity, and even, according to Charcot, the importance of the family in its genesis and in its treatment.
3. That the disease began to slowly increase throughout the twentieth century, experiencing a sort of boom in the sixties and continue increasing, although more slowly, until the present day (Russell 2000).
4. That the disease primarily affects young women. The cases of male with AN absolutely represent the exception. From this, we can infer that in its essence, this suffering has to do with the woman's condition per se.
5. The patients search relentlessly not only to lose weight (as occurs in bulimics) but also the female forms and with it the possibility of being mothers and of having a satisfying erotic life. The rejection of corporal maturation and sexuality was also indicated in the first descriptions.

7.2 More About the Psychopathology of Anorexia Nervosa

The first descriptions by Gull and Lasègue, completed by Zutt (1948), provide an adequate list of most manifestations of this disease. However, there are some elements, in our opinion essential, that do not appear or are not sufficiently highlighted in these descriptions, as, for example, the following:

1. **Intellectualization:** the disdain of the body is accompanied by an excessive valuation of all what is intellectual. They are always the best students, debate very well, and show an extraordinary ability to lie, to elude monitoring, and to attain their purpose of continuing to lose weight. Their style of communication is

merely intellectual and they refer to their own affectivity as "from outside" (alexithymia). In a study about anorexia and family carried out by one of us (Doerr-Zegers et al. 1985), we found this characteristic in 18 of the 20 patients studied, while in ten families, 50 %, an overvaluation of everything that was intellectual and cultural absolutely prevailed.

2. **Disturbance of the body image:** the patients experience themselves as thick and disgusting, even when they are cachectic. They look at themselves in the mirror and they see themselves as fat. It has been spoken of "addiction to thinness" or of "phobia of fatness," but the problem seems to be more complex. In an elaborate phenomenological analysis, Héctor Pelegrina has concluded that in anorectics, there is not only a desire to be thin but "to be continuously losing weight," since the immediate and ineludible presence of their ("voluminous") bodies is lived as a permanent threat. Thus, they have no other way but "removing volume from the body they have," as physical structure, which is not a living body in vital relation with the lifeworld. They perceive this body they have, as something strange to their Ego, obscenely invading both the social external world and personal intimate space. A double threat!
3. **Eagerness to control:** just as they do with their bodies, tyrannizing it to the point of not allowing it to satisfy any of its basic needs, namely, feeding and sexuality, they do with their environment; they dominate parents, siblings, caregivers, and therapists. The obsessive features attributed to them by current psychopathology (DSM V, p. 341, for instance) are nothing but ways of trying to control the world and, in particular, this body they want to mold at their discretion and even make disappear. This characteristic was found in all individual cases studied by us. Now, the anorectic tries to control not only her instincts, her needs, and the environment but also physical and symbolic space. She searches to create a space of her own that protects her body from the common space, lived by her as an enemy. At the same time, he searches to construct a cognitive, symbolic space, in which she exercises her absolute empire, to the point of allowing herself all types of transgressions, among others, kleptomaniac acts. These last represent an exercise of power over all limits. This exercise of spatial power has two functions: first, to control that public space she experiences as a perpetual threat and, second, it has a vicarious and compensatory function of her inability to order her life toward an end extending beyond her body. She experiences her privacy as lacking all value and completely subjected to the opinion of others, hence her well-known dependence and panic lest she be rejected or abandoned.
4. **Fragmentation of the body:** from Gabriel Marcel (1935), we distinguish the body I have or object-body (e.g., the eye) from the body I am or subject-body (the look). But I am object-body only for the other, in its maximum expression, for the surgeon, not for myself. In the anorectic, there is a split of these two bodies, and she tries her lived body as object-body as a fetish, as something that can be manipulated at will. It is probable that this split also has to do with the distortion of the body image, in the sense that for her, every mass (even her cachectic body) is volumetric and disgusting. In the anorectic patient, the own

body becomes a "thing" separated from the Ego itself. This is no longer an incarnate subject, and the body acquires the character of mere object, whose only value is the appearance of the design, as if it were a utensil to contemplate, a pure "public image." Anorectics live the external manifestation of their privacy as something obscene and impudently exposed to the looks of others. They seek an existence that is simply ideal without flesh palpitating with desires and moods, an existence with no secret intentions. This anorectic phobia to the corporal manifestation in the exterior space, crystallizing in phobia to be a volumetric body, that is, expansive and expositional, determines that implacably ruthless and endless war between the Ego and its body. For the anorectic, her body is the biggest enemy. It is an inappropriate body, another body, extreme in its personal dimension. And at this point, fragmentation combines with eagerness to control, because when living the alienated own body full of animosity against its owner object-body, the anorectic needs to establish a continuous and total control over this enemy body. Instead of livelily conducting the living body that they constitute, from within toward the world, they try to control it from outside.

5. **The paradoxes of anorexia nervosa:** The number of paradoxes in which the existence of the anorectic patient evolves is surprising. The Chilean specialist in this field, Rosa Behar (1988), referring to it, has spoken of "the antithetic in anorexia nervosa." We will describe the most characteristic features, some of which were also highlighted by the same specialist.
   (a) The *first paradox* observed in anorectic patients is the coincidence between an extreme thinness, which can develop till **cachexia**, and marked **hyperactivity**. This last already became noteworthy in the early descriptions and contributed, in the case of Lasègue, to consider this syndrome as an independent illness, when comparing it with cases of extreme emaciation as a consequence of the shortages of the Franco-Prussian War in which passivity predominated. Pelegrina maintains that this hyperactivity is not explained only by a desire to lose weight, but rather it is the expression of eagerness to construct a personal space, as a kind of island tolerating and protecting their bodies. With this type of actions, they seek to forge a space there where they feel there is nothing but emptiness and desolation. But this is a manufactured space, not a space constructed in the world with the other and in the framework of an appropriative activity. It does not really constitute an own space, quietly welcoming them. The inherent restlessness of life is not fulfilled as an expression in the world and as appropriation of it, so that instability and unrest appear.
   (b) The *second paradox* is revealed in the contradiction between their tremendous affective **dependence** on others, particularly her mother, and the **rejection** of every real affective bond. Thus, anorexics generally do not have partners or friendships, and in the psychotherapeutic relationship, the rational moment widely rules over the affective one. Much has been said about the alexithymia characterizing these patients. In our experience, this inability to establish adult affective relations can bring them to complete loneliness when the only being with whom they have been able to bond

with, generally the mother, gets sick or goes missing. At least three of our patients ended up abandoned for months, even years, in clinics or hospitals.

(c) The *third paradox* appears as the contradiction between their great **intellectual maturity** and a great **emotional immaturity**, manifested among other things as desire to not grow, to remain preadolescent, and to not join the adult world. Though in fact they are neither in the adult nor in the adolescent world, not in the former because they do not want to accept the challenges, this implies marriage, maternity, professional life, etc. and not in the second either, because they consider adolescents to be intellectually very immature. It is as if they wished to live in an adult world, but with infantile dynamics. This feeling of being thrown outside the child world and not being able to partake of a mature interpersonal encounter is one of the reasons their lives end in great loneliness.

(d) The *fourth paradox* is revealed in the fact that the anorectic has the need to **make her body disappear** (a phenomenon that Pelegrina has called "ex-corporation of the Ego"), to not be seen by others in its volume and, at the same time, she feels the desire to **draw attention** to herself, even to provoke others by exhibiting her extreme thinness. She wants to be absent and at the same time makes herself starkly present, even in sexual relations. In actual fact, very soon after the disease has begun, her whole family begins to worry about her.

(e) The *fifth paradox* can be appreciated in the framework of treatment and rehabilitation. The attitude is completely ambivalent, because on the one hand she is interested in treatment, regularly attends the sessions, smiles at the physician, calls him her "savior," expresses her desire to get better, etc. But, as Rosa Behar points out so aptly, the problem lies in the fact that for them well-being is always associated with low weight, so that any success of the treatment expressed as a weight increase is going to mean for them unease and unhappiness, first, and then the confirmation that their fight to lose weight must continue whatever the cost.

7.3 Family and Anorexia Nervosa

It is interesting that the role of the family in the origin of this disease has been highlighted from the beginning of the explosion in the incidence of this disease starting in the sixties.

Thus, already in 1965, the Japanese Ishikawa describes certain peculiarities of these families. The **father** is generally a weak or absent person, has a good intellectual and financial level, and is unsociable. This author refers also to a fact we have seen repeated in our own clinical practice that the father pulls out or even kidnaps his daughters when they are hospitalized. The **mothers** are active and ambitious but at the same time unstable people and frequently suffer from "anxiety neurosis." The **family** looks very normal seen from outside, but they usually hide obscure conflicts.

Another characteristic observed by the Japanese author is that in these families, the daughters predominate over the sons and the ill daughter is, generally, the second. I cite this author because his observations are identical in every respect with what we found in our investigations about the subject starting in the decade of the seventies (Doerr-Zegers et al. 1976, 1985; Doerr-Zegers 1988, 1994).

In 1965, in the same Göttingen symposium, the German author E. Sperling also makes a contribution to the subject of the role of the family in this illness, warning that there were not yet systematic studies with respect to this, but indeed repeated observations, as, for example, that the mothers shared with the daughter a denial of the gravity of the disease and they help the patient reject the treatment. In fact, from the totality of patients treated in the Psychiatric Clinic of Göttingen University, 50 % did not accept treatment, and of those who did, only one-third completed it. The fathers not only do not support the treatment, but—just as Ishikawa observed—they pull them out of the clinic, sometimes by force. According to Sperling, they maintain a strange relationship with the patient. Typical phrases of anorectic patients with respect to her father are, for example: "I have to work for him..." and "I have to return him the life he gave me." But perhaps the most interesting observation of Sperling refers to the part a grandmother frequently plays, both in the genesis and in the evolution of the illness, the grandmother is in general a person of very strong character and much money, with which she manipulates the whole family. From the 16 families studied by Sperling, this was the combination of circumstances in 12 of them, eight cases on the mother's side and four of them on the father's side. Sperling also observed in these families the systematic rejection of sexuality and praise of everything that had something to do with intellectual performance. Finally, this author also mentions another fact of observation coinciding with what we saw, which is the frequency with which the father becomes ill around the time the anorexia begins.

One of the authors (O. D.-Z.) studied throughout 8 years 35 cases of anorexia and their families (op. cit.) and our observations with respect to the personality of these patients and to the family dynamics widely coincide with what was described by the abovementioned authors, except some new elements that we will describe later. Perhaps what is still more surprising, for its so empirical character, is the wide predominance of the daughters in these families: 69.7 % in our study and 72.5 % in Stoeffler and collaborator's study (1978), practically at the same time as ours. I have no explanation for this phenomenon. But there are other coincidences between the above quoted works about family and anorexia and our studies of the seventies and eighties. Thus, for example, we find the observation of Ishikawa that the mothers frequently suffered from "anxiety neurosis" (very broad concept involving many of the syndromes we call today "major depression" or "anxiety disorder"). We found this type of mothers in 40 % among our patients, and we were able to confirm in 70 % of the cases that the fathers were weak with absent personalities. On this point, it is necessary to point out that this "weak or absent" category of the Japanese author had in our study a slightly more specific nature, since the "weak" father was almost always affected by a chronic disease (coronary insufficiency, crippling arthritis, cancer, etc.), condition in 30 % of the families, while the "absent" one corresponded to fathers who had extramarital affairs or sexual encounters (40 %). It is curious that this apparently anecdotic fact has been mentioned in a footnote by Manfred Bleuler in his book ["Endocrinological Psychiatry" (1956, p. 337)].

Our studies coincide also with some of the observations of Sperling (1965) about the fathers' personalities, but perhaps the more interesting—given its surprising character—is the presence of a dominant grandmother. In 35 % of our study, we find the figure of the overwhelmingly domineering and rich grandmother. In our studies, above all the one in 1985, we arrive a little beyond the mentioned characteristics of parents and grandmothers, establishing three types of anorectic families: (1) with dominant mother and weak or ill father (30 % of the cases), (2) dominant father with weak or ill mother (35 %), and dominant grandmother with weak or ill mother and absent father (35 %). Another Sperling observation showing a high coincidence with our investigations refers to the overemphasis on study, performance and culture, and the rejection of sexuality. He does not give numbers, but in our study, we find the first characteristic in 90 % of the families and the second in 80 %. Finally, we would like to address a subject that was crucial to us in the family dynamics of anorexia nervosa and that does not appear mentioned by the previous authors, but indeed later, by Mara Selvini-Palazzoli (1978, 1982): the topic of sacrifice. In these families, we observe a tradition of sacrifice for others that might go back several generations. Or as Héctor Pelegrina (2006) has suggested, they are families structured from the "must be," as a collection of obligations and not of manifestation of intimacy, where there is no clear boundary between each family component and their roles. This brings the future patients, in their adolescence, to perceive the body they have as a "productive machine" and not as manifestation of life per se. And outside the family, it brings them to pretend to be themselves at the margin of the lived encounter, in the purely rational space. Given the importance and relative originality of this issue, we will deal with it as a separate chapter.

The **tradition of sacrifices** *in the family of anorexia nervosa and its importance for the genesis of the disease:*

In the first place, we will illustrate this phenomenon, observed by us in 70 % of studied families, with some examples:

Case 1 (Ana): the maternal grandmother becomes widowed at 30 years old with nine children, she does not marry again out of a "sense of responsibility" and works all day in occupations linked to food production and/or manipulation that enabled her to raise and educate them the best way possible. In the family, she is remembered as a sort of "heroine." The father of the patient had done something similar. He was Italian, his mother died young, he did not get along with the stepmother, and he emigrated to Chile, where he installed a little chocolate factory, which over the years would be transformed into a big company. Shortly after arriving and having his first job, he began to bring one by one all his brothers from Italy, whom he educated and transformed into successful merchants, industrialists, or professionals. With respect to the fact that his mother worked in restaurants, it seems of interest to us to mention that in 40 % of the families, the parental figure who maintained the household worked in direct relation with food processing or manipulation (pastry chef, butcher, cook, etc.). In another 40 %, the relation was indirect, as, for example, farmers or industrialists who produced food (wheat, potatoes, pasta). Only in 20 % there existed no relationship. We think this is a factor that in some way contributes to making food an object of permanent concern in the anorectic family.

Case 2 (Gloria): in this case, the phenomenon of sacrifice appears even more impressively. The father's family was full of tragedies: his mother, that is, the patient's grandmother, had died, as had three of the father's six brothers; the grandfather did not marry again, because "he had to support" the three remaining children, but when these essentially grown up, he committed suicide. There was a family tradition that "some have to die in order that the others live." Gloria will later become ill when her mother enters a serious depressive state.

Case 3 (Christa): it is one of the first we treated in the seventies and it is also one of the cases of late beginning; besides, she was one of the few patients who got married. She is German and arrived in Chile when she was young, accompanying her Chilean-German husband, whom she had met in the university. Her mother lost her husband in the war; she married again apparently quite in love and had a happy life, but always felt in some way guilty for raising her daughter with a stepfather. Ten years after the war ended, the father, who had been a prisoner all those years in the Soviet Union, reappears, and she ends the relationship with her second husband and accepts the missing one back. According to the daughter, her reason is to give her the experience of growing up with her true father.

Case 4 (Alicia): this case is found in one of the few families of scarce resources within our study. The father suffers from severe rheumatoid arthritis and cannot work. The mother works until late at night in a cafeteria-restaurant, because they had to feed eight children. Suddenly, her sister dies of a brain aneurism, and she decides to adopt her three nephews, at one point having 11 children in the house, with all the effort and personal sacrifices this entails.

Case 5 (Verónica): the father is an outstanding dentist and the mother was dedicated to housework. They have ten children, from which three suffer from a severe cognitive impairment, a genetic disease that at that time had not yet been identified. This disease came from the mother's side, her family of origin having had similar cases. Even though they could have afforded a maid, the mother decided to completely dedicate herself to the care of her ten children and in particular, of the three ill ones, refusing to keep them in adequate institutions. These children had destroyed a good part of the furniture and the house was a real chaos. Only when the youngest of these children grew and began sexually and aggressively harassing his sisters, they agreed to put him into a nursing home. All the healthy children became professionally successful, got married, and have had many children. The father lives today with the two oligophrenic daughters, who are already around 50 years old. The illness of the fifth of the daughters brought several changes in the family: the entire household began to revolve around her, the mother began to worry more about food and not only about the sick children and the father to be more present, and the most problematic of the ill children was put in hospital. This is one of the cases that, analyzed in detail, allow us to illustrate in what way the anorectic act is not only a whim, but many times it has a deep experiential sense: the search to construct a welcoming life world in a reality lived as desolate and stark.

This conduct of sacrifices almost without limits, including the renunciation of love, of sex, of food, and even of life, characterizing for generations the members of these families, gives our patients' fast a quality transcending mere neurotic psychodynamics toward spheres of humanity bordering on ethics and religion. We do not deny that the classic psychoanalytical interpretations (Thomae 1961; Selvini-Palazzoli 1965, 1970; Feldmann 1965; Bruch 1974) can partially account for the etiopathogenesis of this disease. For these authors, they are preadolescent unconscious conflicts worsening when adolescence arrives. These are, according to these authors, the fixation on the oral stage, the repression or negation of every form of sexuality and oral ambivalence. The adolescent changes trigger anxiety linked to repressed sexuality, which is, according to the theory, transferred to orality. The anorectic lives hunger as a threat and source of guilt, against which she is going to fight through the ascetic ideal of the Ego: to be a being without sex, without instincts, and beyond good and evil. And that is obtained by ceasing to eat. But one could ask if the oral fixation and the exacerbation of the instincts that adolescence carries with it will be enough for a girl to begin a voluntary and suicidal behavior like so extreme a fast. How to establish the bridge between these psychodynamic mechanisms and anorectic behavior? We think that the psychoanalytical interpretation is insufficient and that to approach an understanding of this strange disease, we should analyze more in detail the triggering factors, those preceding the beginning of the fast because it is not always the irruption of adolescence that triggers this disease. This requires detailed biographical analyses, which we have also carried out in previous research studies (1972, 1976, 1985, 1988, and 1994).

7.4 The Premorbid Situation

Both the psychoanalytical and anthropological interpretations have sought to find the roots of this illness in the psychological and existential changes of this maturational crisis. However, if we observe the life history in more depth, we find family events preceding the start of the illness and which one should take into account. These are seen both in the anorexia's dating way back and coinciding with the beginning of adolescence and in those of late onset. Here, there are some examples of cases of the former:

- *Case 2 (Gloria):* the adolescent changes coincide with the mother's depression requiring hospitalization, being replaced in the household by the patient. A short time after, the father suffers a severe accident with brain injury, endangering his life. Gloria completely dedicates herself to his care.
- *Case 5 (María Luisa):* the mother dies in an accident. The father, baker, leads a secret life of extramarital affairs and does not marry again. His own mother, who plays the role of the "powerful grandmother," takes care of the house. When she becomes seriously ill, María Luisa takes the role of housekeeper and tyrannizes her younger sisters, making them eat too much, and she begins to fast, until she weighs only 32 kg.
- *Case 7 (Irma):* the mother discovers an extramarital relation of the father. Irma's reaction is of rejection of men and asks to be changed from a coed school to one for girls only. The parents reconcile and the father changes his attitude toward Irma and begins to regularly visit her at school. In this moment, Irma has her menstrual cycle and begins to fast.
- *Case 10 (Regina):* She had a very well-constituted and apparently harmonic family; suddenly, it is discovered that the father has had a second home for a long time. A great family crisis is resolved through the reconciliation of the parents and a change of attitude of the father toward Regina, until then the neglected daughter.

It is noteworthy that all these preadolescent situations have some elements in common. In the first place, it deals with situations in which the above mentioned family tradition of sacrifice is fulfilled in the sense that the patients react in front of death, disease and scandals with this strange behavior of fasting *ad outrans*, but having the unmistakable seal of deprivation, of self-punishment, and of sacrifice. In the second place, we observe a change in the father-daughter relationship, in the sense of an approach and proximity until then nonexistent. This could have to do with the psychoanalytical hypothesis of a preadolescent conflict between the Ego and the instinctive forces, reaching its maximum intensity with the sexualization of the adolescent body, to the point of causing a split between the "ideal Ego" and the "corporal Ego" and the subsequent denial of the latter.

Some examples of late onset:

- *Case 1 (Ana)*: the illness begins coinciding with the end of university studies, a trip to Europe accompanying the father in the capacity of "secretary" and in which she gains much weight and a serious disease of the father (brain hemorrhage) immediately after returning. Ana abandons all her activities to dedicate herself to his care and at that moment begins fasting.
- *Case 4 (Alicia):* she had always had a tendency to put on weight since adolescence. The family lived in a city of the south of Chile. She was very inclined to eating candies and paid for it with her weight. A brother of the father, who lived in the capital, becomes seriously ill. The father with the future anorectic moves to Santiago to take care of him. He dies and the father is hospitalized with

bronchopneumonia. Now fully dedicated to caring for the father, Alicia begins the fast.

- *Case 9 (Digna):* she had had since adolescence a particular preoccupation for the topic of food: she was very fond of the kitchen and liked very much to make others eat, and she suffered from periods when she was overweight. The fast begins when she is 18 years old and in relation with a series of tragic events: her oldest brother dies from a brain tumor, the mother falls into a deep depression, but in spite of it, she adopts the three children of her recently dead daughter, and the father becomes crippled by a deforming arthritis. Digna dedicates herself to his care and begins to fast.

Unlike the previous group, in the patients beginning recently, a group from which we have shown only three examples, the background is observed of an excessive oral activity, preceding anorectic behavior by several years. Very early there begin to happen unlucky or tragic situations (disappearances, deaths, diseases, disabilities), but they do not quite trigger anorexic behavior. It is as if these patients were more "resistant" to misfortune than the others, those beginning early. The girls deal with these situations from an oral point of view by first eating excessively and then protect themselves from the weight gain by going on a diet. In most of the cases, we observe that the fast as such begins in relation with two circumstances: a maturational stage (end of university studies, beginning of the first job, or, in one case, marriage) and severe disease of a loved one, generally the father, to whose care the future anorectic dedicates herself completely.

7.5 Attempt of a Dynamic Interpretation of the Anorectic Act

We speak of an "initial anorectic act" to refer to this first stage of the disease, when the patient manages to bring her appetite under control and begins the fast she has decided to undergo and that will bring her cachexia and other known symptoms. Since Zutt's description in the decade of the 1940s, it is well known that these patients do not really suffer from anorexia, but only behave as if they do. Moreover, the descriptions of oral fantasies and of an uncontrolled appetite outbreak are frequent. To stop eating in those circumstances can be nothing short of an act of great sacrifice. Sacrifice has had since ancient times a double meaning, offering something to get something in exchange and of purification: whoever makes a sacrifice is cleaning, purifying himself through this act. For reasons difficult to understand, there have existed in these families a tradition of mutual sacrifices and offerings between their members, a sort of ascetic spirit (very evident in the mothers) which is in the air and which makes even more shocking the frequent parallel life of the father. The future anorectic has been taught from early infancy to have no more instinct than oral, because all others and in particular sexual are forbidden. She feels very dependent on the mother, but at the same time experiences hostility toward her, since she does not give her the dedication she required, either because she is too worried by the very difficult or unfriendly son (another subject which has been also indicated by other authors, but which we have not mentioned) or by her frequent depressive states. Her father is, by contrast, a very distant soul, who she tries to attract through obedience, achievements, and performance, without ever being able to do it. The brusque, endogenous, and unexpected sexualization of her body with adolescence accentuates her unconscious conflicts, in particular the oedipal theme, but in the measure that the father maintains himself far and the mother near, there is no real threat and she will accompany her pains and joys by eating more or eating less.

And then the situational change happens where, following an unfortunate event (illness of the father, of the mother, or of the grandmother), the daughter and the father meet, know, and love each other. This situation means for the girl the simultaneous discovery of love and death, the first as realization of an old admiration for that unattainable being and the second through the *threat* of the illness (e.g., cases 1, 2, 3, 4, and 9) or of the *loss* in the arms of other women (e.g., cases 5, 7, and 10). But this situation does not only represent the long-desired approach to the paternal figure but also a demand. Love must be *manifested* and the loss (by disease or abandonment) *avoided*. The answer is imposed on the patient from the family tradition and her own life history with perfect naturalness: *sacrifice*, the renunciation of her appetites and her studies and the total commitment to her sick father, in some cases, or to replace the sick mother, together with the father, in others. With this act the girl obtains a new balance, by which she avoids the threats of the internal (instinctive) world and neutralizes an external world by demanding more and more independence. Through sacrifice, she *saves* her father and *purifies* herself of her love for him. Being ill allows her to maintain the situation of dependence on the mother and at the same time to punish herself by not receiving the food her mother offers her. But the balance reached is very precarious, since the threats needing to be overcome afflict her mercilessly: hunger in the form of compulsions to eat and oral fantasies, while the inexorable passage of time pushes her toward the assumption of her role of a woman. Any "relapse" in eating will mean a weight increase and reappearance of the feminine forms with subsequent anxiety. There is no other solution but to repeat the fasting act until eternity, repetition that tells us that the course of this disease is well underway a process character in the sense of Karl Jaspers (1959).

We think these observations referring to personality, family, and preadolescent situation of the young anorectic can contribute to an enrichment in the understanding of the pathogenesis of this mysterious illness, in the measure that they establish a bridge between the unconscious preadolescent conflicts studied by psychoanalysis (Thomae 1961; Feldmann 1965; Selvini-Palazzoli 1965, 1970, 1978) and anorectic behavior, stemming from will. This bridge is nothing but the phenomenon of *sacrifice* which, for the reasons stated, present the patient as the only possible solution for a life crisis characterized by the coincidence of a maturational step—with the consequent instinctive exacerbation—and a tragic circumstance demanding from her an act of love unknown to her.

7.6 Anorexia Nervosa and Postmodernity

Which is the relation between anorexia nervosa and Postmodernity, besides the fact that it just appears in late modernity and in the beginning of the time we are living? To answer this question we should have to review some of the characteristics of our time.

The **first** characteristic of Postmodernity we would like to outline and that also belongs to the previous period, modernity, is **the dominion of technique**. In modernity, the extraordinary development experienced by natural sciences brought to creation more and more complex instruments, which have made human life easier and which have made man progressively more independent of his environment. In Postmodernity, this reaches its real paroxysm with the invention of the computer and its derivatives, through which absolute immediacy and total ubiquity have been achieved, in a certain sense, that is to say, the overcoming of time and of space. The final consequence has been the advent of a more and more virtual world. There even exist online (virtual) romantic relationships! The philosopher Martin Heidegger and the poet Rainer Maria Rilke have warned us with much lucidity about the dangers of the technique. Thus, in his essay, "The question about the technique," Heidegger tells us: "The unveiling which dominates modern technique has the character... of provocation. This happens in such a way that the energy hidden in nature is discovered; what is discovered is transformed; what is transformed is accumulated; what is accumulated is in turn distributed..." (1978). And on another occasion, he brutally states: "(For man in the technical age) nature has become one bigone-stop 'gas station', a mere source of energy for modern industry" (op. cit.). Rilke, for his part, denounces power and the alienating character of the technique in the Sonnet No. XVIII, First Part of the Sonnets to Orpheus:

"Do you hear the New, Lord,
rumbling and shaking?
Prophets are coming
who shall exalt it.

Truly, no hearing its whole
around such noise,
and get the machine's part
too will have its praise.

See, the machine:
how it turns and takes its toll
and pushes aside and weakens us.

Though it draws energy from us,
It, without passion,
drives on and serves."

"The New" evidently represents the technological revolution, praised by all from the middle of the nineteenth century and until at least the discovery made by Heisenberg of the "uncertainty principle" in 1927, according to which we will never be able to get to know reality as it is, because the act of knowing it already modifies it. This glorification of science and progress ("Prophets are coming/who shall exalt it") persisted, however, for decades and in a certain way until the present day, while the doubts stated by the same modern physics were forgotten in the rapture produced by continuous technological advances. For Rilke, this world of machines and their unlimited power appears essentially linked to noise, to the absence of silence, and, consequently, to the absence of peace. And thus, in the first stanza of this Sonnet, the poet defines "the New" as that "rumbling and shaking," and in the second, he reminds us that nobody is "truly, no hearing its whole." Man has no place to hide from noise in the modern world and this is produced almost exclusively by machines: in cities by the vehicles providing transportation, in factories and their surroundings by industrial machines, noise in the airports by airplane motors, noise in houses by multiple domestic machines, etc. Further down in the poem, the poet warns us harshly about the danger which technique brings to human beings as the machine will end up "taking its toll" on us, because it will "push aside and weaken us." With respect to the first consequence of this revenge, it is enough to think of the worrying deformation of the mind of adolescents and children produced by television and computers. The "weakening" that the poet foretells us could be perfectly identified with the worrying increase in depression-type illnesses in the last 50 years. At the end of the poem, the poet accepts that machines have been freely invented by man ("Though it draws energy from us") and that they have made life easier for us in many respects ("it. . . drives on and serves"), but at the same time, he asks us not to forget that they work "without passion," that is, that by lacking feelings, it is very likely that one day they will be transformed into instruments of destruction and predatory activities. It is enough to think of atomic weapons, the destruction of native and tropical forests, the temperature increase on earth, and the gradual death of our cities as a result of air pollution, garbage, and noise accumulation, for not having other possibilities as to find the reason to the poet in his prophetic apprehensions (Rilke 2004, 2010).

The anorectic patient is an extreme example of this predominance of image over reality. And we say extreme, because it is no longer the space nor time nor the objects surrounding us, which have been transformed into illusory artifices, but the body itself, that is, the closest and most private thing a person can possess. In the anorexic, the body becomes a "thing" separated from the Ego itself, which then ceases to be an incarnate subject. The body is transformed into a thing as "something in front of the eyes" (in the sense of Heidegger's *Vorhandenheit*), with the character of being a mere object, whose total value would be in the appearance of the design, as if it were a utensil to contemplate, dimensioned as pure public image. The anorectic suffers an alienation of her own body, which she experiences not only as inappropriate but as an alienated body, another body, which is external to her personal dimension, a body which puts her intimacy at the reach of the humiliating and annihilating look of the other. This is what brings her to try to establish a continuous and total control over her "enemy" body (see Pelegrina 1996).

Just as Postmodernity has manipulated reality through technique to the point of making it almost completely artificial (the virtual world and city of Las Vegas are two near caricature examples of the aforesaid), the anorectic tries to construct herself a body without volume, a body also in a certain way virtual, and a body which does not occupy space and which feels nothing, not even instincts. Now this manipulation of the body is also found in other expressions of Postmodernity, as, for example, in the vast increase of plastic surgery operations and of tattoos. One dramatic case of the consequences which the manipulation of the body of this kind can have is the famous singer Michael Jackson. These behaviors have in common with anorexia nervosa the taking of the body as object and the excessive importance given to appearance, to that which is shown, but they differ in an equally important way: the anorectic girl risks her life in her delusional determination to make her object-body disappear and be transformed into pure spirit.

We would like to mention a **second** characteristic of Postmodernity intimately related with anorexia nervosa, although strictly it is not, as we will see, completely separable from what was previously mentioned, that is to say, from the extreme intervention in objective reality we are carrying out and over the body in the case of anorexia. We refer to **obscenity**. It is not only the progressive tendency to eliminate every form of shame, something appearing every day in the form of nudity, of advertising, and of show business which, to tease its audience, uses bodies or borderline pornographic scenes or even those explicitly pornographic movies shown in the cinema, on television, or in the Internet. It is rather so that our world, so dominated by the sense of sight, desperately searches to look at the objects in the most minute detail, from all possible angles, repeating the contemplation again and again, by means of manual film cameras or video apparatus, for example. Obscenity begins when there is no spectacle or scene anymore, when there is no theater or illusion, and when everything has become immediately transparent and visible, subjected to the crude and inexorable light of information and communication. The French philosopher Jean Baudrillard (1988) has described this phenomenon brilliantly: "In many cases our erotic and pornographic imagery, all that panoply of breasts, buttocks and sexual organs, has no more sense than this: to express the useless objectivity of things. Nudity only serves as a desperate attempt to underline the existence of something... The sexual is nothing but a ritual of transparence. Before it was necessary to hide it; today, by contrast, it serves to hide rickety reality." (p. 27) And further he adds: "In order that a (true) look exists it is necessary that an object be veiled and unveiled, disappears at any time; for that reason the look manifests a sort of swing. By contrast, these images (of Postmodernity) are not taken in a play of emergence and disappearance. The body is already there without even the spark of a possible absence, in a state of radical disappointment, which is the state of mere presence." (p. 28)

Nothing can be more obscene than the body of the anorectic. And it is obscene both when it is shown and when it is hidden. It is well known that some patients like to hide her bodies with wide clothes, while others experience pleasure scandalizing other people by showing them their bones. The case of anorectic models is a good example of this latter. But in both cases, be it when they hide their body with enormous gowns or when they show it discarnate, in the literal sense of the word, there is a human being in a scene, and there is a predominance of the appearance, an empire of the image, that is to say obscenity. Let us remember that "ob" in Latin means being in front and in sight and "scenity" naturally derives from scene. The anorectic has this obscenity in common with the obese and perhaps also the absurd attempt to make the body disappear.

A **third** characteristic of Postmodernity which also has to do with the emergence of this disease in our time is the **loss of religious sense of existence**. This strong linkage of man with the divine, which held him for centuries and millennia, has been replaced first by the good reason and, then by science and in recent decades, by money and pleasure, this last being named in its most ephemeral and decadent sense. The vanishing of the past and of the future, so much a part of the current hedonist attitude and one of whose typical expressions is the consumption of drugs (Doerr-Zegers 1980, 2007), also has made untenable an authentic religious life, since this requires both of the sacred narrative, of myth which illuminates and helps (coming from the past), and of hope in a life beyond death, which gives meaning to our earthly life (the future). The forgetfulness of pain and suffering, which have always constituted the via regia for reaching the transcendent dimension, is also closely related to it. Pain has been anesthetized and suffering denied by tranquilizers, antidepressants, or drugs. Rilke, as in so many other things, anticipated the times and denounced this phenomenon way back in 1922, when in the last stanzas of his famous Sonnet No. XIX of the First Part of Sonnets to Orpheus, he says:

"Sufferings have not been seen,
Love has not been learned,
and what removes us in Death,

has not been revealed.
Only the Song over the land
hallows and rejoices." (Rilke 2004, 2010)

Without a doubt, we have forgotten pain and one does not love anymore as in other times. Death, for its part, is simply denied, as is observed in a form almost bordering on caricature in the rites of the funeral homes in the United States. But faced with these three elements of the drama of our time, not recognizing pain, not learning love, and not accepting death, the poet shows us a way: "Only the Song over the land/hallows and rejoices." The word is, according to Heidegger (1959), "the dwelling of being," but at the same time, it is the bridge uniting earth and heaven, mortals and gods, while music—the highest product of the human spirit—was born, according to Rilke himself, as a trail of vibrations left by the death of the demigod Linus, another son of Apollo, in the middle of the emptiness of primal space, "vibration that charms and comforts and helps us now" (end of the First

Elegy). Heidegger (1980), when commenting on the two last stanzas of the already mentioned Sonnet No. XIX, says: "The time has become precarious not only because God is dead, but because mortals are scarcely able to recognize their own mortality... death has retired toward the enigmatic. The mystery of pain remains hidden. Love has not been learned, but mortals are and they are in the measure that language exists, because the song still prevails on the precarious earth and the voice of the one who sings still keeps the trace of the sacred open... Time is precarious, because the essence of pain, death and love have not yet been exposed This precariousness is precarious, because that essential condition, in which pain, love and death co-belong, has disappeared. There is concealment in the measure that the condition of this co-belonging is the abyss of the being. But the song calling the land still remains. What is the song itself? How does a mortal become able to sing? From where does the song sing? How far into the abyss does the song go?" (translation from German into English by O. Doerr-Zegers).

We think that anorectics represent an extreme example of this loss of religious sense characterizing our time. They live in pure immanence, in the immediate itself of that prison which is the object-body and trying to make it disappear. They are not interested in anything beyond dominating it or occupying themselves, paradoxically, with the subject of food, which is precisely what they hate and love at the same time. They spend hours forcing others to eat to look at them eating as if they were voyeurs. The other is not of interest. It is a world which does not know love, forgetfulness of oneself and needless to say, the search for a transcendent sense. And for this reason, there could not have been anorectics in the Middle Ages or in the Renaissance, let alone in the Romantic period. In those centuries and in previous ones, the human being lived himself as welcomed in God's arms, and everything had a sense from divine Providence, birth, disease, and death, both joys and pains, and the body did not only have value in itself, but it was sacred, sacredness which reached its greatest height in the sacrament of Communion. The body of the anorectic, on the contrary, is the opposite of the sacred body and is very close to the obscene body of Postmodernity that is so well described by Jean Baudrillard in the following words: "...(this body), by being object of that obscene look which denudes everything, loses its dignity and is transformed into a variety of surfaces, crawling with multiple objects, where its finitude and its seduction are lost: metastatic and fractal body, no longer called to any form of resurrection." (op. cit., p. 38)

References

American Psychiatric Association. (2013). DSM V. Washington: American Psychiatric Association.

Baudrillard, J. (1988). *El otro por sí mismo* (pp. 27–28). Barcelona: Anagrama.

Behar, R. (1988). Lo antitético en la anorexia nerviosa. *Revista Chilena de Neuro-Psiquiatria, 226*, 201–204.

Binswanger, L. (1957). Der Fall Ellen West. In: *Schizophrenie* (pp. 56–188). Pfullingen: Neske Verlag.

Bleuler, M. (1956). Psiquiatría Endocrinológica. Buenos aires: Ed. M. Finchelmann y Cía., p. 337.

Bruch, H. (1974). *Eating disorders*. London: Routledge and Kegan.
Charcot, J. M. (1886). Neue Vorlesungen über die Krankheiten des Nervensystems, insbesondere über Hysterie. Dtsch. Übersetzung von S. Freud. Leipzig und Wien, p. 194s.
Doerr-Zegers, O. (1980). Adicción y temporalidad. *Psicología Médica (Revista argentina de psicología médica, psicoterapia y ciencias afines), V*(3), 381–397.
Doerr-Zegers, O. (1988). La familia de las anoréxicas nerviosas. *Actas Psiquiatrica y Psicologica de America Latina, 34*(1), 33–40.
Doerr-Zegers, O. (1994). Contribución a una interpretación sistémica de la anorexia nervosa. Con E, Morales y G. Hernández). *Actas Luso-Espanola de Neurologia y Psiquiatria, 22*, 26 (261–269).
Doerr-Zegers, O. (2007). La postmodernidad y la pregunta por el sentido. En: La palabra y la música. Santiago: Ediciones Universidad Diego Portales, pp. 165–177.
Doerr-Zegers, O., Petrasic, J., & Morales, E. (1976). Familia y biografía en la patogénesis de la anorexia nerviosa. *Revista Chilena de Neuro-Psiquiatria, 15*(1), 3–26.
Doerr-Zegers, O., Petrasic, J., & Morales, E. (1985). The role of the family in the pathogenesis of anorexia nervosa. In P. Pichot, P. Berner, R. Wolf, & K. Thau (Eds.), *Psychiatry. The state of the art* (Psychotherapy and Psychosomatic Medicine, Vol. 4, pp. 459–465). New York and London: Plenum Press.
Farquharson, R. F., & Hyland, H. H. (1938). Anorexia nervosa: A metabolic disorder of psychological origin. *Journal of the American Medical Association, 111*, 1085.
Feldmann, H. (1965). Zur Frage der psychodynamischen Faktoren bei der Pubertätsmagersucht. In J. E. Meyer & H. Feldmann (Eds.), *Anorexia nervosa* (pp. 103–108). Stuttgart: Georg Thieme Verlag.
Freud, S. (1947) Aus der Geschichte einer infantilen Neurose (1918). In Gesammelte Werke, Bd. 12, London, p. 141.
Galeno, cit. por H. Schadewaldt. (1965). Medizingeschichtliche Betrachtungen zum Anorexie-Problem. In J. E. Meyer & H. Feldmann (Hrsg.). *Anorexia nervosa* (S. 1-14). Stuttgart: Georg Thieme Verlag.
Gull, W. Citado por Thomae, H. (1961). *Anorexia Nervosa*. Bern-Stuttgart: Huber-Klett Verlag.
Heidegger, M. (1978). Die Frage nach der Technik. En: *Vorträge und Aufsätze* (pp. 9–40). Pfullingen: Neske.
Heidegger, M. (1980). Wozu Dichter?. En: *Holzwege* (pp. 265–316), 6. Auflage. Frankfurt am Main: Vittorio Klostermann.
Hipócrates, cit. por H. Schadewaldt (1965). Medizingeschichtliche Betrachtungen zum Anorexie-Problem. In. J. E. Meyer & H. Feldmann (Hrsg.). Anorexia nervosa (S. 1–14). Stuttgart: Georg Thieme Verlag.
Ishikawa, K. (1965). Über die Eltern von Anorexia-nervosa-Kranken. In J. E. Meyer & H. Feldmann (Hrsg.). *Anorexia nervosa* (S. 154–155). Stuttgart: Georg Thieme Verlag.
Lasègue, C. (1873). De l'anorexie hystérique. *Archive of Géneral Medicine, 21*, 385.
Lasègue, C. Citado por Thomae, H. (1961) *Anorexia Nervosa*. Bern-Stuttgart: Huber-Klett Verlag.
Leibbrand, W. (1939) Der göttliche Stab des Aeskulap. 3. Auflage. Salzburg, p. 382 ff.
Morton, R., cit. por Thomae, H. (1961) Anorexia nervosa: Geschichte, Klinik und Theorien der Pubertätsmagersucht. Stuttgart: Ernst Klett Verlag, p. 12.
Pelegrina, H. (1996) Estructura espacial de lo fóbico. *Vertex, Revista Argentina de Psiquiatría*, VII, 23, pp. 5–15.
Pelegrina, H. (2006). Mundo de vida y psicopatología. *Monografías de Psiquiatría (Madrid), Año, 18*(1), 48–60.
Rilke, R. M. (2004). *Los Sonetos a Orfeo. Traducción, Prólogo, Introducción y Comentarios de Otto Doerr*. Madrid: Visor Libros.
Rilke, R. M. (2010). *Las Elegías del Duino. Traducción, Prólogo, Introducción y Comentarios de Otto Doerr*. Madrid: Visor Libros.
Russell, G. (2000) Anorexia nervosa. In M. G. Gelder, J. J. López-Ibor Jr., N. C. Andreasen (Eds.). *New oxford textbook of psychiatry, Vol. 1*. Oxford: Oxford University Press, pp. 835–855.

Schadewaldt, H. (1965). Medizingeschichtliche Betrachtungen zum Anorexie-Problem. In J. E. Meyer & H. Feldmann (Hrsg.). *Anorexia nervosa* (S. 1–14). Stuttgart: Georg Thieme Verlag.
Selvini-Palazzoli, M. (1965). Interpretation of Mental Anorexia. In *Anorexia Nerviosa*. Stuttgart: Thieme Verlag.
Selvini-Palazzoli, M. (1970). The families of patients with anorexia nervosa. In *The child and his Family*. New York: Wiley.
Selvini-Palazzoli, M. (1978). *Self-starvation*. New York-London: Jasson Aronson.
Selvini-Palazzoli, M. (1982). Paradoja y Contraparadoja. A. C. E. Buenos Aires.
Shehan, H. L. (1939). Simmonds' disease due to post partum necrosis of anterior pituitary. *Quarterly Journal of Medicine, 8*, 277.
Simmonds, M. (1914). Über Hypophysisschwund mit tödlichem Ausgang. *Deutsche Medizinische Wochenschrift, 40*, 322.
Simmonds, M. (1916). Über Kachexie Hypophysären Ursprungs. *Deutsche Medizinische Wochenschrift 42*.
Soltmann, O. (1894). Anorexia cerebralis und centrale Nutritionsneurose. *Kinderheilkunde., 38*, 1.
Sperling, E. (1965). Die 'Magersuchtfamilie' und ihre Behandlung. In J. E. Meyer & H. Feldmann (Eds.), *Anorexia nervosa* (pp. 156–160). Stuttgart: Georg Thieme Verlag.
Stoeffler, P. (1978). Die Anorexiefamilie. Promotion zum Dr. med. In *Jahrbuch der Dissertationen der Medizinischen Fakultät*. Heidelberg: Universitätsverlag.
Thomae, H. (1961). *Anorexia nervosa: Geschichte, Klinik und Theorien der Pubertätsmagersucht*. Stuttgart: Ernst Klett Verlag.
Schenck von Grafenberg, J. cit. por H. Schadewaldt (1965) Medizingeschichtliche Betrachtungen zum Anorexie-Problem. In J. E. Meyer & H. Feldmann (Hrsg.). *Anorexia nervosa* (S. 1–14). Stuttgart: Georg Thieme Verlag.
Fabry von Hilden, W., cit. por H. Schadewaldt. (1965). Medizingeschichtliche Betrachtungen zum Anorexie-Problem. In J. E. Meyer & H. Feldmann (Hrsg.). *Anorexia nervosa* (S. 7). Stuttgart: Georg Thieme Verlag.
Walker Bynum, C. (1987). *Holy feast and holy fast*. Oakland, CA: The University of California Press.
Zutt, J. (1948). Das Psychiatrische Krankheitsbild der Pubertätsmagersucht. *Archives of Psychiatry 180*, 776 ff.

Alcohol-Induced Psychotic Disorders

8

M. Musalek, O. Scheibenbogen, and A. Schuster

8.1 Introduction

Alcohol use disorders (DSM-5), which in ICD-10 are divided into alcohol abuse and alcohol dependence, are among the most common psychiatric disorders. In terms of 12-month prevalence, alcohol use is already the most frequent mental health disorder among men and among women the most frequent after anxiety disorders (Wittchen and Jacobi 2012).

50 % of individuals suffering from substance use disorder develop symptoms of alcohol withdrawal when they reduce the quantity or frequency of their alcohol consumption. In approx. 3–5 % of cases, severe withdrawal symptoms such as grand-mal convulsions or delirium occur (Schuckit 2014). Despite the prevalence of the underlying dependence disorder, alcohol psychoses are relatively rare, but very severe, and frequently life-threatening phenomena.

Strictly speaking, acute intoxication already constitutes a "reversible exogenous psychosis with impaired self-control and self-criticism, stimulation and disinhibition as well as euphoria or also depression" (Bergmann and Ferbert 2012).

Nowadays psychotic disorders encompass above all delirium tremens (alcohol withdrawal with delirium), alcohol hallucinosis [alcohol-induced psychotic disorder (AIPD)] as well as the very uncommon alcoholic delusional jealousy (Soyka et al. 1991), the epidemiology, phenomenal picture, progress and treatment of which will be described in more detail below.

Below are two case vignettes, one of pre-delirium and one of alcohol-induced delusional jealousy.

M. Musalek (✉) • O. Scheibenbogen • A. Schuster
Anton Proksch Institute, Vienna, Austria
e-mail: michael.musalek@api.or.at; musalek@api.or.at

G. Stanghellini, M. Aragona (eds.), *An Experiential Approach to Psychopathology*, DOI 10.1007/978-3-319-29945-7_8

Case Study Pre-delirium

Mr. L is a 34-year-old patient who was admitted to the hospital in a state of drunkenness and with a blood alcohol content of 1.7 as measured by a breathalyser. He was unclean and unkempt and said that in the last few days he had been drinking up to 2.5 l of vodka a day. Even during admission, he was unsteady on his feet, drowsy and then alert but restless and anxious. He seemed disorientated, above all, with regard to time (clearly confused not just about the day of the week but also the month) and initially thought he was actually at a different clinic. However, he had an adequate understanding of the situation (admission for treatment for alcohol dependence) and also seemed orientated with regard to himself. In conversation, his level of attention fluctuated significantly. In the final analysis, an inability to concentrate and lack of retentiveness could not be determined but were probably present. The same was true with regard to long-term memory loss. In his manner, the patient appeared energised, with thought disorder, on occasions he was incoherent, although he was usually able to follow a train of thought to a logical conclusion. Occasionally, he lost his train of thought. In contact with others, the patient appeared wary and suspicious. There were no indications of panic attacks, health-related anxiety or compulsions. There were no symptoms of delusion (although it was not possible to verify some of the things the patient said) and the presence of ego-disturbances and hallucinations was doubtful (it was conspicuous, however, that the patient repeatedly stared at certain places in the room but when questioned was unwilling to say whether he saw anything). His mood was tense and dysphoric; his mental state was described as very negative in tone. A pronounced psychomotoric agitation was observed, and drive appeared significantly increased. No psychomotoric abnormalities in the sense of mannerisms or stereotypes were observed. The patient denied having thoughts of taedium vitae, specific suicidal fantasies or plans and was also capable of reaching agreements in this respect. Appetite was described as severely reduced and recent sleeping patterns as very irregular, sometimes with day-night reversal. The patient stated that he had on several recent occasions been beaten up, mishandled and even raped, although he did not wish to go into further detail. A recent CT of the skull indeed showed a depressed fracture of the bridge of the nasal bone but no further indications of recent craniofacial traumata. There were no signs of recent intracranial bleeding, the cerebral parenchyma showed no infra- or supratentorial abnormalities, the inner and outer cerebral fluid interspaces were normal for the age of the patient, and there was no midline shift. The clinical examination revealed no pathological findings; apart from a folic acid deficiency, lab tests merely revealed slightly elevated transaminases. During the first few days of treatment, the patient repeatedly experienced severe motor agitation, severe vegetative symptoms (hyperhidrosis, hand tremor) as well as difficulty falling and staying asleep. On one occasion, he vomited. The day after he was admitted, the patient said he had felt threatened by certain gestures made by fellow patients and on at least one occasion had been the victim of verbal abuse. In this situation, he was persuaded to take aripiprazole and quetiapine as medication against his tension, although he categorically refused to take other neuroleptic drugs such as haloperidol.

Treatment was started with the intravenous administration of fluids (3 × 500 ml Ringer's solution), combined with thiamine (one 100 mg ampulla per day), as well as the administration of oxazepam (initially 50 mg 1-1–1-2, with a gradual reduction of the dosage). To prevent cramps, the patient was given valproate (500 mg 1-1–0-1) and to treat his insomnia prothipendyl (80 mg 0-0–0-2). From the second day of hospitalisation onward, medication was supplemented by an antipsychotic therapy with aripiprazole (initially 10 mg) and seroquel (100 mg 1-1–1-1). From the fourth day of treatment, the administration of thiamine to treat the vegetative symptoms, which had by now abated significantly, was switched to oral administration, and the dosage of oxazepam was gradually reduced. Within two and half weeks, it became possible to discontinue treatment with oxazepam completely, although the patient continued to receive valproate, not least of all because of his history of epileptic seizures. Treatment with aripiprazole and quetiapine was also continued. By the time the patient stopped taking oxazepam, he no longer manifested any vegetative symptoms. His sleep patterns had normalised significantly, although he did occasionally experience problems with interrupted sleep. Although the patient's inner tension receded markedly during the first week of treatment, it did not disappear completely, and he continued to display distrust of his fellow patients. However, he was able to remain in an in-patient setting, and no open conflicts with fellow patients were reported.

Case Study Alcoholic-Induced Delusional Jealousy
Pat was admitted to our institute for the second time following a massive relapse but was not under the influence of alcohol when he arrived. He reported that he had previously been admitted to the acute psychiatric unit as an in-patient for 6 weeks and to a rehabilitation centre for 10 weeks. The reasons for these previous hospitalisations were chiefly his bipolar disorder and alcoholic delusional jealousy. At the time of anamnesis, Pat was alert and fully orientated with clear consciousness, mnestic unremarkable, his manner was well-ordered, and he was able to follow a train of thought to a logical conclusion. His mood was normothymic; his mental state was slightly negative in tone. Affectability was present on both scale ranges; affect was flat, drive unremarkable, although Pat was somewhat slower due to the medication. He had no acute suicidal thoughts and no explorable psychotic symptoms.

Pat reported a 38-year history of problematic alcohol consumption. Even as an apprentice aged 15, he had become so drunk at the first company Christmas party that his father had to come and take him home. Generally speaking, large quantities of alcohol had always been drunk at home, and looking back he said both his parents had been dependent upon alcohol but had significantly reduced their alcohol consumption in the last years of their lives. Even then, he and his three brothers had been badly affected by the conflicts between his parents. This was where he had first come into contact with jealousy. His mother had always suspected his father of having an affair with his secretary. As the latter also worked in the family home as a nanny, his father had regularly driven her to work in the morning. Pat's mother had often vocally accused her husband of having improper relations with the young woman and on several occasions had moved out of the family home for short periods. Looking back, Pat was unable to say whether his father really had been unfaithful or not.

Pat recalled that he had experienced jealousy at a very early age. He had always had very smart and attractive girlfriends who had been regularly admired by his friends who had also made sexual advances to whichever girlfriend he had at the time. Even then, he had regularly consumed large quantities of alcohol resulting in verbal, and on one occasion physical, conflicts.

In summer 2014, he had suffered an alcoholic relapse after having been treated for several months at the psychosomatic rehabilitation centre. Pat reported that he had been consuming 10–15 cans of beer (0.5 l) plus 0.5 l of wine and 7/10 l digestive liqueur five times a week. As a result, he had also experienced an episode of pre-delirium with visual hallucinations, during which he had seen small animals scurrying about and books and office material moving on the table. The most conspicuous sign, though, was the refrigerator, which was sometimes suddenly full of alcoholic drinks and then later on almost empty. However, at no time was his consciousness clouded and he was still aware that what was going on was actually impossible.

It was during this period that his delusional jealousy peaked with images of his wife engaged in sexual intercourse with other men repeatedly intruding into his mind. These images were very specific and detailed, rather like a cinema film. Pat had been married since 1994 and had 2 children aged 19 and 11. Since the birth of the first son, one child had always slept in the marital bed, making it difficult, if not impossible, to satisfy his sexual needs. Driven by frustration, he had often got up at night and gone to sit outside on the terrace and have something to drink, after which his sexual appetite receded. Alcohol increasingly began to affect his relationship with his wife. Feelings of guilt about drinking and strong cravings for alcohol often led him to neglect the relationship. This in turn often acted as the driver for renewed delusional processing of the situation. If in the morning his wife spent more time than usual in the bathroom, dressed up more or left the house a few minutes early, he would fall into a jealous rage and often accused her of infidelity. His perception increasingly focused on finding "proof" of this, although he was never able to find conclusive proof either one way or the other.

The more the relationship deteriorated as a result of his dependence on alcohol, the fiercer his jealousy became, as whenever his wife reacted by becoming more distant, he always reinterpreted it as an interest in other men—a self-reinforcing mechanism that ultimately led to his wife leaving him.

Pat is now back at home with his family but feels like a "guest". Although he and his wife still share the house, they are no longer a couple.

During anamnesis, Pat described his situation with regard to his delusional jealousy as follows: "It's my own fault that the relationship ended. I have to accept that and that it was largely because of the alcohol. My wife is entitled to have affairs with other men if she wants to; we're no longer together. Generally speaking, in future, I want to develop a much more liberal attitude. I only want to have open relationships where both people can do whatever they want. And if my partner is unfaithful, that's her right!"

In this situation, Pat is finding his way towards a juxtaposition, in which the world of delusion and reality can coexist without influencing one another. For him, this opens up a strong chance that in the future he will be able to shape relationships constructively and find fulfilment.

8.2 History

The association between increased alcohol consumption and psychosis was documented by Marcel as early as 1847. Even then Marcel, but also Kraepelin (1913), differentiated between alcohol hallucinosis and delirium tremens. In the 1970s, alcoholic psychoses, according to Bonhoeffer (1917) a form of exogenous type of reaction, included delirium tremens, alcoholic Korsakoff's psychosis, Wernicke encephalopathy, alcohol hallucinosis, chronic delusional jealousy, dipsomania and alcoholic seizures (Grünberger 1977). Even then, there were discussions as to whether dipsomania and endogenous mood disorders (Schröder 1912), which lead to a pathological, addictive craving for alcohol accompanied by a massive loss of control, does indeed constitute a separate entity. Today there is a broad consensus that alcohol hallucinosis, delirium tremens and alcoholic delusional jealousy do indeed constitute alcoholic psychoses.

In the interests of clarity, Wieser (1962) suggested that psychotic manifestations be classified as hyperaesthetic-emotional (pre-delirium), delirious-amential (delirious) and depressive-dysphoric syndromes (Kryspin-Exner 1966).

The term alcohol hallucinosis was coined by E. Bleuler (Soyka 1999). In his "Textbook of Psychiatry" 1983, first published in 1916, he wrote the following about inebriation: "...the acute effects of alcohol are individual and very different according to chance circumstances. They depend on the personality of the patient and on the physical and mental disposition at the time alcohol is consumed. In some patients neurological symptoms of poisoning, in others psychological symptoms come to the fore, soon taking on the character of excitation, soon that of drowsiness, and among the emotions, soon euphoria, soon unkindness, soon maudliness ('drunken misery')". He referred to pathological states of drunkenness as a symptom of "chronic alcoholism" and as a severe and appalling disorder, which he says "... is often provoked by very small quantities of alcohol, which would not be able to trigger ordinary inebriation... The patient first begins to be irritated or anxious in order to rave and storm against persons and things about him, breaking dishes and furniture. The paroxysm is sometimes set free by an exchange of words, an attempt to direct. Under the influence of fury, anxiety and illusions and hallucinations, the conditions of their surroundings are mistaken and the patients are markedly disoriented. Nearly always the scene is ended by a protracted narcotic sleep, from which the patient awakes with a dizzy head, but as a rule without any recollection of what has happened. There are people who have such attacks only once in their lives, others, may be so afflicted very frequently. But the above described alcoholic effects are always the exception in the same individual; he also experiences spells of normal drunkenness. To be sure there are drunkards who, finally, in nearly every drunken spell get 'drunken hallucinations' sometimes in the sense of delirium tremens, sometimes more in the sense of alcoholic insanity or of alcoholic jealousy, but here the reaction is usually a much milder one..." (Bleuler 1983).

In pathological drunkenness, also known as idiosyncratic alcohol intoxication[1] (Feuerlein et al. 1998), a specific cascade of effects of toxicity and neurotransmitters occur.

In this relatively rare disorder, inebriation occurs when a small quantity of alcohol is consumed that would not produce any degree of intoxication whatsoever in most people. Patients suffering from this syndrome become verbally aggressive or physically violent (Dilling et al. 1993). The symptoms of intoxication manifest themselves within a few minutes of alcohol being consumed. Typically, symptoms include impaired consciousness and impaired cognitive abilities, perception, judgement and behaviour. However, this violent behaviour is not typical for patients and is not part of their behavioural repertoire when they are sober; they appear to have undergone a change of character.

The ICD-10 classification distinguishes between the following:

- Alcohol psychotic disorders ICD-10F10.5
- Schizophrenia-like ICD-10F10.5
- Predominantly delusional ICD-10F10.51
- Predominantly hallucinatory (including alcohol hallucinosis) ICD-10F10.52
- Predominantly polymorphic ICD-10F10.53
- Predominantly depressive psychotic symptoms ICD-10F10.54
- Predominantly manic psychotic symptoms ICD-10F10.55
- Mixed ICD-10F10.56

8.3 Neurophysiology of Alcohol Use

Alcohol depresses the central nervous system. The initial slightly euphoric and stimulating effect of small quantities of alcohol can be explained by the fact that alcohol first suppresses inhibitory nerve pathways and only suppresses excitatory nerve pathway activity once larger amounts have been consumed. Like benzodiazepines and barbiturates, alcohol rapidly increases the release of gamma aminobutyric acid (GABA) with a clear effect on GABA type A receptors. In addition, it also inhibits *N*-methyl-D-aspartate glutamate receptor activity. Chronic alcohol consumption results in changes to the receptors and the development of

[1] The word idiosyncrasy is derived from Old Greek, and is made up of ίδιο- ("ones own-"), *συν*- ("with-") and κράσις ("mixture") and indicates the complexity of things up to and including radical individual characteristics.

alcohol tolerance with increasingly large quantities of alcohol required to achieve the same suppressant effect.

8.4 Alcoholic Delirium: Alcohol Withdrawal Delirium (Delirium Tremens)

Although alcohol delirium usually occurs as part of a withdrawal syndrome, in patients with enduring and chronic alcoholism, it can occur as a reaction to any change in the pattern of drinking. Approximately 15 % of persons with alcohol use disorders are affected by delirium tremens, which is preceded by a pre-delirious state characterised by disturbed dreams and insomnia, vegetative symptoms and in particular hyperhidrosis and tremors. Untreated, the pre-delirious state develops into an alcohol delirium, which in addition to an intensification of the symptoms of the pre-delirium also manifests itself in a clouding of consciousness. This disorientation is shown with regard to time, place and situation but not, however, to the person. In addition to severe agitation, the most prominent symptoms are perception disorders with usually visual hallucinations.

The patient will hallucinate small moving objects (seeing white mice). Their mood is often lighter but frequently coloured with anxiety. Patients also present with coarse tremor (hence delirium tremens). The vegetative disturbances can be substantial with sweating, palpitations and fever as the main symptoms. An untreated delirium will last for between 4 and 10 days. The condition is serious (Uhl et al. 2009).

Left untreated, a delirium leads to death in 15–30 % of cases. Older people and patients who suffer from repeated episodes of delirium unfortunately have a poorer prognosis.

In addition to the vegetative symptoms of alcohol withdrawal syndrome (pre-delirium) such as hyperhidrosis, tachycardia, hypertension, tachypnea and insomnia, other symptoms associated with discontinuing alcohol use include gastrointestinal complaints such as nausea and diarrhoea. Other symptoms occur in the central nervous system, such as hallucinations (usually visual), perception disorders, generalised seizures, tremor, dysarthria (motor speech disorder) and ataxia (lack of coordination of muscle movements); the mood is depressed, dysphoric and/or anxious. There is a conspicuously increased level of energy and inner restlessness. Generally speaking, pre-delirium lasts for between 3 and 7 days.

The symptoms of alcohol delirium (delirium tremens) are much more marked than those of pre-delirium. The most conspicuous psychopathological symptoms here are a clouding of consciousness and disorientation and an inability to recognise situations and people. The visual hallucinations can be very strong and differentiated; even auditory hallucinations in addition can occur. Furthermore, patients no longer realise that they are hallucinating and believe that what is happening is real. Paranoid experiences, hyperactivity with fidgeting and looking around for things and increased suggestibility occur. The case fatality rate of untreated delirium tremens is approximately 25 %, which is largely due to the

Table 8.1 DSM-5 criteria for withdrawal delirium (delirium tremens) according to Schuckit (2014)[a]

Criteria for alcohol withdrawal
Cessation of or reduction in heavy and prolonged use of alcohol At least two of eight possible symptoms after reduced use of alcohol: • Autonomic hyperactivity • Hand tremor • Insomnia • Nausea or vomiting • Transient hallucinations or illusions • Psychomotor agitation • Anxiety • Generalized tonic-clonic seizures
Criteria for delirium
• Decreased attention and awareness • Disturbance in attention, awareness, memory, orientation, language, visuospatial ability, perception or all of these abilities that is a change from the normal level and fluctuates in severity during the day • Disturbances in memory, orientation, language, visuospatial ability or perception No evidence of coma or other evolving neurocognitive disorders

[a]The criteria are based on the *Diagnostic and Statistical Manual of Mental Disorders*, fifth edition (DSM-5). A patient who meets the criteria for both alcohol withdrawal and delirium is considered to have withdrawal delirium

severity of vegetative symptoms and symptoms affecting the central nervous system. Statistics in respect of epidemiology vary, and 5–15 % of all alcohol-dependent individuals will experience withdrawal delirium.

The triggers are varied, frequently "occasional causes", such as infections or accidents, which as a rule make it impossible to continue consumption. After 3–5 days, the symptoms usually begin to recede, although clinical courses vary widely. Table 8.1 lists the DSM-5 criteria and Table 8.2 the methods of treating delirium tremens.

8.5 Alcohol Hallucinosis

Alcohol-induced psychotic disorder, AIPD, also known as alcohol hallucinosis, is a rare complication of chronic, severe alcohol misuse or substance dependence disorder. In contrast to alcohol delirium, the disorder is characterised by predominantly auditory hallucinations (hearing voices) and only very rarely by visual hallucinations. Patients' consciousness usually remains clear, and mood is extremely anxious and tense. The auditory hallucinations are usually abusive in nature and are therefore perceived as threatening and trigger persecutory delusions. These are usually pseudo-hallucinations as patients know that they are hallucinating. They react to these ideas of persecution with restlessness and marked escape tendencies and an inclination to violent outbursts. A further difference to

Table 8.2 Suggested treatment of alcohol withdrawal delirium (delirium tremens) according to Schuckit (2014)

Suggested treatment of alcohol withdrawal delirium (delirium tremens)
• Provide care in an inpatient setting, preferably an intensive care unit
• Perform a workup to rule out medical conditions and measure values such as the levels of electrolytes and pancreatic enzymes, haematocrit and platelet counts; perform liver-function tests
• Provide supportive care by monitoring vital signs frequently (e.g. every 15–30 min) in a quiet, well-lit room. Reorient patient to time, place and person
• Administer thiamine intravenously at a dose of 500 mg once or twice a day for 3 days; monitor patient for over hydration
• Provide medications to control agitation, promote sleep and raise the seizure threshold
• Administer primary pharmacotherapy with the use of benzodiazepines, preferably intravenously, in doses high enough to achieve a lightly dozing but still arousable state, while monitoring the patient's vital signs until delirium abates (approximately 3 days). The dose on day 1 is the amount needed to control target symptoms (e.g. diazepam at a dose of 15 mg) – Examples of diazepam regimens: Regimen 1: administer 10–20 mg intravenously or orally every 1–4 h, as needed Regimen 2: Begin treatment with 5 mg intravenously (2.5 mg/min) If needed, repeat 10 min later If needed, administer 10 mg again 10 min later If needed, administer 20 mg 10 min later Continue to administer 5–20 mg/h, as needed – Examples of lorazepam regimens: Regimen 1: Administer 8 mg intravenously, intramuscularly or orally every 15 min, as needed. After the patient has received 16 mg, if delirium is still severe, administer an 8-mg bolus intravenously. Then administer 10–30 mg/h Regimen 2: Administer 1–4 mg intravenously every 5–15 min, as needed Alternatively, administer 1–40 mg intramuscularly every 30–60 min, as needed Continue dosing every hour as needed to maintain somnolence
• In addition to benzodiazepines, administer adjunctive mediations such as the antipsychotic agent haloperidol for uncontrolled agitation or hallucinations (0.5–5.0 mg intravenously or intramuscularly every 30–60 min as needed for severe agitation or hallucinosis—not to exceed 20 mg or 0.5–5.0 mg orally every 4 h up to 30 mg)

delirium lies in the vegetative symptoms, which are far less pronounced, and the absence of tremor.

The hallucinosis is acute but may persist for weeks or even months. If it lasts for longer than 6 months, then it is regarded as chronic hallucinosis. If persecutory delusions predominate in the hallucinatory state, clinicians also refer to "alcohol paranoia" (Uhl et al. 2009).

The differential diagnosis distinction between alcohol hallucinosis and other psychiatric disorders, such as alcohol-induced withdrawal delirium and schizophrenic disorders, is important because alcohol hallucinosis requires a different form of treatment. In the acute phase of alcohol-induced psychotic disorders, antipsychotics or major tranquilizers are usually prescribed. However, abstinent patients do not usually require any long-term treatment with antipsychotics, and furthermore, the prognosis is extremely favourable provided that abstinence is maintained.

The distinction between alcohol hallucinosis and schizophrenic disorders remains a subject of heated controversy in the scientific literature, and to date only a very small number of methodologically correct studies have been conducted in respect of the differential diagnosis of alcohol hallucinosis. One reason for this is the high level of coexistence of schizophrenia and alcohol dependence and the problems associated with tracing back the symptomatology to the schizophrenic disorder or the alcohol dependence.

Genetic studies emphasise the existence of alcohol hallucinosis as an independent disorder (Schuckit and Winokur 1971). In their comparative study of the characteristics of alcohol hallucinosis and schizophrenia, Jordaan et al. (2009) reached the following conclusion: AIPD is a discrete diagnostic entity. Patients with AIPD have less severe psychotic symptoms compared with patients in the schizophrenia group. The key symptoms of AIPD are hallucinations, particularly auditory, and to a much lesser extent delusions. Additional features are depression and strong anxiety symptoms and frequently suicidality (Table 8.3).

Table 8.3 Differential diagnostic criteria to distinguish alcohol hallucinosis from paranoid schizophrenia [according to Soyka (2009)]

Criterion	Alcohol hallucinosis	Schizophrenia
Onset	Acute	Often slow
Age at onset	Approx. 40–50 years	Usually before the age of 30, rarely after the age of 40
Prognosis	Usually good (80–90 %)	Often chronic course
Alcohol anamnesis	Positive over many years	Can be positive
Family history of schizophrenia	No increase	Significant increase
Family history of alcoholism	Significant increase	No increase
Psychopathology hearing voices	Obligatory	Frequent
Visual hallucinations	Sometimes	Rarely
Thought disorders	Very rarely	Absent mindedness
Affective disturbances	Anxious, depressive No parthymia	Parthymia
Ego-disturbances	Very rarely	Very frequent
Structural imaging	Possibly cerebral atrophy (cerebellum, frontal lobe, global)	Usually normal Possibly slight expansion of ventricles
Neurology	E.g. polyneuropathy, cerebellum symptoms	At most “soft signs”, rarely catatonic symptoms
Somatic	Adverse effects of alcohol, e.g. liver	No findings

8.6 Epidemiology of Alcohol Hallucinosis

Whereas the lifetime prevalence for alcohol dependence is 10–15 % for men and 3–5 % for women (Schuckit et al. 2005), only 2–3 % of alcohol-dependent patients develop psychotic symptoms (Victor et al. 1953). The majority of psychotic symptoms occur with withdrawal delirium (delirium tremens), with approximately 1/3 of patients developing alcohol hallucinosis (AIPD). Soyka et al. (1988) found prevalence rates of AIPD among patients who had been hospitalised in Germany of 0.4–0.7 %, whereas Finnish studies reported 4 % (Perälä et al. 2010). Furthermore, the Finnish study reported a lifetime prevalence in the general population of 0.41 %. Tsuang et al. (1994) found no significant differences in the sociodemographic data (such as age, education, marital status and employment) between alcoholic patients with and without a history of psychosis. While the age of onset of psychotic symptoms was significantly later compared to schizophrenia, patients who later developed alcohol hallucinosis were found to have begun consuming alcohol at a significantly earlier age (Jordaan and Emsley 2014). In these cases, the duration of alcohol abuse probably constitutes at least a moderating variable.

Key differential diagnoses of alcohol hallucinosis (Soyka 2009) are hallucinations arising during "simple" withdrawal syndrome, alcohol delirium, other forms of delirium, (paranoid) schizophrenias, alcohol/drug intoxication, drug-induced hallucinosis (e.g. cocaine, hallucinogens), alcohol-induced paranoia and alcohol-induced delusional jealousy. Somewhat less common and hence of less differential diagnostic relevance are affective psychoses, in particular mania, organic hallucinoses of varying aetiology, auditory hallucinoses with deafness, epilepsy, endocrine disorders, brain tumours and dementia.

8.7 Delusional Jealousy

If delusional jealousy exists independently of the basic psychosis (delirium) and persists during periods of abstinence, we refer to alcoholic delusional jealousy (paranoid disorder). This type of jealousy can take on delusional characteristics. The term alcoholic paranoia is no longer used today.

Delusional jealousy is encountered predominantly and indeed almost exclusively among men; the dominant symptom is the unshakeable belief that a partner is being unfaithful or wishes to end the relationship. If delusionally jealous ideas occur during alcohol hallucinosis or delirium, they are usually quickly reversible. Persisting delusional symptoms are far less common and are often associated with the occurrence of other paranoid symptoms and hallucinations.

Monosymptomatic delusional jealousy that develops slowly and which does not manifest itself with other psychotic symptoms is encountered much more frequently (Soyka 2009).

Kryspin-Exner (1966) reported that alcoholic delusional jealousy recedes quickly among one third of patients during abstinence. The cause, however, is still largely unclear; earlier assumptions that only impotent alcoholics or individuals with sexual function disorders are affected by delusions have not been proven. In English-speaking countries, the term Othello syndrome is often used.

8.8 Summary

Withdrawal delirium followed by alcohol hallucinosis and alcoholic delusional jealousy are the most common psychotic disorders, even though they occur very rarely relative to the frequency of alcohol dependence syndrome. Alcohol-induced psychoses are a discrete entity which must be differentially diagnosed from schizophrenic conditions and require a specific treatment. Owing to their severity, the complications which often occur during alcohol withdrawal can under certain circumstances present a life-threatening scenario for the patient, whose psychopathology is hugely important for early diagnosis.

References

Bergmann, L., & Ferbert, A. (2012). Alkoholfolgeerkrankungen. In P. Berlit (Ed.), *Klinische Neurologie*. Berlin, Heidelberg: Springer.

Bleuler, E. (1983). *Lehrbuch der Psychiatrie*. Berlin, Heidlelber: Springer.

Dilling, H., Mombour, W., & Schmidt, M. H. (Hrsg.) (1993). Internationale Klassifikation psychischer Störungen ICD-10 Kapitel V (F). Klinisch-diagnostische Leitlinien. 2. Korrigierte Auflage. Bern, Göttingen, Toronto, Seattle: Huber.

Feuerlein, W., Küfner, H., Soyka, M., Dittmann, V., & Haller, R. (1998). *Alkoholismus - Missbrauch und Abhängigkeit: Entstehung - Folgen – Therapie*. Stuttgart: Thieme.

Grünberger, J. (1977). *Psychodiagnostik des Alkoholkranken*. Wien, München, Berlin: Maudrich.

Jordaan, G. P., & Emsley, R. (2014). Alcohol-induced psychotic disorder. A review. *Metabolic Brain Disease, 29*, 231–243.

Jordaan, G. P., Nel, D. G., Hewlett, R. H., & Emsley, R. (2009). Alcohol-induced psychotic disorder: A comparative study on the clinical characteristics of patients with alcohol dependence and schizophrenia. *Journal of Studies on Alcohol and Drugs, 70*(6), 870–6.

Kraepelin, E. (1913). Lectures on clinical psychiatry (translated by T. Johnstone). London: Bailliere Tindall.

Kryspin-Exner, K. (1966). *Psychosen und Prozessverläufe des Alkoholismus*. Wien: Ueberreuter.

Marcel, C. N. S. (1847). De la folie causee par lábus des boissons alcooliques. Thesis (Paris, Rignoux, imprimeur de la faculte de medicin).

Perälä, J., Kuoppasalmi, K., Pirkola, S., Härkänen, T., Saami, S., Tuulio-Henriksson, A., Viertiö, S., Latvala, A., Koskinen, S., Lönnqvist, J., & Suvisaari, J. (2010). Alcohol-induced psychotic disorder and delirium in the general population. *British Journal of Psychiatry, 197*, 200–206.

Schröder, P. (1912). Intoxikationspsychosen. In: Aschaffenburgs Handbuch der Psychiatrie. Leipzig Wien: Deuticke.

Schuckit, M. A. (2014). Recognition and management of withdrawal delirium (Delirium tremens). *The New England Journal of Medicine, 371*(22), 2109–2113.

Schuckit, M. A., & Winokur, G. (1971). Alcoholic hallucinosis and schizophrenia: A negative study. *The British Journal of Psychiatry, 119*(552), 549–50.

Schuckit, M. A., Smith, T. L., Danko, G. P., Kramer, J., Godinez, J., Bucholz, K. K., et al. (2005). Prospective evaluation of the four DSM-IV criteria for alcohol abuse in a large population. *The American Journal of Psychiatry, 162*(2), 350–360.

Soyka, M. (1999). *Optimierte Arzneimitteltherapie: Alkoholabhängigkeit*. Berlin: Springer.

Soyka, M. (2009). Psychotische Störungen durch Alkohol. *Nervenheilkunde, 8*, 533–538.
Soyka, M., Naber, G., & Völcker, A. (1991). Prevalence of delusional jealousy in different psychiatric disorders. An analysis of 93 cases. *British Journal of Psychiatry, 158*, 549–553.
Soyka, M., Raith, L., & Steinberg, R. (1988). Mean age, sex ratio and psychopathology in alcohol psychosis. *Psychopathology, 21*, 19–25.
Tsuang, J. W., Irwin, M. R., Smith, T. L., & Schuckit, M. A. (1994). Characteristics of men with alcoholic hallucinosis. *Addiction, 89*, 73–78.
Uhl, A., Bachmayer, S., Kobrna, U., Puhm, A., Springer, A., Kopf, N., Beiglböck, W., Eisenbach-Stangl, I., Preinsperger, W., & Musalek, M. (2009). *Handbuch: Alkohol - Österreich: Zahlen, Daten, Fakten, Trends 2009. Dritte überarbeitete und ergänzte Auflage*. Wien: BMGFJ.
Victor, M., Hope, J. M., Adams, R. D. (1953). Auditory hallucinations in the alcoholic patient. *Transactions of the American Neurological Association, 3,* (78th Meeting), 273-275.
Wieser, S. (1962). Zur Theorie und Klinik der Alkoholpsychosen. In: Arbeitstagung über Alkoholismus (Kryspin-Exner, K., Wien).
Wittchen, H.-U., & Jacobi, F. (2012). Studie zur Gesundheit Erwachsener in Deutschland. DEGS im Auftrag des BMG vom Robert Koch-Institut, Berlin durchgeführt. Die Zusatzuntersuchung "Psychische Gesundheit" wird zusammen mit dem RKI (Dr. Ulfert Hapke) durch das BMG und die Stiftung der DGPPN gefördert. Studienleiter, zusammen mit der Prof. Dr. W. Gaebel (Düsseldorf), und Prof. Dr. W. Maier (Bonn). http://www.degs-studie.de/deutsch/ergebnisse/degs1/symposium-2012.html

"Synthetic Psychosis" by Novel Psychoactive Substances: A Psychopathological Understanding of a Clinical Case

9

G. Di Petta

I moved, and could not feel my limbs:
I was so light—almost
I thought that I had died in sleep,
And was a blessed ghost
S.T. Coleridge

9.1 The Postmodern Emergency of "Chemical Madness"

In clinical practice today, psychopathological syndromes are ever more frequently characterised by psychiatric symptoms and poly-abuse of new psychoactive substances (NPS[1]). This trend common among young people, with or without a precedent vulnerability, can strongly influence the clinical form of the consequent psychiatric disorders. With our current clinical and gnoseological criteria, we are not able to understand and diagnose these new and hitherto unknown NPS-induced clinical situations. What about prognosis? What is the role of the precedent vulnerability? What are the guidelines in order to treat these new patients, called "psychonauts"? Can we still consider delusions in these new patients as a primary disorder? What is, instead of the primary process, the psychopathological core of their symptomatological cluster? In order to respond to these questions, it is crucial to try to understand—through Jaspers (1913), Schneider (1959), Bonhoeffer (1917)

[1] An increasing number of unregulated websites are dedicated to the dissemination of novel psychoactive substances, which include plant-based compounds, synthetic derivatives of well-established drugs, as well as "designer medicines".

G. Di Petta (✉)
Santa Maria delle Grazie Hospital, Psychiatric Ward, Pozzuoli (Na), Italy

Mental Health Department, ASL Naples 2 North, Naples, Italy

Italian Society of Phenomenological Psychopathology, Florence, Italy
e-mail: gilbertodipetta@alice.it

G. Stanghellini, M. Aragona (eds.), *An Experiential Approach to Psychopathology*,
DOI 10.1007/978-3-319-29945-7_9

and de Clerambault's (1994) models of psychopathology, as well as through the work of Cargnello (1958), Morselli (1935) and Callieri (1956)[2]—how the developing psychosis bases itself on the addiction background.

The crucial questions about this discussion are:

1. To identify a particular state of consciousness, the twilight state, as the switch/crossing point between the toxicomanic experience and the psychotic experience
2. To identify the fundamental sensorial patterns severely compromised/modified by NPS abuse
3. To identify and to define a specific mental automatism as the elementary phenomenon and to consider the consequent thought disorder as only a secondary (interpretative) phenomenon

These patients are not as a rule completely involved in the psychotic process, like schizophrenic patients, and for the clinician to get in contact with their critical ego is crucial in order for him to be able to help them. For example, to recognise the border between the exogenic symptomatology and the personal reaction is a baseline of any subsequent treatment. A good knowledge of the traditional psychopathology and structure of endogenic psychoses along with solid background in clinical practice are necessary and useful in order to recognise the presence of "psychome", i.e. the chemical-induced extraneous (exogenic) part of their mind derived from the NPS abuse. Many of the symptoms present in these patients are only reactive to this extraneous-exogenic part of their mind. Their *sensorium* has been modified so much and for so long by NPS that, consequently, their state of consciousness has also been modified becoming what we call a twilight state. It is through this twilight modification that they arrive at a new delusional perspective based on the delusional interpretation of their now completely altered sensations. It is completely wrong to diagnose these patients as schizophrenic, as is frequently the case in clinical practice. Instead, the risk of these people being diagnosed as schizophrenic patients is elevated using DSM-V criteria. Consequently, the remaining lifetime treatment is strongly influenced by this misdiagnosis.

9.2 "We Are Living Strange Days"[3]: The Case G.

9.2.1 Attempted Suicide and Admission of the Patient to the Psychiatric Ward

On 29 March 2014, G., who was born in 1986, was admitted to a psychiatric ward and diagnosed as being in a suicidal state of "psychological and physical agitation", the patient having threatened to throw himself off the balcony at home. G.'s family

[2] See "Le psicosi sperimentali", Feltrinelli, Milano (1952) which contains the main reference works of Cargnello, Morselli and Callieri.

[3] These are the first words of the patient's transcript of his experiences prior to our first meeting.

belongs to the upper class, and he has a perfectly healthy elder sister, born in 1980. One of his father's cousins and one of his mother's cousins suffer from a not otherwise specified "psychosis and substance abuse". On 10 January 2013, G. had already thrown himself out of a window and fallen 10 m breaking several bones. As soon as he arrived at the hospital, G., who claims to be an expert online poker player, appeared to be agitated and very nervous. He resulted positive to the THC drug test. A neuroleptic therapy was adopted, and a few days later, G. appeared to be in a much calmer state and able to verbalise delusional magical, mystical ideas, delusions of greatness and persecution, full of bizarre details. He recounted that he had been living in a nightmare for several years. This started in 2006 when he was living alone and studying at university in Milan. Like a superhero he was left on his own to fight the forces of evil which controlled the world and had organised themselves into a System. *Chips* had been implanted into his body. He broke down crying because he had irredeemably lost a normal life and because he had never felt loved. He admitted to having used various drugs (cannabinoids, *Spice,*[4] cocaine, salvia divinorum,[5] ketamine, efedrina) since his adolescence. On 07 April 2014, at about 10 p.m., G. attempted to choke himself to death in the ward with a plastic bag. After being revived he was transferred to intensive therapy. The writing "Satan suck!" was found on the walls of his room. He is readmitted to the ward on 14 April 2014. He told stories of external powers that had induced him to try to take his own life. He feels himself to be an angel near to God fighting against Satan. During his recovery in the ward, he has practically no contact with the other patients. Sonorization of his thoughts occurs. After having had X-rays, he was afraid that the implanted *chips* had been discovered and consequently was about to be transformed into a cat. Because of this he had decided to die, since in doing so, he would be transformed into a demon. Demons are different from devils. His house is full of satanic symbols. The sect known as The Enlightened controls the world and has set up a strict hierarchy. He is the alien, the illegible (citing from the films Matrix and Scrabs). As the antipsychotic treatment continued, the patient's health improved and the influence of the drugs decreased. The *chips* remained embedded in his body but no longer obeyed commands from an external source. Their function was reduced to only identify his whereabouts. On 09 May 2014, G. was discharged and assigned to his family. However, he kept visiting the ward on a monthly basis to receive second-generation long-acting psychotic drugs and to attend weekly psychotherapy sessions.

---

[4] Smoking blend containing synthetic cannabinoids, e.g. JWH-018. It appeared in or around 2004; now some 140 plus different "spice" drugs are available.

[5] Aka: *Ska Pastora, Shepherdess' Herb, yerba de Maria, Magik Mint*; the active constituent is salvinorin A (k opioid receptor agonist) and an intense and short-acting hallucinogenic plant. Intake: smokable (pipe, bong). Historical use: shamanic inebriant (Mexico).

9.2.2 The Unbelievable World of G.

After the accident in 1980 in which all his mother's family were killed, G.'s family was replaced because new souls substitute traumatised souls in a continuous system of transmigration. G. has always been special. The kidnappings began when he was in his early teens, and he became aware of them when on waking up, he found his bed full of blood caused by the implantations of *chips* into his body. Sometimes he found himself naked or in a different position. They had even opened his skull and planted chips inside his brain. In 2013 when "the accident" happened, G. was thrown off the roof of his parent's house by external powers. In the days before this happened, strangers would come up to him; machines had been following him and he felt he was being controlled by something. He received lots of messages from various people. All his neighbours were standing on the pavement and watching him. A boy who belonged to the organisation had talked to the caretaker of the flats and he had bumped into him and he had gone away. Then he had received a strange phone call from a private number: "I am the cock that will fuck you!" He wrote a message to his father: "We'll meet in another life where we will both be kittens". If the attempted suicide had been successful, he would have kept his special powers which would have accompanied him into the afterlife. Before falling G. saw five red roses—the five lives which had been lost.[6] A red rose is the death of someone. The organisation was responsible for those deaths. Only divine intervention had saved him. From 2006 to 2009, he had been continuously using cannabis, cocaine and synthetic drugs. He diagnosed himself as suffering from Morgellons[7] syndrome in 2006. At that time he was subjected to a genic transposition. He was shocked to see a little metallic insect, like a *cyborg*, emerging from inside his body (an episode which he believes is mentioned in the Bible). He could feel or see other insects under his skin. The insect that came out of his body disappeared and entered a different dimension. Some of these insects had been implanted into his body when he had been kidnapped; others were produced by chemtrails which are in the sky and all around us. Apart from the little being that came out of his knee, there were lights under his skin, illuminated symbols, shining, like burns, which have left scars. Starting from these sensations, G. began the laborious task of trying to find out exactly what was happening to him. Through the Internet, which helped him identify some of his physical problems (itchiness and various illnesses), he came into contact with various people. He spent time surfing the net and visiting all the conspiracy sites. This is where he came into contact with the sect of the Enlightened—one of the most powerful sects that controls the capitalist world.

[6] The five members of his mother's family who died in the accident in 1980.

[7] Also known as Ekbom Syndrome; it is characterised by hallucinations containing dermatozoic, zooptic, zoomorphic and zooaptic elements (B. Callieri 2001); even while he is walking, the patient takes off his clothes or shoes or trousers to scratch himself. He also sees animals and insects in general not only on his body but also on other objects. Skin lesions caused by the persistent scratching are present on his limbs and over his torso, while imaginary spots on his face are squeezed (dermatozoic illusions).

9.2.3 "I Could Feel Them Moving...": The Rime of the Ancient Mariner[8]

I am 24 years old...as many of you already know, certain information about the truth of human nature has been deliberately kept secret for thousands of years up to today's disgusting scenario in which even the poorest countries are caught up in the failed capitalistic system which devours our souls on Earth...stealing away our lives...transforming our lives into something different from the original intentions of He who created us...The first important episode happened when I was about eight years old[9]...one morning I woke up and found myself covered in blood and lying in a different position from when I had fallen asleep...but I couldn't remember anything... apart from the tormented sensation of having spent an uneasy night full of nightmares... I thought I must have bashed my head against the wall and turned around in my sleep..,this happened more than once and they often took me away at that time ...when I was young I didn't know aliens existed[10]...I didn't realise immediately the connection between my strange nightmares and the scars (or the implantations) which I could feel during the day[11] ... there's a big scar on my right foot... I remember it happened overnight... this scar thing...but I just couldn't figure out where it had come from...sometimes I ask myself how it was possible for me to have ignored or misunderstood so much... and I don't know why...maybe it had been decided that I wouldn't think certain things, or maybe I just wasn't quick enough to understand from the very beginning what was going on...in the end they woke me up ... Morgellons... the unknown...everything began in 2006[12]... I didn't know what was going on... I started having various problems, especially during the night... I could feel something moving above my head...or more exactly I should say inside my head... I could feel them moving...

---

[8] Samuel Taylor Coleridge. These autobiographical sketches of the patient are taken from a longer account written by the patient in 2010 and handed to the author during the interviews with the patient after his stay in hospital (2014). In the text the patient is addressing the invisible people of the web.

[9] Evident hallucinations begin at this point in the patient's recollection of events.

[10] Hallucinations of the memory, or retrospective inclusive delusions, which allow for a global reinterpretation of one's own existence based on a new world of meaning.

[11] At this point the patient reveals the interpretative key to his own delusional construction, that is, the connection between the dermatozoic illusion (the animal inside the living body) and the implantations which refer to an external manoeuvring.

[12] The patient started using cannabis, cocaine and mescaline during a trip to Mexico when he was 17 years old. Referring to mescaline, which derives from the peyote cactus, Cargnello (1958) wrote "The most important thing to point out and to remember is that the whole hallucinatory state takes place without any serious repercussion on the person's awareness. In fact the peyotl eater remains almost perfectly aware of all that is happening to him, to the incredible phenomena in which he participates, all of which he is able to describe lucidly—this is possible because of an increased ability to be introspective and communicate. Furthermore, once the effect of the drug has worn off it leaves no unpleasant after-effects and doesn't lead to dependence. Those people who use peyotl hardly ever become addicts". The patient had already been suffering from the effects of continuous poly-abuse of NPS for 3 years when what he calls Morgellons syndrome first appeared.

they were very uncomfortable but I couldn't see them let alone try and catch them... I don't remember if I thought about trying to photograph them at that time... they tickled me and I felt itchy but I never found anything... I felt them moving inside my body... I could see my hair move[13]...eventually every part of my body became itchy... I haven't been able to prepare any exams since Morgellons began... I always felt as if there was something distracting me... I couldn't remember what I had been studying... although I was having enormous difficulty with my studies at university, it never crossed my mind to give up[14]... it would have been a complete failure. It all began with this ray of light that blocked me... then many things started to happen around me... which I can't remember and I couldn't remember... what I do remember is that I was terrified when these things started to happen... I suppose most of the kidnappings were carried out by the greys... though I don't remember ever having seen one... (I remember that aliens usually remove the memory of these kidnappings... I have never been hypnotised)[15] ... at that time I started to lose my hair and I realised that my hair had changed a lot[16] ... my new hair was much thinner, much lighter in colour and brighter... it looked transparent and artificial...it got electrified very quickly[17]... I've always been very particular about my hair so when I realised what had happened I was very upset.[18] I heard loud noises inside my body...they were being caused by something happening inside of me... something was changing me from the inside[19]... once I was sleeping with some friends and when I woke up, my back was full of round red marks that looked like insect bites... it was as if something from inside my body had been giving me mini-injections... I could often feel little pricks coming from under my skin.[20] As my "illness" progressed, things

[13] Seeing and feeling are the two senses which are very powerfully involved in the synostosis which fundamentally influenced the patient's delusions.

[14] The taking control of his internal space by this increasingly invasive complex reveals itself to be unstoppable.

[15] The logical sequence is the following—I discover "objects" that are inside my body; these things are clearly not part of me and are extraneous to my body; therefore they have been implanted into my body by someone, why have they done this? The reasoning follows the pattern—what is happening to me? Who is causing this to happen? And why?

[16] Dermatozoic illusion introduces the sense of believing in the presence of numerous extraneous objects present inside one's own body. Both the boundaries of the self and the physical barrier of skin have been violated. The next stage is the idea that one's own body is transformed since its very boundaries have been infringed upon. This violation has resulted in the patient no longer recognising his own body as such.

[17] These details indicate the passage from a human body to a post-human body or a "synthetic" body.

[18] See Fig. 9.2.

[19] The modified body is open to passivity and is easily influenced (*Gemachten*). Anything is possible inside this body.

[20] The dermatozoic illusion is increasingly losing the connotation of being the result of parasites and has become something even more disturbing—extraneous objects have entered the body and are modifying it. It is no longer a parasitic infestation.

started to get better and I began to show some interest in the world around me...in life...I was still very emotionally unstable, but my recovery had begun...slowly...Spring 2009...at that time Morgellons continued... then I felt something quite big[21] ...moving inside my body[22]...I could feel it in my veins...I could feel it moving quickly and once I managed to trap it as it was moving inside my arm and I was able to see its shape...but I thought I must have been spooking myself...but in August (I don't remember the exact day but it was near the end of the month), I was in my house in Naples...lying on the bed when suddenly I felt something like a very strong pinch... a slight pain that lasted only a couple of seconds... I turned round to see what had caused the pain and saw a little being... at first sight it looked like an insect... there was a scratch on my leg but no blood... it was about two centimetres' long, completely black and very thin...I noticed its tail... the tip of its tail was cone shaped and seemed to have blades[23] (or something similar) all over it... this mechanism on its tail couldn't have been there when it passed through my veins quickly; otherwise it would have destroyed them... I realised then and there that it must be something very highly technological[24]... its head was similar to a man's head...a stylized man which was definitely highly intelligent and reactive...in those handful of seconds during which I was looking at it, it moved madly around on top of my leg...it looked like it was tearing off pieces of my skin...that's when I picked it up because I was afraid it would go back into my leg again (I thought it had come out of my leg by mistake—but I was wrong!) and I was surprised that it wasn't at all slimy as I had expected...it was made of carbon fibre and it was so light I could hardly feel it in my hands...I don't remember noticing any wings, but I'm not sure how it managed to stay on my leg...maybe it did have wings, but I just couldn't see them...anyway it was well attached to my leg even if it didn't seem to have any legs...just when I let it go and put it on top of the bed to get a better look...just when I let go...it disappeared, dissolved in a cloud of smoke right in front of my eyes...I couldn't believe it...all of this only took about ten seconds.[25] And you can imagine how I felt...I nearly had a heart attack...I wandered around the room asking myself about what had just

[21] The symptoms appeared in 2006 and the transformation happened after 3 years of preparation in 2009.

[22] The size of the animated extraneous objects changes from microscopic to macroscopic.

[23] In patients suffering from Ekbom Syndrome caused by intoxication, the description of small lanceolate corpuscles is quite frequent. They are scales of skin uncovered through continuous scratching.

[24] At this point the patient's interpretation has advanced and the appearance of the extraneous body has changed from zoomorphic to anthropomorphic; the machine-like technology of the object is a clear psychotic indicator.

[25] The detailed description is not typical of schizophrenic hallucinations which tend to be filled with atmosphere and contain landscapes (Straus 1930). What we have here is, on the contrary, a very minutely detailed and geographical description of a disperception which now contains all the elements of the successive delusional interpretation. Rather than being a delusional perception, this is a delusional hallucination. The extremely perceptive vividness is maintained by the use of hallucinogenic substances (salvia divinorum, spice, efedrina, ketamine).

happened. . .I just couldn't believe it. . .another episode the next day. . .I felt something moving under my skin on my left side. . .I went over to the mirror and could see a flashing green light. . .you could make out a symbol under my skin. . . it was a triangle with two dark circles inside it. . .it remained bright for a few seconds. . .then a scar appeared in front of my eyes, something like the burn of a cigarette. I had ignored my nightmares for years. . .the visions. . .the premonitions. . .the implants. . .the scars. . .but this was a bit more difficult to ignore[26]. . .at first, though, I managed. . .I told a few close friends what had happened, but nobody believed me. . .but it was impossible not to think about what I was sure I had seen and above all I wanted answers. . .so I kept looking . . .something similar comes out of Neo's body in Matrix. . .then I came across crop circles that were very similar shapes, but it was what I found in the Bible that struck me most[27]. . .After what they had done, they must have continued working on me during the night. . .my daily routine changed. . .I remember going to bed for a week at 11 pm and getting up at 7 am which might seem normal to you, but since Morgellons began in 2006, I hadn't gone to bed before 5 am sometimes I even went to bed at midday. . .but during that week, I always went to bed at the same time[28]. . .I had just got to know Malanga, though not personally. . .he helped me find lots of implants. . .but his studies didn't answer all the questions I was asking myself. . .I was terrified by everything that had happened to me. . .and Malanga had convinced me that they wanted to steal my soul. . .so I was worried. . .it was only a lot later that I realised that that was not possible because we are our soul. . .I forgot to mention that since the Morgellons started, some marks "appeared" on my head. . . I've still got them. . .and I often found little scabs on my head. . .always in the same places. . .During the night between the 19th and 20th of September 2009, I was at my computer in my house in Milan when suddenly I "decided" to take the car and drive out to a place I didn't know. . .I didn't know what I was doing. . .I felt a strong attraction. . .it

[26] Here it is evident just how strong the need to interpret is and how over the years the intense evidence felt and perceived by the patient's senses of the modifications in progress have inevitably led to the necessity of finding a meaning to somehow explain them.

[27] Ap 9, 1-6. 9-11 "Then the fifth angel sounded: And I saw a star fallen from heaven to the earth. To him was given the key to the bottomless pit. [2] And he opened the bottomless pit, and smoke arose out of the pit like the smoke of a great furnace. So the sun and the air were darkened because of the smoke of the pit. [3] Then out of the smoke locusts came upon the earth. And to them was given power, as the scorpions of the earth have power. [4] They were commanded not to harm the grass of the earth, or any green thing, or any tree, but only those men who do not have the seal of God on their foreheads.[5] And they were not given *authority* to kill them, but to torment them *for* 5 months. Their torment *was* like the torment of a scorpion when it strikes a man. [6] In those days men will seek death and will not find it; they will desire to die, and death will flee from them.[9] And they had breastplates like breastplates of iron, and the sound of their wings *was* like the sound of chariots with many horses running into battle.[10] They had tails like scorpions, and there were stings in their tails. Their power *was* to hurt men 5 months. [11] And they had as king over them the angel of the bottomless pit, whose name in Hebrew *is* Abaddon, but in Greek he has the name Apollyon".

[28] The transformation of the patient into a completely controlled being is now complete. He is like a programmed robot now that the he feels sure that he is being controlled from inside.

wasn't an unpleasant feeling...they were leading me somewhere[29]...I continued driving towards Novara on a main road when I noticed a UFO right above me[30]...I slowed down (nearly causing an accident) and tried to take a picture of it...it had four lights and was the shape of a pentagon...I couldn't stop the car and I drove on...that's when I saw a ball of fire in the sky...it looked like a shooting star but only much brighter...shortly after that the same thing happened again...it lasted the same time (about 10 s but I didn't manage to take a picture)...that's when I noticed two balls of light...first one then another...we chased each other for about a minute ...after that I found myself on a lonely country road...I got out of the car carrying my digital camera. I wasn't afraid...there was an extremely bright ball of light...almost blinding...all I could see was white light...I couldn't make out any shape or distance from me...after this I felt a little disoriented but without missing time (the sensation that time has passed but you can't remember what happened)... the ball of light waved goodbye to me in a friendly way as it went away...with a ray of light...then I couldn't see it any more...I didn't realise at first that they had kidnapped me...but when I got back to the car I noticed that my eyes were strange...as if I had been hypnotised...and strange things happened to me in the following days...I'm sure they were all caused by my being kidnapped...everywhere I went I noticed that my presence always seemed to influence what was happening around me...it wasn't a very nice feeling...at that time I still knew nothing about aliens though that thing had come out of my body and I was a little afraid about it all...I'll tell you what happened...I was in a field...I could hear a lot of noises around me...coming towards me...in my car...I could hear the same noises coming out of the engine, metal parts moving...the same thing at home...things that dropped to the ground...the next day I was walking past a pile of dry leaves...there was no wind at all, but the leaves started to fly up and whirl around my legs...I don't know if it's all something to do with radiation I'm sure they are beings which are very different from us...I don't think they have a body...maybe it's lux? It might be...(...). One evening while I was sleeping, I could see myself being sucked up to the ceiling by a ray of green light...the next day I thought I had been dreaming...but I remembered what had happened...it had been a very physical sensation...I don't understand how it works...sometimes I can still remember something about what had happened...who knows?...maybe they leave me those memories on purpose...During the following months, I started to notice some changes inside

[29] The external interference is the cause of the three successive suicide attempts. G. has lost control of himself and is at the mercy of his enemy who can do whatever he wants with him. G. at times identifies himself in this enemy, while at other times, he fights against it. However, he is no longer able to control his own actions. Even when he fights against the system perceived as an enemy, he is only acting in consequence to external forces.

[30] The appearance of UFOs underlines the atmospherisation of the hallucinations in which the extraneousness expands from the intrapersonal and intracorporeal space towards an immediately pericorporeal and peripersonal space and ultimately towards an extracorporeal and extrapersonal space.

of me. . .I was able to feel what other people were feeling, in their hearts. . .I began to really understand people and the world. . .sometimes negative vibrations would block me. . .at the same time, I started to notice things that I'd never seen before. . .our world was starting to appear less solid than before. . .furniture began to move from side to side. . .the walls, too. . .sometimes I felt myself swaying. . .and I saw orb UFO more and more. . .I started to get to know my new body. . .the world. . .the universe. . .I started reading a lot and studying. . .more than I ever had done before. . .for sure more interesting and useful things. I began to meditate. . .and it was around this time that I started going in to trances very easily. . .I just shut my eyes and let myself go. One day I woke up at 4 pm, but I didn't want to get up. . .there was no reason for me to get up. . .I felt emotionally exhausted. . .suddenly I heard quite a loud noise in my head. . .something changed after that noise. . .and I could feel my body was as light as a feather. . .and I began to levitate above the bed with the quilt still covering me. . .I could just make out a blue light but I don't know where it was coming from. . .I don't know if I caused it, but the blue light made me think something else was causing this to happen to me. . .I stayed suspended in the air for about ten seconds and I was a bit afraid of what was happening to me. . .but if I think about it now, I remember it was quite a nice experience. . .I was a little afraid of hurting myself when I came down but I didn't. . .I stayed horizontal and the blue light was like that colour over there. At that time a strange thing happened to me that has never happened again—at least I don't think it has. I was sleeping when something woke me up. . .I opened my eyes but I couldn't see anything. . .I could feel something heavy on my chest. . .I felt that there was someone right in front of me, but I wasn't afraid. . .though I could feel that the person in front of me was nervous. . .after a couple of seconds, I heard a loud click. . .and I found myself tied to something. . .I was no longer in my bed but somewhere else. . .it was as if I was flying through space. . .I could see lots of instructions being given. . .in fact I was giving those instructions; I was piloting the spaceship. . .I was attached to it and it was only for one person. . .I can't remember much else, but I'm sure it was real. . .when I woke up the next day, I couldn't remember anything at all. Everything they did to me changed me completely. . .I discovered that I was living in a magical and mysterious world. . .the TV disturbed me. . .this had happened before but not like this. . .all TVs emit a signal that disturb the pineal gland. . .I can feel it when my next-door neighbours turn their television on (I'm proud of the fact that I don't have one) and it doesn't make any difference if the sound is turned down. . .a noise comes into my head. . .it's not very loud, but it's acute and doesn't go away[31]. . . mobile phones disturb me, too. . .they give me a headache so I've had to stop using them. . .I have one only for emergencies. . .it's switched off. My Internet connection is always being interrupted; I just can't keep it connected. . .it doesn't matter where I am . . .(. . ..). It took me a long time to get used to a new function of my body. . .some substances. . . when I breathe, drink, eat, smoke,. . .my body doesn't want to, can't keep it in. . .it rejects them. . .I wasn't used

[31] The perceptive-sensorial participation is particularly powerful.

to spitting...I never used to...I would just swallow...I slowly realised that there was something wrong inside my body...it was as if there was a decomposing corpse inside my body...I didn't understand...then my body helped me to understand what was going on...for a few successive nights, I woke up all wet...this liquid was coming out of my mouth...I can't tell you what kind of liquid it was, but I'm sure it was something that was bad for me and my body was getting rid of it...I haven't had this liquid properly analysed but I'm sure it's something very heavy[32]...heavier than water...leaving it to dry, I noticed it left a yellowish mark...A lot of people find this disgusting...I just want to say that I find it disgusting just thinking that the stuff I spit out they keep inside their bodies...because I see what I spit out every time I eat or have a cigarette (I've given up smoking now)...or even just when you breathe...and I'm happy it doesn't stay inside me...(...). The itchiness, I discovered, was caused by little animals which I managed to photograph...the itchiness disappeared and so did the insects but fibres still come out of my body[33]...these fibres are of different colours...they look artificial...white, red and blue...they haven't caused any problems...of course at first, it wasn't very pleasant...the Bible says the same thing...it says that smoke blocked out the light of the sun and the atmosphere...Chemtrails from the locusts of the apocalypse...apocalypse means revelation and it also tells us how long it will stay in men (5 months) and it explains what they're for...talking about the seal of God on your forehead (the third eye)...it mentions men being tormented by stings...men who implore death...all these words apply to me too exactly just to be a coincidence...the other theories about what the locusts of the apocalypse really are very unconvincing...I hope it's clear to anyone reading that Morgellons isn't a disease (and if it's not clear yet, the other parts will convince you)...I don't want to persuade you that Morgellons is good...or the aliens are good...but this is what happened to me...I think it's a complicated process that they have carried out to help us evolve...now there are a few things that worry me about Morgellons...about how it controls the mind...and not only...but for now it's just a supposition, whereas the fact remains that I have a completely different body now which is much better than it was before...I have a lot of other things to say and I'll publish them because there is so much incorrect information going about...I have known about these things for a while now...I don't think I'm wrong...I haven't spoken about it up to now because I thought the truth would have come out eventually...Carlo Saito's indigo-crystal transition explains the whole process very well...I recommend you take a look at it...it's interesting even if I think it's kind of taking the piss...because it never once mentions aliens or nanotechnology...as being responsible for these changes...I don't understand why there is so much interest in chemtrails and so little interest in Morgellons since it is the only reason they produce chemtrails...I don't understand why I seem

[32] Here the sense of corporeal transformation is quite obvious.

[33] The transformation from organic to inorganic is part of the patient becoming psychotic.

to be the only person who's got Morgellons. . .when there are chemtrails all over the world. . .are you sure you don't have it? Someone in your family? Your children?

9.2.4 Psychopathological Understanding

The psychopathological elements of this case suggest that the patient is suffering from "synthetic psychosis" (a different diagnosis from schizophrenic psychosis). This conclusion is based on the following psychopathogenic elements:

1. The first elements that are affected in the patient are all sensorial and perceptive, thus altering his field of awareness. This is a direct result of patient G.'s prolonged use (since 2003) of hallucinogenic, dissociative and stimulating drugs. G. began to feel itchiness, skin irritation, pain and burning sensations in various parts of his body which he self-diagnosed as being caused by parasites after having read about Morgellons disease on the Internet.[34] The discovery of Morgellons enforced G.'s belief in the scientific existence of patients suffering from the parasitosis of microorganisms and delusional skin parasitosis. The sensations that G. feels are so strong that, on the one hand, they completely modify his coenesthesis, while on the other hand, they give way to the eruption outwards from within of something extraneous and repugnant. In this case we can see how parasitosis hides or camouflages a corporeal transformation which after an appropriately lengthy incubation time "gives birth" to the little carbon fibre being which seems to be G.'s synthetic alter ego, and which, when it disappears, seems to take with it G.'s very human nature. This transformative passage is supported by Beringer's so-called Verbindungen[35]—that is, the tactile-visual synaesthesia which Callieri (2001) has examined in great detail. Revisiting the sequence of events in slow motion, G., tormented by itches, begins to scratch himself, to touch himself persistently, to film himself and to take pictures (see Figs. 9.1 and 9.2). What is happening is the patient's first perception of the interface between the body and the rest of the world, the dermic-hypodermic layer or stratum, the perception of extraneous little bodies,

[34] It is well known that this syndrome is frequently encountered in drug-addicted patients ("tactile hallucinations caused by external drugs: alcohol, cocaine, sympathetic-mimetic amines", Callieri 2001) and, because of this, is considered to be of organic nature. Bruno Callieri in his memorable paper "L'animale nel vissuto corporeo", published in "Quanto vince l'ombra: problemi di psicopatologia clinica" (1 ed. 1980, La Città Nuova, Roma; 2 ed. 2001, Ediz. Univ. Romane, Roma), examines in great detail Ekbom Syndrome and dermatozoic delirium. Callieri had already written on this subject in 1958 ("Considerazioni su un caso di deliroide dermatozoico", Il Lavoro Neuropsichiatrico, 22) and later with G. Vella in 1960 ("L'esperienza tattile nel deliroide dermatozoico, Il Lavoro Neuropsichiatrico, 27) considering the delusional formation absolutely "secondary" and at this point explaining the meaning of the term delusion. Callieri was interested in what he called the "plurivoiced perceptiveness", or the "haptic and optic synaesthesis" (the experience of the I feel-I see).

[35] K. Beringer, Der Mascalinrausch, Springer, Berlin, 1927.

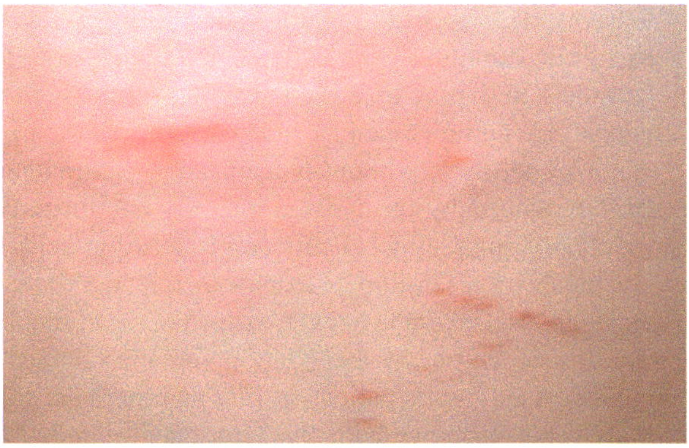

Fig. 9.1 Morgellons disease. This picture of the patient's skin was taken by himself. G. being convinced that his skin was infested with parasites

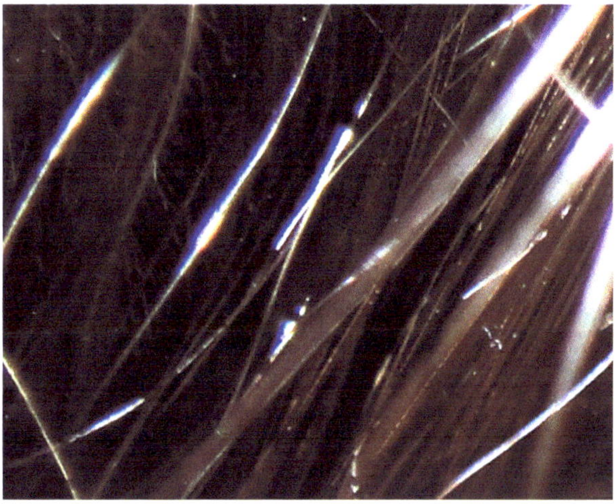

Fig. 9.2 Morgellons disease. This picture of the patient's hair was taken by himself. G. being convinced that his hair was infested with parasites

which constitute the violation of a *self-not self*-barrier, the overcoming of a frontline. At first G. is convinced the cause is insects or parasites. This induces him to find out more, and since he is an expert navigator on Internet, he soon comes across Morgellons syndrome, as it is known in America, or Ekbom syndrome, as it is known in Europe. G. has been using drugs since he was a young teenager. Not only has he been regularly taking synthetic cannabinoids (Spice) and alcohol, but he has tried cocaine, efedrina, ketamine and salvia divinorum. The combination of sensorial irritation and crepuscular awareness causes G.'s internal experience to become a stable "psychoma". Currently for psychoma we intend a series of disorders of the patient's coenesthesis which appear both in de Clerambault's model of mental automatism and in the base symptoms of Huber and Gross. "We should, first of all, make it clear that every different psychotomimetic drug affects people in a different way, having its own particular psychopathological picture and "physiognomy"—the different early symptoms, the various specific effects and the different way each drug generally behaves. This specific picture—specific for every particular psychotomimetic exogenic stimulus—was called "psychoma" by Hellpach. Psychoma, or the "absolute new psychopathological element" which the substance causes in the person it is administered to, independently of their pathoplastic disposition. We can assume, then, without fear of being contradicted, that psychomas derived from/produced by the most commonly administered substances in pharmaco-psychiatry (mescaline, diethylamide lysergic acid, psilocybin, adrenochrome) are much more similar to each other than they can be similar to any other endogenous psychoma or even exogen of the clinical practice" (Cargnello 1958).

2. The insistence on the localization somatic polycentric, including the scalp, is characterised by the patient feeling that there are foreign bodies inside his own body. This, together with the subsequent detailed observations, leads G. to a basic experience, in which he observes a strange little being (which G. calls a "cyborg") coming out of his knee. Apparently it is not an organic parasite. It is an electronic gadget, a receptor and a transmitter, clearly the result of advanced nanotechnology, which has put his body online. At this point we can interpret a sort of atmospherisation of the event (the incorporation of an external object, its coming out into the world). This is possible thanks to intense crepuscular states of conscience. It is at this stage that a range of phenomena—subcontinuity as well as continuity—of mental, ideo-verbal, sensorial and perceptive and motorio automatisms set in, which leads to delusional state and which in turn develops into reseau, destroying G.'s experience and causing his repeated attempts at suicide or rather putting G.'s newly transformed mental state in to a position which is incompatible with life.
3. G. is controlled and influenced by an articulated system of persecution, the sect of the Enlightened, who want to dominate the world sub-satanic specie. G. sees UFOs. He is even able at times to travel through space thanks to his mobile phone. His phone contained maps that allowed him to be transported immediately all over the world (substances induced space displacement). G.'s relation with the persecutory system is completely embodied, since G. is physically connected to the system through the microchips implanted under his skin. And even if this means that he is manoeuvred and monitored by the system, he is also able at the same time to remain to some extent against the system. G.'s delirious reconstruction (or reinterpretation or *nachtraglichkeit*) of all his previous life predates the presumed episodes of being kidnapped by aliens to his childhood. G. had remained for years a prisoner of time travelling, though in a more or less stable time, crystallised into a continuous, eternal instant—this is a typical example of the addicts' perception of time. Drug addiction is a severe Time disorder, which leads to a profound crisis in the basic structure of subjectivity, selfhood and one's sense of reality. Without time it is impossible to feel oneself at home in the world. A moment or an instant perceived by someone under the effect of drugs is completely different from the everyday present of lucid consciousness. "As soon as the drug addict achieves a moment of pleasure this moment suddenly vanishes and he is condemned to impulsive repetition. The addict is trapped in this repetition with no chance of moving forward" (von

Gebsattel 1954). Drug abuse is a trip in a time machine. G., under the influence of drugs, cannot decide when or where to stop or when or where to go. He loses the control of time during the chemical trip. He becomes unable to stop this chemical roller coaster. G. becomes a passenger in this time machine, a prisoner of a ride which is out of his or anyone else's control (internal or external), like a child alone and left to himself in the fairground rides. Being here and now but being separated from the past and the future, G. loses the passing of Time, becoming a mere bystander (onlooker) who cannot take part in the passing of Time because he has been removed. G. has lost the ability of anticipating Time.

4. G. is engaged in his own personal fight. He is fragile and at the same time a special superhero, a half divine angel that gets his power from knowing the phenomena in play and from his having been chosen as a hostage of the system. Bit by bit he is separated from his ordinary daily existence and he sets out to find out the truth, accompanied by the continual use of drugs. He tries to inform his parents of the tragic truth of his discovery, but they don't appreciate its importance. It is only on the web that he finds some answers to his questions, and after eliminating all the people who think he's mad, the answers he finds here become an important part of his understanding of the new world order.
5. In December 2012 G. returns to Naples to attend his uncle's funeral, and it is on this occasion that he is induced to commit suicide (as he himself later explained) because he feels as if he is caught in a vice that is closing tightly around him. The only way to remain eternal and to keep his superpowers is to kill himself, thus killing the derivation of the system of evil that has so perniciously taken control of him from inside his body. The development of this delirious system shuts out everything else, and G. eventually arrives at abolishing death itself and as a consequence not fearing death; on the contrary he even courts death seeing it as an experience denied to common mortals. In his case he believes that it gives him the chance to finally become a bodiless soul.

9.2.5 G.'s Present State: A Fallen Angel

The following information is based on a period of just over a year during which the patient was treated as an outpatient after he was dismissed from the hospital. As well as having been given a phial of paliperidone (second-generation long-acting antipsychotic, 150 mg once a month, intramuscular), he was obliged to visit the hospital as an outpatient once a week. He was always punctual and well dressed for the weekly appointments and seemed to have orientated himself. He passed the admission test to the Faculty of Biology in September 2014, thus turning his back on Business Studies which seems to have been more his father's wish than any real interest in the subject. On the other hand Biology and Chemistry are more in line with G.'s need to understand and explain the details of the metamorphosis that he has undergone—within the world's chemical-physical framework. The confidential nature of our relationship is a result of the many nights we spent together when I was working the night shift and he was a patient in my ward. I was the psychiatrist who wanted to find out more about his personal experience beyond the mere diagnosis of psychosis and the administration of a cure. During our regular meetings, he hands me a memory stick which contains some autobiographical sketches and dozens of enlarged photographs of his scalp and films of his limbs. His special powers have been taken away from him following what he calls "the incident"—the attempted suicide in 2013. He has been put inside a machine that takes his powers, and his soul, away. He had been immortal when he still had his special powers; nevertheless he is happy to have experienced such a unique experience that ordinary people have never felt, even if people who have these special powers are bound together with the devil. Now his life has lost its unique potential. He feels himself to be ill-suited and unfit for this everyday common sense world which no longer interests him. He is a survivor and a veteran, who has experienced things that no one else can understand. He often dreams of huge empty ships in the middle of the sea. He often feels awkward and out of place and constantly dreams about the System that has tried to kill him, that controls him, and that keeps him prisoner. His own personal war is not over yet. However, the System reveals some anomalies. Even if he feels that he is now sitting on the sideline, he still has dreams about being a superhero saving the world in the struggle between good and evil. All in all he is nostalgic about the world which has so terrorised him. It is not easy to keep G. anchored to reality and the common sense of ordinary life. He keeps on playing online poker with mixed results; he sometimes wins and sometimes loses up to hundreds of euros. He also continues to use cannabinoids on a daily basis. His therapy continues with the administration of a second-generation long-acting antipsychotic (LAI-II G). He is not able to examine critically the hallucinatory events he has experienced and is convinced that they represent the proof that all that has happened to him really did happen.

9.3 The "Addicted" Consciousness: The Crossing Twilight

For psychiatry the psychopathology of consciousness has always represented a sort of final frontier. From Janet's studies on the splitting of consciousness to Ey's studies on the de-structuring of the field of consciousness, there is no psychiatric disorder which cannot be collocated on the ground of consciousness. According to Jaspers (1913), the ego-consciousness can be understood in four different ways: (1) the sense of activity, (2) the sense of uniqueness, (3) the sense of identity and (4) the sense of oneself. It is very clear how subjective consciousness here limits the field of experience of one's being-at-the-world-with-others, the dramatic change of which indicates the beginning of psychosis. The assessment of a state of consciousness is fundamental when the psychopathologist is face to face with addicts under the effect of drugs. In this kind of encounter, the clinician perceives the boundaries between the areas of consciousness where there is attunement and the areas of consciousness where there is no attunement (i.e. psychoma).

For example, if we assume that depersonalisation, derealisation and dissociation are global experiences of the formal de-structuring of the field of consciousness and not simple symptoms, we can find them also in a broad spectrum of psychiatric disorders, from schizophrenia to panic attacks, from phobia to dissociation, from post-traumatic stress disorder to somatic disorder and from addiction to withdrawal. The twilight state of consciousness is the common background of all these psychopathological dimensions. What do the addicts mean when they say: "I am high"? What is the psychopathological meaning of this state of consciousness (*highness*) which for them represents a sort of steady state of daily living existence? Probably the experience of *highness* is an equivalent of a *twilight state* of consciousness (*Zwielicht-Daemmerung-zustand*). This modification of the state of consciousness is well represented by many current expressions: numbness, clouding and drowsiness. In the classic description of Jaspers (1913) and Schneider (1959), a *twilight state* of consciousness is a restriction of the field of consciousness. In the *twilight state* of consciousness, there is no dramatic alteration of arousal. The field of consciousness, furthermore, can still spread itself (Fig. 9.3). The *twilight state* of consciousness is a sort of threshold between the light of reality and the shadow of dream and psychosis. The *twilight state* of consciousness promotes illusions, delusions, visual or auditory hallucinations: the patient may respond to them with irrational behaviour. The person may be unaware of the surroundings at the time of the experience and have no memory of it later, except perhaps to recall a related dream. Depersonalisation and derealisation are normal experiences in the *twilight state* of consciousness, in which it is easier that Klosterkotter's transitional phenomena take place, from basic symptoms towards final phenomena. NPS addicts experience this vulnerable condition everyday, every month and every year, over a prolonged period of time. The perception of reality in addicts is discontinuous and incomplete and this *twilight state* becomes a sort of normal way of life. Their state of consciousness is like a display that is continuously turned on and off; short flashes appear and disappear. Being instable the *twilight state* becomes a transitional state, like a *funnel*. When the *funnel* is upside down, the addicts lose touch with reality and fall into delusions (Fig. 9.3).

At this point we come to the following conclusions:

1. Consciousness is a field with formal and fundamental characteristics, and there is no psychiatric disorder which doesn't find its background in modification and de-structuring of consciousness.
2. The causes of disease which produce the modification of the ordinary state of consciousness, especially substances, strongly influence the development of psychiatric disorder, touching many aspects of psychopathological vulnerability.

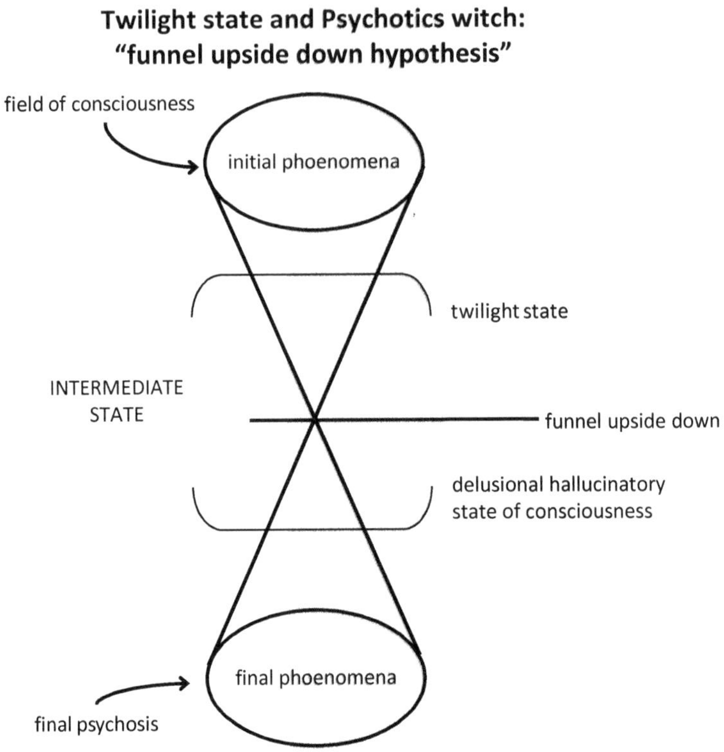

Fig. 9.3 This figure shows how the initial field of consciousness reduces itself until the crossing point, after which the field of consciousness is inside out and instead of looking out is polarised on psychotic phenomena

3. The twilight modification of consciousness NPS induced is the principal gate for the link between the sensorial modifications and the delusional interpretation.

9.4 The Synthetic Psychosis of G. or the "Alice in Wonderland" Syndrome

Seeing something out of the ordinary visual field; seeing an unreal (inexistent) landscape, a bizarre environment and geometric forms; and seeing bi-dimensional and flat images added to the ordinary visual field: all these are common visual perceptions induced by hallucinogenic drugs. It is not easy even for a general psychiatrist, even one well versed in all things medical and psychopathological, to deal with these emerging (chemical) hallucinatory-delusional patterns. The diffusion of NPS in young people is responsible for a new pattern of mental disorders induced by substances: chemical psychosis, which can be also called "synthetic psychosis", a sort of "Alice in Wonderland syndrome".[36] This is the paradigmatic speech of Stefano—"I have to say that I have been hearing voices ever since I was a young child though I only started to have visions after the breakdown I had when I was twenty. I remember the first time I heard voices. I was two or three years old and I was sitting in my high-chair and I could hear them talking to each other but I couldn't understand what they were saying. Then the voices noticed that someone was listening to them. Now I can say that those voices already knew the meaning of everything that has happened to me since then. When I was four years old I was in the front yard of my house and I heard the female voice that I already knew and then three aliens came out of a hole in the ground and I walked towards them and I was ready to throw myself into their arms not knowing that they were the incarnation of evil. As I have already said I was four when the aliens took me with them on a journey into another reality controlled by a different logic from ours. I was there for an indefinite time which might have been all of eternity, though compared to time on Earth it was just a moment". Stefano has retrospectively modified what he remembers to such a degree that he has built up an authentic hallucination of memory on which he has built up the story of his life. Surprisingly, however, his relation with everyday reality has not been adversely affected, and even if he lives a quiet and retiring life, he has never had to undergo any hospital treatment. The typical deterioration common to many forms of schizophrenic psychosis is altogether absent. In spite of the evidently severe hallucinatory dimension causing delusional interpretations, there is no evidence that shows NPS is able to induce thought directly. However, NPS severely compromises the reality testing. How are criticism and judgment really effective in the reality testing? NPS probably compromises human *sensorial* knowledge, in order to explain that the classic consciousness philosophy, based on Descartes' and Kant's conception, is no longer a good model for NPS-induced synthetic psychosis.[37]

"The man thinks, not the brain" was the conclusion of E. Straus (1891–1975), the author of "The Sense of the Senses" (1930), in which sensorial consciousness is common to animals and human beings. From the perspective of these authors, the world of life is embodied, there is a logic of living, we can find an a priori structure of feeling, there is a spatial-temporal horizon of feeling, the sensorial experience is active and cognitive and the *pathic* dimension of existence has a communicative structure. In Straus's theory (1930) *seeing* is the immediate consciousness of spatial distance. It is a sort of temporal scanner, and *touching* is the nearness receptor.

[36] The "Alice in Wonderland Syndrome" was described by Todd, Lippman in migraine and epilepsy, and is characterised by morphological fluctuation, like metamorphopsia, micropsia, macropsia, temporal distortion, temporo-occipital lesion and parieto-occipital lesion.

[37] The idea of the Gestalt's cycle (*Gestaltkreis*) by Victor Von Weizsacker (1886–1957), instead, is the better model in order to understand NPS psychosis. The cycle "perception-movement" is probably the first and the principal target of NPS. H. Plessner (1892–1985) and M. Merlaeau-Ponty (1908–1961) give a strong contribution to identify and to define this perception/sensation area. Also J. Zutt (1893–1980) wrote about this aesthetic field of lived experience (*Das aesthaetisches Erlebnisbereich*).

Aesthesiology ("Theory of Feeling") by Straus allows us to understand that the approach to reality is based on and guaranteed not by criticism and judgment but by preverbal, pre-reflexive ground and that the perception-movement cycle is crucial in the structure of common sense. As a consequence, drastic modifications of perception-movement cycle (von Weizsaecker 1968), caused by NPS, can influence (though only in a secondary way) both criticism and judgment. Therefore chemical delusions are not primary, but secondary to strong modifications of relationship with reality, based on perception-movement distortion induced by NPS. Various typical psychopathological signs of schizophrenic syndromes are unknown in these synthetic psychotic syndromes (e.g. the crisis of "me-ness" and the invasion of "relationships that concern me" (Schneider 1959), the crisis of "basic trust" (Husserl 1907), perplexity (Callieri 1997), the "exclusion of casuality" (Berner 1981), the "loss of overall perspective" (Conrad 1958)). Where, then, are the classic psychopathological signs, like delusional atmosphere or delusional perception, in these postmodern *chemical* patients? How is countertransference or attunement possible in these postmodern psychonauts? Is it still important to understand life history versus the hallucinogenic power of the "plants of God"?[38] In chemical delusions, for example, we do not have:

1. Delusional atmosphere
2. Delusional perception
3. Primary delusions

The NPS are not really able to induce thought disorders. Chemical delusion of G. is characterised by *confirmation* and *interpretation*, not by *revelation*, and by fantastic contents. NPS delusions are like paraphrenic delusions,[39] with a feeling of unreality while at the same time maintaining the ability to analyse this feeling (Callieri 1962). On these differential signs, it is possible to set a precise distinction between chemical delusions secondary to NPS sensorial modification and primary delusions of classic endogenic psychosis. The core gestalt of these contemporary psychonauts' psychosis is far from the classic naïve psychotic patients. For the

[38] These are often sold as something else, e.g. mystical incenses, plant chemicals and bath salts and herbal smoking blend (synthetic cannabinoids, Spice drugs, mephedrone).

[39] Illusions, as well as, acoustic, olfactory, gustative and coenesthetic hallucinations, and chronic delusion in particular—where imagination and fantasy lead to bizarre and unrealistic situations—are all fundamental. Another common case is the feeling of being persecuted by strange electronic machines. Other cases include patients who believed they were without vital organs, responsible for "the end of the world", the son of famous historical figures, protagonists of epic events and in communication with aliens. In differential diagnosis with schizophrenia, the personality cohesion and the affective participation in these cases are not completely damaged and social skills and personal autonomy are well maintained. The patient lives two lives at the same time (one real and another imaginary and delusional), which, however, do not completely compromise his behaviour and his relation with reality.

acute syndromes, the exogenic psychosis (Bonhoeffer 1868–1948)[40] is still a good model. Many acute clinical conditions in these "chemical patients" are brain organic syndromes (*Durchsgangsyndromen*). After acute symptomatology a differential diagnosis is often possible between naïve patients and chemical patients. De Clerambault's concept of delusion,[41] based on the mental automatism syndrome,[42] is a very good model in order to understand this synthetic psychosis. In this atypical psychosis, a part of the patient's ego remains a critical spectator of his or her own pathology (a spectator of the internal/extraneous psychoma, Cargnello et al. 1962). The ego goes mad in its desperate attempt to "synthesise" (to repair) the profound wound opened by dissociative drugs,[43] and this causes the "psycho-motrice attitude" that is the *primum movens* of delirium (Morselli 1935).

---

[40] Toxic psychosis, traumatic psychosis, brain disease psychosis, delirium, progressive paralysis and withdrawal psychosis: these are the exogenic psychosis described by Bonhoeffer in 1914.

[41] G. de Clerambault was the Director of the Special Infirmary for the Insane (prefecture de police, Paris, 1905). He described a lot of patients intoxicated by absinthe, clorhalius hidratus, ether, hashish and alcohol.

[42] The mechanisms generated by psychosis hark back to automatism, or rather the triad of mental, sensitive and motorial automatisms. Among the phenomena that characterise automatism, which when taken together can be considered as being a little mental automatism, are verbal phenomena, word games, nonsense, foolish aspirations and lack of abstract thought. On top of this, we have to add the effects of reactive delirium and the consequences of sensitive automatism which represent the initial tribulations brought on by chronic hallucinatory psychosis. The construction represents an attempt to interpret the sensorial phenomena and is based on (a) the affective form of the patient, which we can sum up as pessimism, optimism or hostility; (b) the intellectual form, for example, an interpretive or imaginary tendency; and (c) on the concordance between the hallucinatory tendency on one hand and the affective-intellectual dispositions on the other. The ideo-verbal type of automatism is characterised by its anideic form (syllable games), ideo-verbal phenomena (thought echo) and negative phenomena (no longer being able to think), all of which have a mechanical origin. This division in which the patient finds himself has been described by De Clerambault with the metaphor of the two personalities where the second one receives sensorial data and the first one elaborates the data coherently with its own intellect and its own character: every psychosis is like a kind of double or two-piece delirium in which the psychisms are united in the same brain and where one dominates the other because it is more inventive and persistent, dominating it with mechanically derived laws. He goes as far to say that it isn't the persecutory idea that creates the hallucinations, but, on the contrary, the hallucinations that create the very idea of persecution.

[43] Five years previously, in 1930, the Rivista Sperimentale di Freniatria published Morelli's "*Sulla dissociazione mentale*" better known as "Il Caso Elena" where he affirms that even if nothing specific can be argued about the nature of the dysfunction, we can venture to say that any suspicion that Elena's sensorial motility, apart from being damaged indirectly by dissociation and by intrapsychic reactions, represents very real disorder caused by an unknown organic "process". See the article in Rivista Sperimentale di Freniatria, vol. CXXXV, N. 3, 2011, Franco Angeli Editore, Milano.

9.5 "Synthetic Psychosis" Versus "Classic" Schizophrenia: The Differential Diagnosis (Fig. 9.3)

The conventional diagnosis of G. on dismissal from the psychiatry ward was "paranoid schizophrenia", because this satisfied the diagnostic criteria of DSM-V (2014). The patient's experience of being controlled, being influenced, along with the apparently bizarre nature of his behaviour and his ideas has apparently convinced the doctors to diagnose schizophrenia:

1. G. maintained an adequate behaviour, good logic, personal autonomy and the ability to communicate even during the most intense moments of his symptomatology, for example, those immediately before he attempted to commit suicide.
2. G. suffered the long prodromal phase when he was living alone in Milan which meant he did not receive any help from his family at that time. Nevertheless he never looked for psychiatric help, he never took any medicine and he was able to clearly observe his own symptoms distonically.
3. The hallucinations began when he had already been taking drugs for a long time and have always been so vivid that they were immediately accepted and encouraged him to try and find an explanation for them. G.'s delusion is not born as a revelation (Conrad 1958); rather it is a confirmation based on the consequent interpretation of very strong sensorial events. "We could say that the psychosensorial disorders dominate the psychoma, so that often the substances in discorso are defined hallucinogenic and classified among the "fantastic" just for this fundamental action of theirs. Talking about frequency and number, psychosensorial disorders of the exogenic (toxic) psychosis are incredibly more frequent (and it should be remembered) than endogenic psychosis. But that is not all. Putting aside the quantitative criteria, in drug-induced psychosis, it is the visual field that is the most frequently affected by hallucinations and sound the least; in endogenic psychosis and especially schizophrenia, visual psychosensorial disorders are much less frequent, whereas sound disorders are more frequent. Furthermore psychosensorial disorders, in the case of experimental psychosis, are more often very close to/similar to hallucinations (a strong sensorialisation of the lived experience, a net objectivisation of space, an awareness of the pathology, etc.); on the contrary in schizophrenia, they are very similar to/close to pseudo-hallucinations, another critical observation that is difficult to refute" (Cargnello 1958). Callieri (2001) about Ekbom syndrome (toxic substances induced) wrote "… from a phenomenological point of view the abnormal tactile experiences felt by schizophrenics reveal something different from analogous experiences in patients suffering external (exogenic) intoxication…The tactile hallucinations of the schizophrenic are something more complex, more organised and much more integrated into that particular modality of existence. In other words the schizophrenic's tactile hallucinations are very closely related, both formally and thematically, to the primary psychotic process, precisely in Jaspers' sense".

4. After being released from hospital and in the following months, G. showed no sign of his intelligence being in any way impaired—in fact he managed to pass the entrance test to the faculty of Biology. His delusional interpretations become weaker, but the overall picture remains the same since it is supported by the subjective certainty afforded by his senses: foreign bodies ("the carbon-fibre cyborg") were inside his own body and they had been put there after he had been kidnapped. The fibre-carbon cyborg that emerged during a hallucination from his own body with receiver/transmitter was the element of contact between the animal in the lived body and the persecutory System.
5. G. describes what happened to him extremely accurately and ego distonica, outlining a condition of psychosis viewed from the point of view of a spectator. This is contrary to what happens in patients with schizophrenia where the "I" narrator very often founders along with the delirium and when it does re-emerge is profoundly defective. "In induced psychosis the intoxicated patient passes through very many and quite extraordinary psychopathological experiences which he identifies as happening inside him, but with which he does not usually identify himself. The patient takes part in these experiences (at times amused, amazed surprised, astonished, even terrified, etc.) preserving almost intact his own deeper self to the extent that he is induced to bear witness to those events as if he were separate from them" (Cargnello 1958).
6. The tone in which G. recounts the incredible events that he has witnessed is detached almost as if what he is saying has happened to someone else and not him. On the other hand, the extremely precise details of the events he describes could only be the result of a first-hand experience. He is at the same time a spectator and an actor (Table 9.1).

Table 9.1 Classic schizophrenia symptoms compared to synthetic psychosis symptoms

Endogenic psychosis (classical psychosis)	Exogenic psychosis (synthetic psychosis)
Lucid consciousness	Twilight consciousness
Thought	Sensory perceptions
Self-concerning ontological insecurity	Object-concerning instability
Delusion: primary, metaphysical, systematic transcendental ego	Delusion: secondary, everyday, phantastic empiric ego
Fusionality, passivity	Insight, agency
Bizarre and inexplicable behaviour	Impulse discontrol and aggressivity
Autism	Anaclitism
Progression	Basic and germinative
Distance/apathy	Overexcited/excessive emotivity

9.6 Conclusion and Perspectives

"Synthetic psychosis" in NPS addicts is characterised by an induced hallucinatory symptomatology and by a reactive delusional interpretation, which include a relative conservation of the patient's ego for the rest of his or her life. It is not uncommon for a psychiatric diagnosis to hide and even dispel the toxic etiopathogenic nature of the disorder. In this way the patient begins an odyssey in the tunnel of chronic psychiatry, and often the intermediate medical check-ups make him appear indistinguishable from cases of classic psychosis. This is because of the muscular armour resulting from the extrapyramidal collateriality of the neuroleptics, which makes these "synthetic" patients resemble classic psychotic cases. Diagnosing these new patients as classic psychotic cases effectively hides their potentialities and/or resources. If these patients are recognised for what they really are, they reveal a better prognosis since their ego has not been compromised from within by disruptive processes. They suffer neither from a loss of natural evidence (Blankenburg 1998) nor from Bleulerian or Minkowskian autism. Furthermore they are not subject to a Kraepelinian process of deterioration. Synthetic psychosis, if we try to describe it using the terms of classic psychopathology, is a sort of paraphrenic syndrome reactive to a mental automatismus induced by NPS. This clinical form of *nonclassic psychosis* is a pervasive and common disorder in NPS addicts which limits the social functioning of patient and encourages continued addictive behaviour or, as in the case of G., suicidal behaviour. It is important to identify this form of psychosis in NPS addicts in order to treat it adequately. The destiny of an addict today can depend entirely on the recognition and treatment of this disorder. This psychosis can be considered as being a sort of "Alice in Wonderland syndrome". In this case the patient presented (G.) *is not* psychotic, but he *does have* a psychotic syndrome. This form of psychosis is nearer to organic psychosis or to psycho-organic syndromes. This psychotic syndrome is often a nonresponder to traditional antipsychotic treatment. On the other hand, second-generation long-acting antipsychotics are more useful in order to control the main symptoms. However, this does not mean that the patient is impossible to treat. Dasein-analytical treatment is characterised by the constitution of an intense emotional warming.[44] The experience shared by therapists and patients, session after session, is characterised by focusing consciousness on one's own internal experience, searching for the lost structure of one's own *being-at-the-world*, the encounter between one's own self and another and the rebirth of one's own existential movements, finding oneself and losing oneself and finding oneself again, in an

[44] Empathising means "feeling the other from within" (Stein 2012). The "pathicity" of existence is the background of this phenomenological approach (Binswanger 1942, 1957, 1963; Binswanger et al. 1958; Minkowski 1971, 1973, 1980, Von Weizsaecker (1886–1957), Straus (1891–1975)). Every feeling is a *feeling-of-something*: hate, disgust, love, desire, joy and sadness (H. Plessner (1892–1985), Scheler (1875–1928). Our feelings are not senseless state of consciousness or psychic facts, but concrete modes of existence in situations with others (F. J. J. Bujtendijk (1887–1974).

endless game of swapping of changing the intimate parts of oneself. Group experience inspired by the Dasein-analytical approach, characterised by a particular group atmosphere, is made up of the following elements: lack of preselection and free accessibility into the group which is unrestricted by rigid rules; less structured actions; the presence of addicts, psychotics and normal people side by side; and the assumption of the space and time of addicts (here and now) as group time. The desired objective is nothing less than freedom from addiction and the stabilisation of the psychotic syndromes. In many cases the patient must learn that it is possible to survive with the extraneity inside, developing the residual intersubjective part of himself/herself through the therapeutic relationship.

Synthetic psychosis could replace the classic madness described by Foucault and become the typical form of madness in the postmodern age.

References

Anderson, E. W., & Rawnusley, K. (1954). Clinical studies of LSD. *Monatsschrift für Psychiatrie und Neurologie, 108*, 39.

Blankenburg, W. (1998). *La perdita dell'evidenza naturale*. Milano: Cortina.

Berner, P. (1981). The demarcation between schizophrenia and cyclothymia. *Archives of Neurology and Psychiatry, 18*, 147–159.

Binswanger, L. (1942). *Grundformen und Erkenntnis Menschlichen Daseins*. Zurich: Niehans.

Binswanger, L. (1957). *Daseinsanalyse und psychotherapie*. Speer, Zurich: Aktuelle Psychotherapie.

Binswanger, L. (1963). Essere nel mondo, Astrolabio, Roma, 1973.

Binswanger, L., Daseinsanalyse, Psychiatrie, Schizophrenie, Conferenza in lingua tedesca e inglese tenuta a Zurigo al II congresso internazionale degli psichiatri (1958), *Schweizer Archiv für Neurologie und Psychiatrie*, LXXXI, ½, 1958; trad.it. di Esposito S., in Attualità in psicologia, 18, 3–4, 2003, 197–204.

Bonhoeffer, K. (1917). Die exogenen Reaktionstypen. *Archiv fur Psychiatrie und Nervenkrankheiten, 58*, 50–70.

Callieri, B. (1962) Aspetti psicopatologico-clinici della 'Wahnstimmung'. In Kranz, H. (a cura di). *Psychopathologie Heute* (pp. 72–80). Stuttgart: Thieme.

Callieri, B. (1993). L'esperienza del *Leib* sessuale nei tossicodipendenti. *Attualità in Psicologia, 5–9, 8*.

Callieri, B. (1997). Wahnstimmung e perplessità: la sospensione di significato tra gli esordi del delirare schizofrenico, in Psicopatologia della schizofrenia a cura di Rossi Monti M., Cortina, Milano.

Callieri, B. (2001). *Quando vince l'ombra*. Roma: Edizioni Universitarie Romane.

Callieri, B. (2004). *Prefazione a "Il mondo tossicomane"*. Milano: di G. Di Petta, F. Angeli.

Callieri, B. (2006). *Presentazione a "Gruppoanalisi dell'esserci"*. Milano: di G. Di Petta, F. Angeli.

Cargnello, D., Callieri, B., & Morselli, G. E. (1962). *Le psicosi sperimentali*. Milano: Feltrinelli.

Conrad, K. (1958). *Die beginnende Schizophrenie. Versuch einer Gestaltanalyse des Wahns*. Stuttgart: Thieme.

Correale, A. (2006). *Presentazione a "Gruppoanalisi dell'esserci"*. Milano: di G. Di Petta, F. Angeli.

De Clerambault, G. (1994). Automatismo mentale. Psicosi passionali, Metis, Chiesti.

di Petta, G. (2004). *Il mondo tossicomane, fenomenologia e psicopatologia*. Milano: FrancoAngeli.

Di Petta, G. (2006). *Gruppoanalisi dell'esserci: tossicomania e terapia delle emozioni condivise*. Milano: F. Angeli.
Di Petta, G. (2009). *Nella terra di nessuno. Doppia diagnosi e presa in carico integrata: l'approccio fenomenologico*. Roma: Edizioni Universitarie romane.
Gross, G., Huber, G., Klosterkoetter, J., & Linz, M. (1987). *BSABS. Bonner Skala für die Beurteilung von Basissymptomen*. Berlin: Springer.
Husserl, E. (1907), L'idea della Fenomenologia, Il Saggiatore, Milano, 1988.
Husserl, E. (1913–1928). Idee per una fenomenologia pura e per una filosofia fenomenologica, Einaudi, Torino, 1965.
Husserl, E. (1981). *Per una fenomenologia della coscienza interna del tempo*. Milano: Franco Angeli.
Husserl, E. (2000). *Fenomenologia e teoria della conoscenza*. Milano: Bompiani.
Jaspers, K. (1913). "Allgemeine Psychopathologie" . Berlin: Springer, 1973.
Klosterkoetter, J. (1988). Basissymptome und Endphänomene del Schizophrenie. Berlin: Springer. Tr. it.: Cosa hanno a che fare i Sintomi-Base con i sintomi schizofrenici?. In Stanghellini, G. (a cura di): *Verso la Schizofrenia*. Napoli: Idelson, 1992.
Merleau-Ponty, M. (1945). Fenomenologia della percezione, Il saggiatore, Milano, 1965.
Minkowski, E. (1971). *Il tempo vissuto. Fenomenologia e psicopatologia*. Torino: Einaudi.
Minkowski, E. (1973). Trattato di psicopatologia. Tr. it. Feltrinelli, Milano.
Minkowski, E. (1980). La schizofrenia. Tr.it. Bertani, Verona.
Mustata, C., Torres, M., Pardo, R., & Perez, C., The Psychonaut Web Mapping Group., & Farre, M. (2009). Spice drugs: Cannabinoids as new designer drugs [Spanish]. *Adicciones, 21*(3), 181–186.
Schneider, K. (1959). Psicopatologia clinica. Tr. it. Roma, Città Nuova, 1983.
Stein, E. (2012). *Il problema dell'empatia*. Milano: Studium.
Straus, E. (1930). *Vom Sinne der Sinne*. Berlin: Springer.
Straus, E. (1978). *Geschehenis und Erlebnis*. Berlin: Springer.
von Gebsattel, V. E. (1954). *Zur Psychopathologie der Sucht, in Prolegomena einer medizinschen Anthropologie* (pp. 220–227). Berlin: Springer.
von Weizsaecker, V. (1968). *Der Gestaltkreis. Theorie der Einheit von Warnhemen und Bewegen*. Stuttgart: Georg Thieme.
Weizsaecker von, V. (1967). Pathosophie, Vandenhoeck § Ruprecht, Goettingen.
Zutt, J. (1963). *Zur Anthropologie der Sucht, in Auf dem Wege zu einer Anthropologischen Psychiatrie* (pp. 423–430). Berlin: Springer.

Melancholia from the Perspective of the Self

10

Alfred Kraus

10.1 Historical and Methodological Part

10.1.1 The Notion of Melancholia Today and Earlier

The notion of melancholia goes back in history to Greek antiquity. Schmidt-Degenhard (1983), Aretaeus of Cappadocia who lived in the second century AD, described most of the essential symptopms of melancholia. Only in the end of the nineteenth century the notion of endogenous depression came up, whereas until now many psychopathologically oriented authors, particularly those of the Phenomenological-Anthropological Approach, still adhere to the notion of melancholia as a pathological Disturbance Entity. The notion of melancholy (Schwermut), coming up in literature at about the same time, has to be differentiated from melancholia as a clinical term. Already in antiquity, as, for instance, in the writings of Aretaeus, an alternation of melancholic and manic mental states was known. Later on, by Falret in 1854, melancholia and mania were not conceived of as two different syndromes, but as one illness, the "folie circulaire." Kraepelin (1913) coined the term of manic-depressive psychosis. According to elder classical literature, every endogenous depression and manic-depressive illness, particularly in case of delusional ideas or hallucinations, was mostly treated as a psychotic illness. It was particularly Angst and Perris (1968) who, referring to genetic and personality research, pleaded for a separation of unipolar depression with purely depressive states from bipolar states, i.e., manic-depressive disturbances.[1] In the meantime, however, it has been shown that

[1] This separation is also to be found in DSM-5-TM (2013) insofar as "bipolar and related disorders" and "depressive disorders" are separated. We refer to the recently published DSM-5-TM (2013) by the American Psychiatric Association, because it represents the newer version of a diagnostic and categorical glossary, compared to the international glossary of ICD-10-V(F) (2005). But it is

A. Kraus (✉)
University of Heidelberg, Heidelberg, Germany
e-mail: akraus593@googlemail.com

G. Stanghellini, M. Aragona (eds.), *An Experiential Approach to Psychopathology*,
DOI 10.1007/978-3-319-29945-7_10

many of these patients with unipolar depression also developed manic states. Symptoms presented by patients with melancholic states in unipolar and bipolar disorders are practically identical, with just some small questionable differences. On the contrary, as we will show, the type of their personality is partly different.

In the new glossary classification of DSM-5-TM (2013), melancholia is now only given by adding the specifier "with melancholic features" to one of the "depressive disorders," if indicated. But in the traditional understanding, also delusions and hallucinations and so-called bodily feelings like leaden paralysis could be included in what was understood as melancholia. Therefore, if we want to restore, as we do, the former and still ongoing understanding of melancholia, we include also what is now registered by the specifier "with psychotic features" (i.e., delusions and/or hallucinations to be present) and bodily feelings which are now in the specifier "with atypical features" as possible features of melancholia. Even DSM-5-TM (2013) mentions that melancholic features were more likely to occur in more severe major depressive episodes and in those with psychotic features.

10.1.2 Phenomenological-Anthropological Diagnostics as a Supplement to a Criteriological-Symptomatological One

Since their appearance, manuals like DSM and ICD were not only welcomed because of their reliability but also exposed to vivid criticism. Apart from a sometimes missing validity, we mention an insufficient consideration of the subjectivity of the psychiatric patient, particularly with respect to her original experiences of disturbances, as well as the lack of a holistic comprehension of her altered being. The manuals should not only, it was argued, be instruments of communication for an international understanding, but should also be available to the needs of very different groups of users. Moreover, the manuals were expected to be the basis of manifold psychopathological considerations, not only to present ready-made nosology. A one-sided theoretical language of function in the glossaries should not cover a premature nosologization, if not sufficiently justified by respective results. A general lack of psychopathology as a particular basic science within psychiatry nowadays shows itself in the fact that not only in the USA but also elsewhere the notion of psychopathology is often used only as a generic term for psychiatric disturbances and symptoms. It is not always used for basic methodological considerations. Nancy Andreasen (2007) spoke of the death of phenomenology in the USA. She complained that the training and further education in the USA is too much concentrated on operational diagnostics. Complex approaches would systematically be neglected. According to Saß (1987) the development of the diagnostic instruments has reached a border which demands a reflection of the psychopathological basis of diagnostics (see also Mundt (2002)).

planned to bring the awaited ICD-11 in line with DSM-5-TM (2013). In the following DSM-5 and ICD-10 relate to these editions of the manuals.

10.1.2.1 Symptom and Phenomenon

In several articles (Kraus 1991, 1994, 1996a, b, 2005) we not only reflected critically on operational diagnostics and classification but also tried to confront these with a so-called Phenomenological-Anthropological diagnostics as a possible supplement, by taking into account the complex original experiences of the patient. In doing so, we related to different phenomenological approaches (i.e., descriptive phenomenology, phenomenology of essence, transcendental phenomenology, daseinsanalytical and existential approaches, etc.), which can be summarized under the title of a "Phenomenological-Anthropological Psychiatry." Because of our intention to relate particularly to the experiences of melancholic patients, hereby depending on these kinds of methods, we have first to make some comments to these.

Often the notions phenomenon and symptom are used in a promiscuous way. From a methodological view, however, these notions have to be differentiated. In a strict sense, the notion of symptom is defined by that of an illness to which it should point, which as such often does not show itself. For instance, fever only points to the possible presence of a physical disturbance in general and is not a determined one. Jaspers speaks of symptoms, if causes are taken into account, compared to the notion of symptom that phenomenon is much more complex. In Phenomenological-Anthropological Diagnostics and Psychopathology, the notion of phenomenon has at least primarily not a causal or etiological orientation, but is meant in a descriptive sense. Phenomenon (phainesthai = to show itself) is used for that which shows itself by itself. For example, in a diagnostic situation, a phenomenon is what the patient tells the diagnostician about her original vivid experience. In the sense of Edmund Husserl and his followers, a phenomenon is, however, not only the factual thing of an experience, but also comprises the "essence" or "eidos" of what is experienced. This essence in the ideological approach is coexperienced with the experiences of the factual thing which a patient has communicated to the diagnostician. The experience of the essence of something is constituted methodologically by intuitive acts of variation, i.e., comparing the actual experience of an object with other experiences, grasping the necessary invariability ("das invariante") of an object. Jaspers speaks only of empathy of the diagnostician as necessary for the understanding of a psychotic patient. In our view empathy, however, is not sufficient, even if it is necessary and helpful. Apart from an empathic relationship to the patient, also intuitive acts of variation of the experiences are important for the understanding of the essence of what, e.g., the psychotic patient tells the diagnostician. Bearing this in mind, the diagnostician not only has to grasp what the patient factually feels and experiences but also has to try as far as possible to get access to her particular way of being in the world. To describe this particular kind of being, e.g., of a psychotic patient, is, however, a big language problem.

In the contemporary discussion of the question of dimensional or categorical description, particularly of psychotic experiences, we firstly often miss the primary question, whether we have to do only with quantitative or also with qualitative deviances from normality. Secondly, the question what the premorbid and morbid experiences and behavior of a patient say about the particular kind of her being in the (life)world is often not sufficiently considered. In particular, this is the question of the constitution of her altered self.

10.1.2.2 Disturbance Entity and Existential Type

The consideration of the altered being of the Self and the world of the patient, particularly under the aspect of its constitution, i.e., from the view of Phenomenological-Anthropological Diagnostics, allows us to speak of the Disturbance Entities as particular Existential Types of being. Even in traditional classification, Kurt Schneider (1967), as a prominent representative of it, spoke of types not only with personality disorders but also with schizophrenic and manic-depressive illness. Because of the lack of reliable results regarding the causes of these illnesses, he avoided in these cases to speak of diagnoses in the usual sense, but spoke only of types. However, Kurt Schneider (1967) did not explain whether by his notion of type he understood only a correlative type, or an ideal type [in the sense of Karl Jaspers (1997)], or even possibly a type of essence. Anyway, in operational diagnostic entities, the criteria have, apart from a possible statistical correlation, mostly no methodologically justified understandable interconnection. Instead, Existential Types are different insofar as they, as well as the phenomena which build them up, are seen as understandable entities, methodologically entities of essence constructed by intuitive variation. Thus, all parts of Existential Types should have understandable interconnections.

Similar to what Jaspers said about ideal types, Existential Types, even if they are not identical with Disturbance Entities, can function as a complement to a criteriological diagnostics and can thus be an important support in the whole diagnostic process. They can as well as ideal types also be helpful for research in finding causes of psychiatric disturbances. However, the Existential Type is on one hand not developed by real or hypothetical causal construction, like the usual Disturbance Entities, and is on the other hand not taken as a fictive thing like the ideal type of Jaspers, but as an entity of essence. Diagnostics should always be oriented to the whole of the patient, particularly as far as possible to the Self of the patient.

10.1.3 Significance of Anthropology

Often the term of anthropology is taken for cultural anthropology. However, there are many kinds of anthropology, among others biological and philosophical anthropology. We restrict ourselves here to underlining the importance of philosophical anthropology in the context of a Phenomenological-Anthropological Psychiatry. Philosophical anthropology was founded by Max Scheler, Helmut Plessner, Arnold Gehlen, and others and was developed further mainly by existential philosophers. It is often identified with humanistic and ethical approaches and focused on aspects of the individuality, subjectivity, freedom, and historicity of man. Bodily experiences and the corporality of man (biophysiological, biochemical, genetic processes, etc.) are also of importance. As well, philosophical and phenomenological anthropology has great significance for methodological questions in psychiatry. It influences to a high degree what becomes an important object in psychiatric research and by which methods this respective object is seen to be accessible. Thus, it promotes the development of certain scientific and therapeutic methods, but can also prevent the development of others.

Concerning anthropological issues, so-called Anthropological Proportions have become particularly important to us. This concept was described by Binswanger (1956) and further developed by Blankenburg (1971). The notion refers to certain basic structures of man, often standing in an oppositional relationship to each other. Because man has to integrate these structures in his being, they show us in a particular way the existential achievements man has to fulfill. According to Blankenburg a dialectical thinking is needed here in order to grasp these often opposing structures, which are always individually realized in a certain proportion of each other. Such basic structures are, e.g., self-realization opposed to role realization, individuation opposed to being with others and also to the generalized other ("das Man" in the sense of Heidegger), and continuity opposed to openness for development and innovation. In the context of manic-depressive disorders, we introduced further the proportional and oppositional structures of hypernomia and antinomia, hypo-personalization and hyper-personalization, lack of identification and overidentification, subject (or ego) identity and object identity, and identity and nonidentity.

10.2 A Case Report

Our patient H.K. was married and had one daughter. Until his retirement he always worked in the same company. His mother as well as his brother supposedly suffered from depression.

H.K. had his first melancholic phase after moving to live in a much more beautiful apartment at the age of 31. Six years later he was treated with the same diagnosis by me in our clinic. Also, this severe depression occurred in consequence of the restructuring of his company, when he was promoted to be the substitute of the group manager. This meant that he had to leave a big working room with many colleagues and move to a smaller room. Because he now had less work to do, he erroneously experienced this as a professional degradation. He feared that his chief did not trust him to do his work well, and he therefore felt more and more worthless and a professional failure. He even feared he would be dismissed for this reason. All his thoughts now spun around committing suicide, what he attempted several times without success. When brought to our clinic, he was very anxious and agitated. He expressed many self-reproaches, often without any certain content. He also feared that his colleagues would think very badly about him.

Ten years later, H.K. stayed again in our clinic because of depression. He was now in the position of a group leader, but often felt isolated from and not accepted by the group he guided. Often he felt responsible for the failures of others. All tasks which were delegated to him occupied him day and night, also in his free time. In his depression, he brooded about the question which mistakes he could possibly have done in his work. He felt insufficient in his work and often had feelings of guilt, which he mostly could not substantiate. This time he worried much about a planned celebration of his 25th year of affiliation to his firm. He believed this would be the end of him and he would have no future. He became more and more stuporous and even refused treatment, which he considered useless. He was convinced that his wife would never visit him again and that his daughter was starving to death because of the impoverishment of his family. Being asked to control his assumption by phoning her, he thought this would be useless, because he was convinced that she was already dead. Once he even thought all patients in the ward would die or already dead. This feeling of himself, of his daughter, and of all the patients was in our view only partly delusional and much more a "feeling for loss of feeling" ("Gefühl für Gefühllosigkeit") as K. Schneider (1967) put it. During his stay in the hospital, H.K. was severely depressed most of the time with a feeling of not being himself and without the possibility to change his state. He could not react adequately to joyful situations, normally he was a cheerful man, who liked to laugh. Only with high doses of antidepressants and even two electroshocks did his melancholia get better.

Personality: According to his wife, H.K. was always an overconscientious man, who fulfilled all his duties with painstaking care. He could not see something unfinished. Until his marriage he lived with his parents, to whom he had a very close relationship all his life. He liked to be with others but was also very sensitive to criticism and could not stand discordant relationships.

Diagnostically several periods of severe melancholia could be registered, twice with delusions of insufficiency, guilt, and impoverishment and once also with stupor and nihilistic delusion in the sense of a Cotard syndrome. Most of his melancholic phases were precipitated by feelings of not fulfilling the normative expectations of his job, thus being a professional failure. This corresponded in a very typical way with what we will call a hypernomic behavior and an overidentification with the professional role. He also showed symbiotic features in his relations to others and an intolerance of ambiguity, which we will speak about later on. As he was very sensitive to all kinds of changes, he had a marked novophobia.

10.3 Personality and Self of Melancholics

10.3.1 Typus Melancholicus: Clinical and Empirical Studies

From the aspect of DSM-5-TM, our term "melancholia" refers mainly to "major depressive disorder" with the specifier "with melancholic features." In the traditional understanding of melancholia, "psychotic features" and "atypical features" could also be included, as we do it. We will now deal with the question of the personality or self of melancholics outside and inside their clinical melancholic phases. Because of the worldwide intense clinical and objective-empirical research on the personality of unipolar melancholic and bipolar subjects in the last decades, we are today in a much better situation than it was at the time of Emil Kraepelin, Sigmund Freud, and Karl Jaspers. The relatively concurring results of this research are in our view very important for the understanding of the precipitation of melancholic phases as well as of their single clinical phenomena. The bridge between these two issues is for us our orientation to the experience of the Self of the patient in the premorbid state, compared with that in the melancholic phase by means of a phenomenological analysis. A mere orientation to the personality properties or traits of the patient in both of these endeavors is, as we believe, not sufficient. We refer mainly to the concept of the so-called Typus melancholicus ("T. mel.") of Hubertus Tellenbach (1961, 1980). Predecessors of this concept were Abraham (1971), Freud (1967), Bibring (1952), and Shimoda (see Kraus 1971a). Tellenbach described the personality of his "T. mel.," that is, the personality of melancholics, not to be mixed up with the melancholic type of depression, above all under the aspect of extreme diligence at work, painstaking orderliness, and a symbiotic dependence in the relationships with others. According to Fiedler (1995, 2001, 2007), items of the T. mel. in remitted melancholic, endogenous depressive patients were found in up to half of them in empirical studies. Surveys of studies on these patients and other studies using self-rating instruments and informant-rating scales and other methods were provided by von Zerssen (1996b), Sato et al. (1996), Kasahara (1976), Mundt et al. (1997), Kronmüller et al. (2005), von Zerssen (2000), and Kronmüller et al. (2002). Kronmüller et al. (2005) compared four questionnaires on the "T. mel." personality (TMP). The factor analysis of the items of the TMP questionnaires could differentiate four dimensions of the TMP: dependence, intolerance of ambiguity, norm orientation, and perfectionism. von Zerssen (1996b) found TMP traits correlating negatively with aggression and extraversion and positively with conscientiousness and rigidity. Sato et al. (1996) investigated a group of Japanese patients of both sexes with primary major depression, using the Japanese T. mel. scale of Kasahara in combination with the F-list of von Zerssen. They found significantly higher scores in both of these scales than in normal controls, but no difference between mel. and non-mel. subtypes of depression. Clinically many bipolar patients also seem to show personality traits of the "T. mel." (more often and more prominent in bipolar II than in bipolar I patients), who by test did not differ from controls. von Zerssen (1996b) summarized these personality traits oppositional to the T. mel. under the title of a so-called Typus manicus ("T. man."). We will show this later on. It is not possible here to enter into the personality research to its full extent, but we point, in particular, to the research on temperaments of the manic-depressive spectrum by Akiskal (1996).

10.3.2 Typus Melancholicus: Is It Really an Obsessive-Compulsive Personality Disorder?

Many authors as well as Tellenbach (1961) himself at first identified the "T. mel." with anancastic or obsessive-compulsive personality. He later on abandoned the identification of these two kinds of type. Already in our book on *Sozialverhalten und Psychose Manisch-Depressiver* (1977) as well as in an article on *Role Performance, Identity Structures and Psychosis* (1996), we showed a differentiation between anancastic behavior and what we call hypernomic behavior (in Greek, nomos = norm, law, rule) as the main characteristic of the "T. mel.," on principle different from obsessive-compulsive behavior. Among a series of other criteria, hypernomic behavior is in our view mainly oriented to the normative expectations of society, mostly in the context of social roles, with which "T. mel." patients in our view are overidentified. Hypernomic behavior in this way is hypernormality. Stanghellini and Mundt (1997) as well as Stanghellini (2004) and Ambrosini et al. (2011) introduced, besides our notion of hypernomia, heteronomia as an exaggerated receptivity of external norms, concordant with the particular "sensitivity in his conscience" (p. 83) and an "intolerance for being guilty" (Tellenbach 1980, p. 83) of the melancholic patient.

In the following, we will compare the criteria of "T. mel." with those of the "obsessive-compulsive personality disorder" in the DSM-5-TM. Many authors, however, still use the term "anancastic personality" with the meaning of being ego-dystonic at least in some aspects; ego-dystony in DSM-5-TM is (implicitly) now preserved for obsessive-compulsive disorder, but not mentioned in the category of obsessive-compulsive personality disorder, in spite of the same adjectives in both kinds of disorder. In ICD-10-V(F) (2005) the symptom 6 of anancastic personality disturbance "intrusion of insistent and unwelcome thoughts and impulses" still has an ego-dystonic meaning. In fact, with obsessive-compulsive personality disorder in DSM-5-TM, we have now to do with an ego-syntonic structure of obsessive-compulsive character, which in our view is a contradictio in adjecto, misleading and confusing. Most of the criteria of obsessive-compulsive personality disorder in DSM-5-TM have now a strong similarity to the personality traits of the "T. mel.," which in our view can all be addressed as being ego-syntonic, even if sometimes a transition to ego-dystonic behavior is possible. We (Kraus 1996c) showed different items of hypernomic and anancastic behavior on a table (Table 2.1, p. 36), among others: (1) related to social norms vs. egocentric, often antisocial, (2) oriented to standards of society vs. oriented to individual standards, (3) ego-syntonic vs. ego-dystonic, etc. Another important difference is that the first ones are oriented toward interpersonal relationships, whereas the obsessive personality is oriented toward the organization of things (Stanghellini 2004, p. 109). In Japan, Sato et al. (1996), comparing the different items of the melancholic type of personality with the obsessive personality, in concordance with our view, found the following opposites among others (Table 3.1, p. 50): (1) centered on other people vs. self-centered, (2) aggression not likely to appear vs. aggression likely to appear, (3) more guilt feelings vs. less guilt feelings, etc. The decisive difference of hypernomic behavior compared to obsessive-compulsive behavior is, as also Stanghellini (2004) ascertains, "an extreme social adaptation" (p. 104).

In DSM-5-TM, it is said that obsessive-compulsive personality disorder may be associated with depressive and bipolar disorders. As well, there is possibly an overlapping with "type A" personality characteristics (e.g., preoccupation with work, in patients with myocardial infarction). The notion "T. mel." or hypernomic behavior is not mentioned. For the differential diagnosis between major depressive disorder and obsessive-compulsive disorder, the DSM-5-TM (2013) mentions that ruminations in major depressive disorders and in OCD can be differentiated insofar as the first ones are usually mood congruent, not necessarily experienced as extensive or distressing as in the last ones.

10.3.3 Hypernomic Behavior as a Defense of a Threatened Social Identity

Apart from the terminological problem, our main criticism of the concept of the obsessive-compulsive personality disorder in DSM-5-TM is that its single criteria are not oriented to the Self of the patient. This is partly also true for Tellenbach's concept of "T. mel." A first step toward the Self of the melancholic is to speak of the behavior of the "T. mel." as hypernomic behavior, i.e., an overidentification with social norms and also with one's social roles, respectively (Kraus 1980, 2007). This particular orientation to social norms was empirically confirmed by several studies: von Zerssen (1996a, b, 2001), Mundt et al. (1997), Stanghellini and Mundt (1997), Hecht et al. (1998), and Heerlein et al. (2002). Von Zerssen and Pössl (1990) and von Zerssen (1977, 1996a, b) showed that, compared to the "T. mel.," "T. man." patients have traits which are in many respects contrary to the first ones. They can even ignore or oppose to social norms and rules, showing rather hyponomic behavior, but in the basis of their personality, they have often more traits of the T. mel. than what they show. To summarize, the hypernomic behavior of the "T. mel." is in our view a defense against a loss of social identity, whereas anancastic behavior in its elder, particularly psychoanalytic understanding, is a defense against aggressive and sexual drives.

According to DSM-5-TM, an enduring pattern of inner experience and behavior as being "pervasive and inflexible" (p. 645) is characteristic of all personality disorders. On the other hand, to be "inflexible about matters of morality, ethics, or values" (criterion 4) and to show "rigidity and stubbornness" (criterion 8) should be diagnostic criteria of the obsessive-compulsive personality disorder. Tellenbach himself and the following studies describe a particular rigidity of melancholic patients in the way of a fixation to orderliness ("Festgelegtsein auf Ordentlichkeit"), which for Tellenbach is a "constitutive trait of the T. mel." (p. 66). Orderliness in his understanding means being orderly in every respect. Another basic trait of the "T. mel." for him is that the patient conceives the "demands for achievement" much above the average, concerning the quality as well as the quantity of work (p. 66). Orderliness for Tellenbach is on one hand a possibility to protect oneself against the danger of becoming melancholic, but on the other hand paradoxically is also a vulnerability factor leading to the precipitation of a melancholic episode.

10.3.4 Includence and Remanence. High Demands on Oneself: Altruistic or Narcissistic Attitudes?

Particularly important for the understanding of melancholia as well as of mania are Tellenbach's (1980) concepts of includence ("Inkludenz") and remanence ("Remanenz"). With includence, he describes an inclusion in borders which the patient cannot transcend to a regular performance of herself, which for Tellenbach is a decisive pathogenetic aspect of melancholia. Sometimes the patient can be "included" in her demands on herself ("Selbstanspruch" p. 136) of orderliness. This can be the case, if, in certain situations of overdemanding achievements of her environment, she cannot fulfill them all. In spite of all her endeavors, she may get into a situation of self-contradiction with respect to her own demands on herself, with the consequence that she stays back to herself. This staying back to her self-demands is what Tellenbach calls remanence. Because of this remanence, the patient in this situation gets more and more into a situation of desperation (Tellenbach 1980, p. 153). Bürgy (2010) described this situation more extensively.

Relating to Tellenbach's depressive patients with high demands of orderliness, Mundt et al. (2009) wrote an article on altruism vs. self-centeredness in the personality of depressives in the 1950s and 1990s. These authors used case records of depressive patients. They differentiated patients with "high standards for themselves" in those with altruistic and those with self-centered attitudes, classifying the last ones as those with narcissistic personality features. We quote the authors: "Of the 40 patients with early onset of depression 13 (33 %) were classified as narcissistic personalities, whereas only 4 (10 %) late onset depressives fell into the narcissistic personality category. In the 1990th decade, about 29 % of the patients were grouped into the narcissistic personality category, compared to the 1950th decade in which 13 % of the patients were classified as narcissistic personalities" (p. 161). The self-centeredness in part of their depressives, according to the authors, stays in contrast to the altruistic personality features of the "T. mel." described by Tellenbach (1980) and Kraus (1982). With advanced age an increasing of altruism and decrease of self-centeredness could be confirmed. These more self-centered narcissistic personality type patients, according to the authors, are in some aspects more in accordance with the self-centered narcissistic personality view of Kernberg and Kohut. In our view, the two groups of patients, both with high demands on themselves, but one with altruistic and the other one with narcissistic personality features of Mundts' concept, need to be compared by further investigation. Concerning the problem of narcissism in melancholia, see Lang (2003). Some of the features of the narcissistic personality correspond to the symptoms of hypomania.

10.3.5 Sympathetic and Symbiotic Relationships with Others

Another aspect of the T. mel. patient in the sense of Tellenbach is what he calls a sympathetic-symbiotic being with others, particularly in relation to family members, to the partner, and to the children of her family. Her relationship to others, according to Tellenbach, consists particularly of an achievement for others. In this sphere of being with others, he says the patient is particularly sensitive to a disturbance of orderliness. Tellenbach points to the very low rate of divorce in unipolar melancholic patients. We could confirm this in our study of divorce rates, comparing unipolar melancholic patients with bipolars (not yet published). In this study the divorce rate in unipolar melancholics was below the average population, but that of bipolars much higher. Differently from Tellenbach we see not only a sympathetic and symbiotic relationship to others in T. mel. patients but also a strong tendency to identify oneself with others. Thus, we assume that this identification with others is at least partly the basis of their symbiotic relationship to others. In this context, a strong identification with the identity found in the role of being a mother or father and of being a partner (role identity) is also important. Concerning recent empirical research on altruistic features, see Mundt (2011).

10.3.6 What Decompensates in Melancholia?

10.3.6.1 The Typus Melancholicus as a Competence

Coming back to Tellenbach's concept of remanence and of the situation of desperation, he sees the consequence of this situation in the precipitation of an endogenous process, which shows itself in the phenomena, signs, and symptoms of a melancholic episode. What causes this decompensation and makes out of the "T. mel." a vulnerability factor? In Tellenbach's view the rigidity of the "T. mel." is a being fixed to orderliness ("Festgelegtsein auf Ordentlichkeit"). This is the core of all single traits of the "T. mel.," specifying them all from the aspect of their motivation. In this way, orderliness, even if orientation to order is at first only a single trait of the "T. mel.," now becomes a formal or structural quality of all traits of the "T mel." (In empirical research, we often find no differentiation between trait and structure of personality, which we however deem to be important.) It is this structure of orderliness which, according to Tellenbach, is decompensated by "remanence" and "includence." What this fixation really is and how it develops is, however, not explained.

In this context we want to point to a general problem of personality research. As long as important phenomena like "orderliness," "rigidity," "fixation to orderliness" a particular "sensitivity to norms" ("heteronomia"), or "sensitivity in one's conscience" stay for themselves and are not integrated on a higher level of the personality, or in a particular concept of identity or self, they can also be seen as effects of an endogenous process.

Fiedler (1995, p. 348) suggests that the "T. mel." and the "T. man." could both be conceived as extreme variations of normal behavior, which as such can be seen as competences. In his view of a merely one-sided personality, he thinks of the possibility of a further "extreming" of this behavior in order to protect the individual in situations of social difficulties. As a consequence, similar to Tellenbach's view, the structure of the "T. mel." decompensates with the possible issue of a depression or mania. In this case, we would rather speak of the decompensation of an undialectic identity structure (see later!). Orderliness alone as a formal structure of the personality of melancholics in our view cannot sufficiently explain the precipitation of a melancholic episode and particularly not the occurrence of the melancholic symptoms of a deep melancholic mood alienation, not the insufficiency of mourning, and not the delusional ideas in the melancholic episode and so on. Being fixed to orderliness is in our view nothing more than the extreme of the Latin proverb: "serva ordinem et ordo te servabit." This cannot explain a severe pathological state. A mere fixation to competences such as orderliness, perfectionism, and symbiotic relationship is not a sufficient factor of vulnerability. We first have to explain why these competences are so highly needed. And what decompensates? What is their function on the higher level of the Self?

10.3.7 The Self as a Bridge Between Typus Melancholicus and Melancholic Episode

10.3.7.1 Significance of Ego-Achievements

What we miss in Tellenbach's concept is a bridge between the premorbid personality of the "T. mel." and the melancholic disease. The missing link for him is the endogenous process, which for him is the real cause of the melancholic disease. But is this assumption really necessary? A bridge in our view would be if we could proceed from the "T. mel." to an adequate concept of the Self or identity of the patient. But first we have to ask how it is to be understood when in his excellent description of "includence" and "remanence" Tellenbach speaks of a lacking possibility to transcend oneself. In our view, it is the lacking competence of the "T. mel." to use "Ego-Achievements." Only the application of Ego-Achievements could overcome the includence and in this way prevent remanence.

We think the lack of Ego-Achievements should be an important feature in the concept of the "T. mel." The single traits of the "T. mel." as well as its structural aspect of orderliness are only oriented to the norms, or normative expectations of social roles. Ego-Achievements instead are ways of behavior reacting to the norms and normative expectations of the social roles, i.e., the expectations of society. The Ego-Achievements react by interpreting these norms, the normative role expectations, respectively. In this way, they allow a certain distance to these roles. Sociologists speak of a "role-distance" (Dreitzel 1968, p. 212), which as such is also an Ego-Achievement. Role-distance is not a denial of the norms or of the expectations of the role partner by the holder of a certain position. According to

Goffmann (1961) (quoted in Dreitzel p.213), "Role-distance is a behavior which takes a distance to the identity somebody finds in a certain role, which is called Role-identity, in order to realize oneself as a personal, individual identity able to use Ego-Achievements in the performance of a social role." Ego-Achievements originate in the "Subject-Identity," this being an important part of one's identity or self in the sense of G.H. Mead (1934, 1980). The behavior of T. mel. in our view is not as Tellenbach puts it, primary, but mostly secondary to the lack of Ego-Achievements, which compensate this lack. Because the behavior traits of the T. mel. as such are capacities, we cannot consider these as "enduring and pervasive maladaptive" (DSM-5-TM p. 679). For most of their life span, melancholics are well adapted to this lack of Ego-Achievements; only in certain situations, the hypernomic T. mel. behavior alone is insufficient for compensation.

For a better understanding of this and of the clinical aspects of melancholia, we relate to the concept of the Self by G.H. Mead (1980). In this concept, role-distance is the distance between the "I" as "Subject-I" and the "me" as "Object-I[2]." Mead's concept of the Self starts from these two poles of the Self, the "I" and the "me" being the issue of a process going on between these two poles. "I" and "me" thus stay in a dialectical relationship to each other, which means that the "I" as an always anew projecting itself ("sich entwerfendes"), creative, spontaneous Subject-I relates to the "me" as an Object-I, constantly reacting to it. In this way, Mead advocates a processual theory which he opposes to a self-concept which starts from a substantialistic, stable identity which is in itself always the same. The polarity of "I" and "me" as different parts of the Self makes possible a dynamic becoming, which on one hand prevents a mixture of "I" and "me" and on the other hand unites "I" and "me" in the unity of the Self. The polarity of Subject-I and Object-I also enables a certain availability of the two parts of the Self in the respective individual. In our understanding and interpretation of Mead's concept, the Subject-I is in its core something like a "nonidentity" compared to the more substantial identity of the Object-I. We do not know if J.P. Sartre was influenced by G.H. Mead, as he spoke of man as conditioned by one's family and society, i.e., man making something out of what one has made of him or, when he maintains that facticity (in Mead the "me") and transcendence (in Mead the "I") are the constitutive structures of our consciousness (in Mead the "Self"). Sartre here accurately says what Mead means. Interpreting Mead we can say that the "I" as the Subject-I of this moment, unsubstantial to a far-reaching extent, free and oriented to the future is the "me," the Object-I, of the next moment. Thus, the earlier "I" is always present in the remembrance of our experience. But the "me" is also much more than merely our memories, or the past. It is above all the identities we have built up taking over the attitudes of others, of the generalized other, and the "one" (the "man"), which are

[2] The German translator of Mead's text interpreted the "me" as the "I" (which experiences itself as an object). For this reason, we speak of the "me" as an "object-I" and oppose it to the "I" in Mead's understanding as a "subject-I." According to Mead, the self is a reflexive and indicates that it can be both subject and object.

the social norms, to which we react with our "I." Also our social roles, our values, our ideals, our property, our experiences, our lived life, and our body make up the "me" as an Object-I. The Subject-I and the Object-I are normally always an interaction of both, not only given reflexively but also prereflexively. There is, however, a "temporal and logical pre-existence of the social process to the self-conscious individual that arises in it" (p. 186).

We summarize Mead's concept by quoting him: "There would not be an 'I' in the sense in which we use that term, if there were not a 'me'; there would not be a 'me' without a response in the form of the 'I'. These two roles, as they appear in our experience, constitute the personality or self. We are individuals born into a certain nationality, located at a certain spot geographically, with such and such family relations and such and such political relations. All of these represent a certain situation which constitutes the 'me'; but this necessarily involves a continued action of the organism towards the 'me' in the process within which that lies. The Self is not something that exists first and then enters into a relationship with others, but it is, so to speak, an eddy in the social current and so still a part of the current" (Mead 1934, p. 182).

The diminution of the Ego-Achievements of melancholics in the premorbid condition as well as in the melancholic episode shows itself above all in a space-time continuity of their identity, in their lack of flexibility, sensitivity, and vulnerability by any change, e.g., changes in their profession, their dwelling, etc., like in the case study we presented. The melancholic wants to be "lived" by the steadiness of her daily concerns; she has strong ties to her family, tends to conform with the common sense, and shows conventional attitudes. We spoke of a tendency to be "lived" by external representatives of identity. She tries to constitute a sameness of her identity which is not worried by the freedom of new decisions. Stanghellini (2004) spoke of an "overidentification with tradition" (p. 141) as a main characteristic of unipolar melancholics and of a tendency to "submit to the pressure of public opinion" (p. 141), of a "permanence of selfhood," and of a sameness "instead of oneself" (p. 143). All this indicates a diminution of the Subject-I with poor Ego-Achievements, which resemble much of what Freud calls a diminution of the feeling of oneself ("Selbstgefühl"), of the feeling of one's ego ("Ichgefühl") (vol. X, 429).

10.3.8 Intolerance of Ambiguity as an Aspect of Content and Form of the Melancholic (T. mel.) and Manic Type (T. man.) of Personality

Intolerance of ambiguity (Intol. amb.) is not described in the concept of Tellenbach's "T. mel." and von Zerssen's "T. man." This intolerance, as we will see, is particularly prominent in the clinical episodes of melancholia and mania in an inversive way, but can more or less also be seen in an inversive way in the premorbid personality of unipolar melancholics on one hand and of unipolar manics and bipolars on the other hand (Kraus 1988, 1996c, 2013, Heerlein and Richter 1991; Heerlein et al. 1996a, b).

The concept of a Tol. amb. and Intol. amb. was originally described by the social psychologist Frenkel-Brunswik (1948, 1949, 1951) as an emotional, perceptual, and cognitive personality variable. Ambiguity etymologically means double aspects. Tol. amb. enables somebody to have positive as well as negative feelings, perceptions, and cognitions in relation to another person or something. Frenkel-Brunswik defined Intol. amb. as a "tendency to resort to black-white solutions, to arrive at premature closure as to evaluative aspects, often at the neglect of reality to seek i.e. for unqualified and unambiguous overall acceptance and rejection of other people" (1949, p. 115). Tolerance of ambiguity instead allows selectively for different, also conflicting aspects of something or somebody or of the reality as a whole. In this selective, integrating function, Tol. amb. in our view is an Ego-Achievement. In its reaction to the "me," the "I" searches to integrate also different dimensions and aspects of the "me" into the Self.

What is relatively characteristic is that in melancholic and manic episodes, the patients have more or less lost the possibility to have feelings, cognitions, and behavior in a compromising way contrary to what they actualize in each episode.

As Frenkel-Brunswik showed, Intol. amb. can also be seen in normal people.

She studied Tol. amb. and Intol. amb in her works on prejudices, particularly social prejudices, in the personalities of several groups. In these studies she used a rigidity scale, memory scales, and projective tests. As a consequence of Intol. amb., she observed misconceptions of reality and a loss of insight into oneself in the sense of "idioagnosia" (Stanghellini 2004, p. 107) as well as into the personality of others in the sense of alteroagnosia (Kraus, unpublished). Compared to manics and melancholics, Intol. amb. in the groups investigated by Frenkel-Brunswik was oriented to certain complexes like, e.g., racism.

In our view, Tol. amb. should not be mixed up with ambivalence, but sometimes is difficult to differentiate. Ambivalence is defined by the coexistence of certain contradicting feelings, imaginations, desires, intentions, and/or impulses of somebody, e.g., love and hate being present in the same individual in a not integrated way. Tol. amb. admits different feelings, perceptions, and cognitions in oneself in an integrated way. Intol. amb. is on the contrary a restrictive one-sidedness of one's emotions, perceptions, and cognitions.

We introduced and applied Frenkel-Brunswik's concept already in earlier studies on the premorbid behavior of melancholics and of manics as well as on the clinical states of melancholia and mania (Kraus 1977, 1988, 1991, 1995a, 1996b, 2011, 2013). The particular advantage of the concept of tolerance and intolerance of ambiguity is that it not only allows for finding possible new single additional traits of the personality of melancholics and bipolars as well as new symptoms and phenomena of melancholia and mania. Apart from contents also formal aspects are considered. Such formal aspects are the belonging together of personality traits, e.g., under the aspect of orderliness, or norm orientation, temperaments, and clinical aspects of mood congruence, of a dominant orientation to the Subject-I or the Object-I, etc. "Formal aspects to content" are as Frenkel-Brunswik maintains "an important task of psychology" (1949/50, p. 120). All parts of Tol. amb. and Intol. amb. in some way become interconnected to each other and build up a certain "gestalt." Whereas this "gestalt" in Tol. amb. is a more open one, Intol. amb. is always more or less a "closed" one, because it excludes certain emotions, perceptions, and cognitions as well as behavior which does not in a holistic way correspond to the actualized ones. This closure, which is always an exclosure of certain aspects of reality, not only makes up the rigidity of the "T. mel" and "T. man." and of the respective states of melancholia and mania but always also involves the danger of a distortion of reality. It explains as we will see later on not only the experiences of the development of "includence" and "remanence" in the situation of the precipitation of melancholic and manic episodes in the sense of Tellenbach, but also the different styles of experience in the clinical episodes, e.g., the generalized "experience of loss" in melancholia and the generalized "experience of winning" in mania. We want to point to the relationship between the concept of Tol. amb. and the concept of Anthropological Proportions of Binswanger and Blankenburg, which we already extended to some proportions which we deem to be particularly relevant with respect to manic-depressives (see p. 5 of our text). The concept of Tol. amb./Intol. amb. can be seen as a more concrete and testable continuation of the Anthropological Proportions, which as such can also be contradictive like the melancholic and manic states themselves. There may sometimes be a danger of overgeneralization of given phenomena with the concepts of proportions as well as with that of Intol. amb., but in our view, they always have some heuristic value for further investigation.

In the following, we will firstly show Intol. amb. by opposite personality traits in melancholics and manics, as these appear in specialist literature and from our own perspective. These traits are examples of behavioral, emotional, perceptual, and cognitive Intol. amb. We already mentioned some of these opposite traits of the "T. mel." and "T. man." according to Tellenbach and von Zerssen, which von Zerssen (1996b) enriched, opposing these on a table (Table 4.1, p. 69) relating to the research issues of many authors. We only mention consistent vs. inconsistent, dependent vs. independent, conventional vs. unconventional, and imaginative vs. unimaginative. Apart from our book on *Sozialverhalten und Psychose Manisch-Depressiver* (Kraus 1977) and our article on *Ambiguitätsintoleranz als Persönlichkeitsvariable und als Strukturmerkmal der Krankheitsphänomene Manisch-Depressiver* (Kraus 1988) and in other articles, we showed that the opposites of melancholic (T. mel.) and manic (T. man.) behavior from a role theoretical point of view can also be seen under the aspect of an Intol. amb. (Kraus 1996c Table 2.1, p. 36): striving for conformity vs. striving for autonomy, determination by others vs. self-determination, fulfilling the interests of others vs. attending to one's own interests, and recipient vs. sender of norms.

In specialist literature (see Kraus 1996b, Table 2.3, p. 41) we find many references to the circumstance that unipolar depressive patients have a tendency to over-friendliness and goodness, whereas manic-depressives are sometimes the opposite: selfish, reckless, demanding, and violating. Whereas the first ones are often idealizing others, showing a low aggressivity and avoiding conflicts, the last ones are often critical to others, have an increased awareness of the faults and weak points of others, and can also be very aggressive. Intol. amb. like the behavior of T. mel. and T. man. shows a lack of Ego-Achievements, which can have positive as well as negative consequences. Thus, on one hand nonassertive behavior of the T. mel., by making sure harmonious relationships to others, can compensate the lack of Ego-Achievements. On the other hand, in other situations where assertive behavior would have been needed, even this behavior could have led to intolerable consequences provoking a melancholic episode.

10.4 The Self in the Melancholic Episode

10.4.1 Intolerance of Ambiguity as an Aspect of Content and Form in the Melancholic and Manic Episodes

A holistic, one-sided intolerance is particularly prominent in the melancholic and manic episodes. Whereas in the melancholic episode the patient only "must" and "should" and cannot do anything, the manic patient "must" and "should" do nothing and can and may do everything. Feelings of guilt and anxiety of the first ones stay opposite to the lack of guilt feelings and anxieties of the last ones, experiences of the past vs. experiences of the future and relation to objects vs. giving up long-lasting relationships.

We summarize: whereas patients with melancholia are more determined by their Object-I, the patients in mania realize themselves more by their Subject-I and show more Ego-Achievements, more likely Pseudo-achievements at the expense of an orientation to the Subject-I.

The consequences of the Intol. amb. for the perceptions and experiences of others are described in detail in the big psychoanalytic study of Cohen et al. 1954. These authors observed in manic-depressives in general an avoidance of the exchange of complex feelings, combined with a deficit of the perception of others in the sense of recognition and identification of a mixture of attractive and inconvenient traits of others. In the pronounced state of melancholic or manic episodes, we have to do with a holistic change of being, which as an intolerance of ambiguity shows itself in emotional, perceptive, and cognitive alterations of function originating in the respective particular being. For this reason it does not make much sense to speak only of a priority of an alteration of mood, or of affects, or of perceptions, or of drive. There is always a holistic change of all of these functions, which is better explained by a holistic alteration of the Self in the sense of a hypo-personalization in the case of melancholia and of hyper-personalization in the case of mania. This reminds us of what K. Schneider said of psychosis in general: "psychosis is always a totality of alteration, not like a defective stone in an otherwise intact mosaique" (1967, p. 96).

Even since the medicine of Greek antiquity, there was the question whether and how the disturbances of melancholia and mania are connected with each other. With the operational classification, not only more and more divisions of melancholia and mania occurred, but these were also more and more separated from each other. In the glossaries, there exists only an additive correlation between the opposite symptoms or phenomena within these entities of melancholia and mania, and both episodes are only interconnected in a sequential way. With our introduction of the two nonmedical concepts of a Tol. amb. (ambiguus = zweiseitig) vs. Intol. amb. by Frenkel-Brunswik and the self-concept of "I" and "me" by G.H. Mead, we want to put the question mentioned above anew. Both concepts not only have each two poles but also integrate both poles. On the basis of the theoretical concepts of Frenkel-Brunswik and G.H. Mead, which we connect with each other, we put the following clinical questions:

1. How far are the single features of melancholia and mania within each state connected in an understandable way in a structure, in an integral way of an entity of being?
2. Can melancholia and mania as opposite kinds of being be seen under the virtual aspect of normally belonging together as a whole, divided in different kinds of being by intolerance of ambiguity?
3. Can melancholia and mania genetically be related to Mead's concept of the Self, the first one more to being a "me" and the second one more to being an "I"?

10.4.2 Precipitating Situations of a Melancholic Episode

Even if there exists an impressive amount of empirical studies on the influence of life events on the precipitation and the course of melancholic episodes, a deficient integration of theoretical considerations and empirical research as well as of the subjective experiences of the patient, those of the therapist and biological findings, has been complained about. A general overview on life event research in depressives and in particular on that in the frame of the Heidelberg study is given by Reck (2001). Phenomenological-Anthropological Psychiatry has in two ways contributed to this research. One is the development of a differentiated concept of the notion of situation [Kraus (1971b), Tellenbach (1980), Schmitdt-Degenhard (2005) and others]; the other one is the influence of the personality of the T. mel. or T. man. on the specificity of the precipitating situation. These concepts have had mainly psychotherapeutical consequences. Some formal specificity of the objective situation of the precipitation of depressive episodes is already obvious in the following terms of depression: bereavement ("Verlustdepression"), uprootedness ("Entwurzelungsdepression"), postpartum ("Wochenbettdepression"), retirement ("Pensionierungsbankrott"), empty nest (depression when children leave home), and promotion ("Erfolgsdepression"). Tellenbach (1980) not only showed the specificity of the precipitating situation consisting in a particular violation of what he calls orderliness but also in an alteration of the situation of the patient by "includence" and "remanence." Includence means being fixed to orderliness, which normally protects one against the danger of becoming melancholic, but now becomes a vulnerability factor if somebody stays back to his demands on himself

("Selbstanspruch") of orderliness (i.e., remanence; see our text p. 11). This in Tellenbach understanding does not only mean becoming guilty, but is also a general stagnation of becoming ("Werdenshemmung"). It is this alteration of the situation of the patient which according to Tellenbach provokes an endogenous process, which for him is responsible for the melancholic symptoms and phenomena. Because of this endogenous process, he rejects every idea of melancholia or mania as being a mere reaction to the outer situation without heed to the personality of the T. mel. and T. man. Melancholia for Tellenbach is not a reactive depression.

For reason of the precarious identity structure of melancholics of a fragile Subject-I, which needs to be compensated by the Object-I, in our view even threat or loss of one of the representatives of the Object-I can precipitate a melancholic or manic episode. We point particularly to losses of social roles by death of an intimate social role partner, the change of one's social roles, and role conflicts. We described such role conflicts as precipitating melancholic episodes more extensively in an article (Kraus 1996b, 2011). Role conflicts, e.g., often result from overdemanding or conflicting normative role expectations within one role, or between several roles, e.g., in the case of somebody who is at the same time superior and in the role of a subordinate or in the case of a housewife who feels overcharged by her roles as a partner, mother, and professional role. Hypernomic behavior in such cases is often not suitable and not sufficient to solve such role conflicts. Here, some role-distance, an interpretation of social roles, and other creative Ego-Achievements are needed. The same is true in a situation of personal conflicts, e.g., of insult or disappointment by a role partner, if a behavior of emotional and cognitive intolerance of ambiguity is not sufficient to cover these negative experiences. This can also lead to a breakdown of one's identity found in such a relationship. A sudden or creeping loss of values or ideals in consequence of the development of society for elder people, or in the case of an emigration to another country, can also cause a weakening or collapse of one's identity. A breakdown of one's role identity(-ies) or of another Object-Identity can have more severe consequences for melancholics because of the deficient activity of the Subject-I, which is especially dependent on the constancy of the Object-I. The deficiency of the Subject-I can be a more temporal or constant diminution of the Subject-I. Freud speaks of an "extraordinary diminution of the feeling of the ego" and of "tremendous impoverishment of the ego" (Freud vol. X, p. 431) in the melancholic episode. In his otherwise excellent description, his assumption of a choice of the love-object on a narcissistic basis, of a conflict of ambivalence to this love-object, and the replacement of the devaluated love-object by internalization as an explanation for the loss of the ego seems to us problematic or as Freud himself (vol. X p. 440) means worth considering. The excellence of his description relates very much to what he says about the difference of mourning and melancholia in the case of the death of a loved person. Whereas in the first case nothing of the loss is unconscious, in the second case, the melancholic, "certainly like the mourner knows, whom she has lost, but not what she has lost with him" (Freud vol. X, p. 431). Not as in the first case, the world became "poor and empty, but in Melancholia it is the ego itself" (p. 431). The "ego" in our understanding here would not be the "I" but the "self." Also Janzarik's (1966) view of emotional and intentional loss of power of the ego ("emotionale und intentionale Entmächtigung" p. 457) in melancholia corresponds to our concept.

10.4.3 "Distinct Quality" of Melancholic Mood

According to the DSM-5-TM (2013) (pp. 160–161), for the diagnosis of major depressive disorder without the specifier "with melancholic features," five or more of nine symptoms have to be present. Of the first ones, no. 1 and no. 2, at least one of them has to be ascertained: it is either depressed mood (no. 1) or diminished interest or pleasure (no. 2). The depressed mood is characterized by persistency and inability to anticipate happiness or pleasure and should be differentiated from grief. The prominent affect of grief is feelings of emptiness and loss. In contrast to ICD-10-V(F) (2005), where depressive mood is not further specified, DSM-5-TM (2013) makes some attempts to differentiate mere depressive mood in major depressive disorder as feeling sad, empty, and hopeless from that in the specifier "with melancholic features" in speaking of a "distinct quality of depressed mood" (p. 185). This distinct quality is "characterized by profound despondency, despair, and/or moroseness or by so-called empty mood" (p. 185). Distinct quality of mood should be understood as qualitatively different from depressive mood during a non-melancholic depressive episode. This distinct quality is not only poorly defined positively but also mostly negatively by saying it should not be understood as being merely depressed, more severely depressed, or longer-lasting, or without reaction to pleasurable stimuli, as already mentioned in the symptom no. 2.

K. Schneider (1967) characterized the melancholic mood disorder in a cyclothymic patient, not to be found in other kinds of depression, in the following ways: (1) The sad feelings come up without reason. (2) They cannot be influenced. (3) They do not flow together with reactive mood. (4) They show a vital character.

We think that the distinct quality of melancholic mood can best be grasped, if we let the patient herself describe it, when exploring her more deeply. Then she will often say that compared to normal mood, or being depressed for some reason, in the melancholic episode, she feels her mood as being forced upon her. She cannot find any reason for being depressed and has in consequence no access to it. She feels to be empty, cannot behave sadly, and cannot weep; instead, she feels blunt, or like a stone. It is not only a loss of feeling and of liveliness but also a feeling of estrangement, which to a large extent is invariable. She cannot take a distance to that state, and it is completely impossible for her to have other feelings and cognitions than those she has all the time. Mostly the patient is not only unable to mourn, but above all not being able to *behave* herself mourning. Normally, a mourning person on one hand has feelings of still being bound to the lost person, but on the other hand, she tries to endure the loss, to achieve a leave-taking. But this last movement for a melancholic person seems to be impossible. She cannot take a distance because she is overidentified with that lost person who as a representative of her Object-Identity is part of herself. For this reason, she cannot tolerate an ambiguity of emotions and cognitions. This intolerance of ambiguity is the opposite of being ambivalent to a love-object, as psychoanalysis maintains. This intolerance of ambiguity in melancholia is expressed in a general inhibition of drive, in feelings of a heavy and weak body as well as localized bodily feelings as the expression of a corporealization of the Self, as we will see in the next chapter. The "distinct quality" of the mood alteration is in our view only one part of a general Intol. amb. and as such an aspect of the lack of the Subject-I, which could not be compensated by the respective representative of Object-I in consequence of the loss. In a note to the specifier "with melancholic features" of DSM-5-TM (2013), it is said that there is "a mere complete absence of the capacity for pleasure." A (scil. complete) "lack of reactivity of mood" can be evaluated if "even highly desired events are not associated with marked brightening of mood" (p. 151). This in our understanding would mean that a complete Intol. amb. is given.

10.4.4 "Corporealization" and Self

Already in Kraus (1995a, b), we wrote an article on the bodily feelings in melancholia. At that time and even today, often bodily feelings in melancholia were and are not discriminated from somatic symptoms, but appear under the heading of "somatic." Real somatic symptoms are a loss of appetite, constipation, rhythmological changes, sweating, palpitations, etc. It was particularly K. Schneider (1967) who pointed to the importance of bodily feelings without somatic findings for the diagnosis of cyclothymic depression. He even took in consideration if it would be possible to compare a "being down in the dumps," feelings of heaviness or elevation, which he called the vital character of mood with so-called first-rank symptoms in schizophrenia. Mostly the bodily feelings, which can also be localized in the throat (globus melancholicus) and as pressure on the breast, are accompanied by psychic feelings. But the last ones can also be missing like in "depressio sine depressione." We think it is mostly not an alteration of mood plus bodily feelings but that the patients themselves localize their being depressed into the body, into an emptiness of their head, into the throat, into the breast, into the stomach, etc. A general psychomotor inhibition is often accompanied by a heavy body, an increased drive by bodily restlessness.

Several philosophers like Sartre, Merleau-Ponty, and Schmitz have given important contributions to the phenomenology of the body in general. Thus, it was said that our body is not only a being thrown in some way ("Geworfensein"), like being an object in a certain place and time but that our body is also a medium for giving access to the world. Because of our being-in-the-world ("In-der-Welt-sein") with our body most of the time, we have only a lateral consciousness of our body. But this is not the case in melancholia, in which the body is not transcended to the world, but is experienced in its weight and as an obstacle. Normally, we do not feel the physical substance and weight of our body or of our organs, like our larynx, our heart, and our chest, but in melancholia we feel our larynx as a "globus melancholicus" and the resistance of our chest in every inspiration. Dörr-Zegers and Tellenbach (1980) spoke of a becoming "chrematic of our experience," with which these authors anticipated the notion of "corporealization" of Fuchs (2000, 2005) and Kraus (1995b, 2014a, b) and of "reification" of Fuchs (2011) and Kraus (2014b). This corporeal feeling of weight cannot be separated from the loss of psychic élan, from the general psychomotor inhibition, immobility, and dropping down of the whole body, particularly if we compare it with the lightness of the body in mania. This heaviness of the body in melancholia is combined with the feeling of a loss of possible being and loss of the future, of not being able to do anything. Here the dialectic ambiguity of having and being a body vanishes for the benefit of being a body. Because we think that the "corporealization of the body" is secondary to a primary diminution of the Subject-I in melancholic mood as well as in melancholic anxieties, we would now prefer to speak of a hypo-personalization. In consequence of the deficit of the Subject-I to react to the "me" in vitalizing the body, the body becomes "corporealized" also with the consequences of an alteration of the normal bodily feelings and loss of transcendence of the body to the world in the psychomotor inhibition. If we speak here of primary and secondary, this is not meant in a temporal sequence or causal relationship, but in the sense of constitution. Being a body and having a body stay in a dialectical relationship to each other. Having a body always involves a certain distance to the body. Otherwise it is not possible to transcend the body to the environment and to others. This distance of having a body is constituted by the Subject-I, by Ego-Achievements, respectively, originating mostly in the Subject-I [more details on bodily feelings, somatic and psychomotor symptoms, on Fuchs (2000) and Schmitt (2015)].

What we said about the distance of having a body and the need of Ego-Achievements is also true in the case of mourning. As we showed, mourning as well as every normal feeling needs the possibility to behave to oneself and to the mourned object. This "behaving to" is an Ego-Achievement which constitutes the normal bodily feelings of a mourner. The loss of Ego-Achievements makes it impossible to have the feelings of a mourner and thus leads to the corporealized ("verkörperlicht") and "distinct quality" of depression and the general loss of feeling for feeling ("Gefühl für Gefühllosigkeit") (K. Schneider 1967, p. 119). Fuchs (2011) instead sees "corporealization" as primary in a partly causal sense to the manifestation of most of the psychic phenomena in depression. These are in his view secondary to the body alterations and to the reduction of vital dynamics, i.e., the melancholic anxiety founded in a fixation of a narrowness of the body, the impossibility or loss of feeling for others in the loss of intercorporeality ("Zwischenleiblichkeit", p. 40), and the impossibility to weep in the impossibility to let oneself "fall in the spontaneity of the body." Fuchs (2000) also derives delusional experiences partly from the bodily restriction and inhibition of drive.

10.4.5 Melancholic Delusions, Anxieties, and Self

Feelings of anxiety in melancholia mostly occur in delusional and agitated states. Only a part of these anxieties are understandable. This is the case, if the patient fears consequences of his/her depression, not to be equal to his/her professional or familial tasks or demands. Partially understandable are also his/her multiple anxieties not to be able to do many things, particularly those which relate to Ego-Achievements, and also fears relating to his/her delusional ideas, as long as the patient is open for arguments and does not show a complete intolerance of cognitive and emotional ambiguity. The border of incomprehensibility is reached and delusional (in the traditional sense), respectively psychotic experience starts when the patient overgeneralizes her anxieties in saying that she never will be able to do anything, never will be healthy again, or making any other a priori assumptions. The last ones are given when the fears not only relate to certain objects, but to the whole being of the patient saying, e.g., my whole being is rotten or guilty. Often in delusional melancholia, we can observe that the patient easily changes the respective object of her delusional ideas, or generalizes the object of these, e.g., if she speaks of a general loss of feeling of the worth of everything in the sense of a nihilistic delusion. Here the patient may also doubt if she ever can have normal relationships to others, to the world, and to herself. These anxieties in our view are different from what K. Schneider (1967) denominates as primary anxieties ("Urängste") or basic anxieties ("Grundängste"). Whereas K. Schneider's basic anxieties, i.e., illness, impoverishment, and sin against anything ("Versündigung"), are related to concrete threats, delusional anxieties in melancholia are in our view not only related to certain objects (contents) but also to the a priori assumption to have lost all conditions of the possibility of being and having as such. In the sense of Husserl, these are anxieties of the loss of transcendental or constitutive possibilities. Insofar as melancholic delusional anxieties can reach to such fundamental anxieties of not being able to constitute, e.g., a self, they are completely detached from every normal experience. We would speak here of melancholic anxieties of constitution, which we deem as being highly specific for melancholic delusion. An overview of different aspects of anxiety is given by Géraud (2011).

Compared to the delusional ideas of schizophrenics, the delusional ideas of melancholics are from the aspect of their contents intra- and transculturally relatively constant. Relatively often we find delusional self-reproaches of guilt, delusions of insufficiency, delusions of inferiority, delusions of an impoverishment, and delusional hypochondria. A basic transhistorical-anthropological constancy seems to exist (Schmidt-Degenhard 2013).

Already K. Schneider (1967) put the question whether the topics of cyclothymic depressives are dependent on the premorbid values of the respective individual. Normally the individual self is mainly determined and definable by its values. Janzarik (1956, 1957a, b, 1966) in several articles with case studies investigated the relationship of central individual values to the individual topics of delusion in melancholic depressives. He could show that topics of delusional guilt are mainly to be found in warmhearted personalities with ties to others. They had also more than other delusional depressives a higher dependency on personal instancies, like God. Delusions of insufficiency ("Insuffizienzwahn") relate to the delusional assumption of not being able to go or to eat. They often show a general assumption of not being able to do anything, which is as such an immediate articulation of what we call an insufficient subject (Kraus 2014a). Delusions of inferiority relate to the worth of one's being. According to Janzarik (1956) delusions of impoverishment are mainly to be found in patients who in a particular way are rooted in their property, like farmers and businessmen, because their profession and keeping as well as increasing their property are equal. Melancholic patients with hypochondria are more centered on themselves than on the world and others (Janzarik 1957a). Here the bodily being of oneself is in the foreground, i.e., "the bodily basis of being a self" according to Fuchs (2011, p. 147). In our understanding the body itself is not a self, because it cannot be an object for itself, which is necessary for the definition of any self.

Kaestner (1947) in his interesting article on the behavior of melancholics in relation to values speaks of a being fixed to their values. In our identity-theoretical understanding, this fixation means a being overidentified with certain values. According to Kaestner on one hand, the conscious knowing of a value is preserved, but on the other hand, there is a fading away of the feeling of values ("Wertverlöschen"). We would say, whereas the identification with one's central values increases, in the same time, these values become devalued, i.e., felt as not existing anymore.

How is this seeming contradiction to be understood with our model of the Self without the assumption of an endogenous process? We already showed how the Self normally originates in a steady reaction of the Subject-I on the Object-I, thus activating the personal values as part of one's Object-I. With the general decrease of Ego-Achievements, in alliance with an insufficient Subject-I, in the melancholic episode, this positive effect of the Subject-I on the Object-I, on one's values, respectively, decreases. This corresponds to Janzarik's structural-dynamic concept of an inhibition of the actualization of values. This inhibition is mainly a loss of the feeling of values or, as Janzarik put it, is an emotional and intentional losing of power ["Emotionale und Intentionale Entmächtigung" (Janzarik 1966, p. 457)].

In the so-called nihilistic delusions, first described by Cotard (1882), all values, even one's being and the existence of the world, are negated. It seems as if the actualization of the whole Object-I cannot be realized, particularly not the lived body. It is possible that the patient maintains not to exist, though speaking with us. According to K. Schneider (1967, p. 122) such claims are only partially delusional, but also hallucinative "alterations of the body" can lead to such experiences. A further development of such a state could be a mutistic stupor. This in our view nearly complete loss of the Subject-I can be called a depersonalization in its highest degree.

Summing up we can say, delusions of guilt are related to a lack of one's identity or self, based in a supposed or real failure in one's relationship to others. Delusions of insufficiency are related to a lack of one's identity felt in the unworthiness of one's achievements and abilities, delusions of inferiority to a lack of identity felt in one's missing worth of one's self, delusions of impoverishment to a lack of identity felt in the unworthiness of one's property, and hypochondriacal delusions to the identity based on the feeling of unworthiness of one's body.

It is characteristic of the contents of melancholic Delusions that these on one hand relate to something which is objectively given, but on the other hand also often to the feeling of an alteration of the Self of the patient. This double orientation is due to her emotional, perceptive, and cognitive Intol. amb. which leads to a holistic, one-sided loss of the (outer) reality (e.g., delusion of impoverishment) as well as a loss of herself (e.g., anxiety of emptiness of one's self). The Intol. amb. in this case results in a hypo-realization of her property as well as a hypo-personalization of the Self. The same is analogously true for other kinds of delusion. The border between anxieties relating to the felt alteration of the Self and their transition to delusional, content-oriented experiences is often difficult to determine by the diagnostician. The informations of the patients about their delusions often have this double structure and only those relating to (outer) objects can be proven and assessed as a false judgment, even if there is no doubt that the feelings concerning the depersonalization of the Self also really exist. Then the informations about the alteration of the Self which cannot be proven by the criterion of reality can easily be taken as mere anxieties by the diagnostician. The presumption of the patient about the (outer) objects might, however, be only a secondary projection of the primary feelings of anxieties and of the alteration of the Self.

Compared to the traditional understanding of delusions, the definition of delusions is now much more strict. In the AMDP-System (2007), delusion is defined by a misjudgment of reality, which is asserted by a priori certainty. If we start from this definition, only the information which the patient gives about the (outer) reality can be judged as delusion. DSM-5-TM (2013) differentiates between mood-congruent delusions and hallucinations and mood-incongruent ones under the specifier "with psychotic features." Mood congruence corresponds to our notion of Intol. amb. Mood congruence is "typical" (DSM-5-TM (2013), p. 186). We do not deal here with atypical delusions.

10.5 Some Remarks on Psychotherapeutic Guidance and Rehabilitation

It is self-evident that our orientation to the Self in the premorbid personality as well as in the melancholic episode is of major importance for the psychotherapeutic guidance of melancholic patients. We cannot enter into details here. The core of what we call "identity therapy" (Kraus 1995a, b in English; Kraus 1998 in French; Kraus 2011 in German) should consider that with the Self of these patients, we have to do with an overidentified identity structure, i.e., an overidentification with certain representatives of identity. In Mead's concept of the Self, consisting of an "I" (Subject-I) and a "me" (Object-I), the Self has a dialectical structure. Insofar as the Subject-I is designing oneself ("Selbstentwurf"), it is constantly producing the Self anew. Because melancholics have a weak Subject-I, they need to compensate this lack by overidentifying themselves with their social roles as part of their Object-Identities (the "me").

Apart from encouraging and fostering Ego-Achievements in "identity-oriented psychotherapy," we should always take into account that the T. mel. and the Intol. amb. should on one hand be seen as competences compensating the lack of

Ego-Achievements, while on the other hand they are also vulnerability factors, insofar as they can also prevent the development and application of Ego-Achievements. This double aspect of these kinds of behavior as well as of the overidentified identity should always be considered, particularly in the melancholic episode, with respect to psychotherapy and rehabilitation. On one hand it is necessary in the first phase of therapy to lighten the load of the duties of the social roles of the patient and, on the other hand, take into account the importance of reconstructing her social role identities in order to prevent a chronification of the depression or even its worsening due to an increasing loss of identities as the consequence of the illness itself. Thus, the knowledge of the dynamics of the Self is very important in order to recognize possible precipitating situations (life events) of melancholic episodes in the future as well as to understand a melancholic phase itself in its social consequences, e.g., as a possible main "event" for a further negative course of the illness. This is one of the most important topics of psychotherapeutic guidance of melancholics.

10.6 Summary

In current manuals of diagnosis and classification (DSM-5-TM (2013)), the notion of melancholia is much more restricted than it was before. This is partly due to methodological reasons or to an operational reductionism, which among other dimensions excludes many aspects of melancholia, with which the methods of the so-called Phenomenological-Anthropological Psychiatry are concerned. With respect to diagnostics, the "Phenomenological-Anthropological" methods can supplement the Criteriological-Symptomatological ones. Thus, criteria and symptoms can be supplemented by "Phenomena of Essence," Disturbance Entities by "Existential Types" or "Entities of Essences" ("Wesenseinheiten"), and "Anthropological Proportions."

Our main aim was to show aspects of the Self of the premorbid personality of melancholics as well as of clinical phenomena of melancholia, which in the manuals as well as in specialist literature are not sufficiently considered. This question of the Self in melancholia has now got a very strong impulse by the worldwide intense empirical research on the melancholic type of personality, particularly in the sense of Typus melancholicus (T. mel.).

We have supplemented the research on the personality of melancholics by three further concepts. The first one is that the behavior in the sense of the T. mel. on the level of qualities of personality with extreme diligence at work, orderliness, and symbiotic features is mainly oriented to social norms and to the needs of others. Hence, it is ego-syntonic and can as such, in our view, be contrasted to dystonic, autistic, and obsessive-compulsive behavior.

Our second concept states that in fulfilling social expectations, the hypernomic behavior helps to build up social identities, in particular role identities. The behavior of the T. mel., thus, compensates a lack of Ego-Achievements, which according to our first concept is primary, so that in our view, the behavior of the T. mel. is not, as Tellenbach put it, primary, but secondary.

Our third concept is that of Intol. amb. Intol. amb. is inverse in the premorbid state of unipolar melancholics to that in unipolar manics and bipolars. Like the T. mel. or hypernomic behavior, it also tries to compensate the primary lack of Ego-Achievements. Similar to the behavior of the T. mel., it describes on one hand content-oriented, single personality traits, but on the other hand, like orderliness in the view of Tellenbach, it is also a formal structure determining the single traits of the T. mel and T. man. as the expression of a particular type of essence.

Intol. amb. as a formal structure is more basic than the T. mel., because it also comprises the T. mel. behavior in its one-sided, pervasive, formal structure of being determined mainly by social norms and by others in contrast to the behavior of the T. man. As a formal structure of a pervasive, perceptive, and cognitive one-sidedness, Intol. amb. determines not only the premorbid personality but also the phenomena of the clinical states of melancholia and mania. The behavior of the T. man. and of Intol. amb. in mania is mostly opposite to that in melancholia. In mania, we have Ego-Achievements, but also Pseudo-Ego-Achievements at the expense of an orientation to the needs of others and also the norms of society.

We use G.H. Mead's concept of the Self built up by the two poles of "I" and "me," by us taken up as Subject-I and Object-I, to show the behavior of the T. mel. and T. man. on the level of Identity or the Self of the patient. Ego-Achievements originate mostly in the Subject-I. T. mel. behavior is mostly oriented to the Object-I., particularly to social norms, showing hypernomic behavior. T. man. instead is oriented to the Subject-I, often ignoring the needs of others and social norms, in this way showing hyponomic behavior. Thus, the behavior, cognitions, and perceptions in the sense of Intol. amb. depend on the melancholic and manic episode with an orientation to inverse extremes.

T. mel. and T. man. behavior as well as Intol. amb. can have a protecting as well as a vulnerating function. We restrict ourselves to T. mel. and Intol. amb., because mania is not our primary topic. T. mel. behavior and Intol. amb. have a protecting function inside and outside of the melancholic episodes, insofar as these kinds of behavior seek to preserve all representatives of identity localized in the Object-I, e.g., by keeping up role identity, by means of fulfilling possibly all expectations of their social roles, by taking overall needs of others, as well as by harmonizing behavior. All these kinds of behavior can however also be vulnerability factors because of the dependency of the melancholic on this kind of behavior. If the protecting function of the T. mel. and of Intol. amb. behavior for the Object-I fails, this can, because of the lack of the Subject-I, have severe negative consequences for the self. The breakdown of the self can precipitate a melancholic or manic episode. The breakdown of the Self and the Intol. amb. describes and explains not only the precipitation of the melancholic and manic episodes, their symptoms, and phenomena, but in particular the "distinctive quality" of the melancholic mood and "corporealization" of the body, the specificity of melancholic anxieties and delusions, and so on. Melancholic delusions in our view are specified, direct expressions of the damage on the respective dimensions of the object-I and of the lack of the subject-I.

Because most of the symptoms and phenomena of melancholic episode are a consequence of the impeded functions of the self, we prefer to speak of melancholia as a melancholic kind of hypo-personalization.

References

Abraham, K. (1971). Versuch einer Entwicklungsgeschichte der Libido aufgrund der Psychoanalyse seelischer Störungen. In *Psychoanalytische Studien*, Bd. 1. Frankfurt: Fischer.

Akiskal, H. S. (1996). The temperamental foundations of affective disorders. In C. Mundt, M. J. Goldstein, K. Hahlweg, & P. Fiedler (Eds.), *Interpersonal factors in the origin and course of affective disorders*. London: Gaskell.

Ambrosini, A., Stanghellini, G., & Langer, A. I. (2011). El typus melancholicus de Tellenbach en la actualidad: una revisión sobre la personilidad premórbida vulnerable a la melancolia. *Actas Españolas de Psiquiatría, 39*(5), 302–311.7.

AMDP. (2007). *Das AMDP-System*, 8. Auflage. Göttingen: Hogrefe.

Andreasen, N. J. C. (2007). DSM and the death of phenomenology in America: An example of unintended consequences. *Schizophrenia Bulletin, 33*(1), 108–112.

Angst, J., & Perris, C. (1968). Zur Nosologie endogener Depressionen. Vergleich der Ergebnisse zweier Untersuchungen. *Archiv Psychiatrie Zentralblatt gesammte Neurologie, 210*, 373–386.

Bibring, E. (1952). Das problem der depression. *Psyche, 6*, 81–101.

Binswanger, L. (1956). *Drei Formen von missglücktem Dasein*. Niemeyer: Tübingen.

Blankenburg, W. (1971). *Der Verlust der natürlichen Selbstverständlichkeit*. Stuttgart: Enke.

Bürgy, M. (2010). Zur Psychopathologie der Ich-Störungen. *Nervenarzt, 81*, 1097–1107.

Cohen, M. B., Baker, G., Cohen, R. A., Fromm-Reichmann, F., & Weigert, E. W. (1954). An intensive study of 12 cases of manic-depressive psychosis. *Psychiatry, 17*, 103–137.

Cotard, J. (1882). Du délire de négation. *Archives of Neurology, 4*, 152–172, 282–296.

Dörr-Zegers, O., & Tellenbach, H. (1980). Differential phänomenologie des depressiven Syndroms. Über melancholische und epileptische Depressivität. *Nervenarzt, 51*, 113–118.

Dreitzel, H. P. (1968). *Die gesellschaftlichen Leiden und das Leiden an der Gesellschaft*. Stuttgart: Enke.

DSM-5-TM. (2013). Arlington VA: American Psychiatric Association.

Falret, J. P. (1854). Leçons clinique de medicine mental, faites à l'hospice de la Salpétière, Paris.

Fiedler, P. (1995). *Persönlichkeitsstörungen*. 2. Auflage. Weinheim: Psychologie-Verlagsunion.

Fiedler, P. (2001). *Persönlichkeitsstörungen* 6. Auflage. Weinheim: Belz Verlag.

Fiedler, P. (2007). *Persönlichkeitsstörungen* 6. Auflage. Weinheim: Belz Verlag.

Frenkel-Brunswik, E. (1948). A study of prejudice in children. *Human Relations, 1*, 295–306.

Frenkel-Brunswik, E. (1949/1950) Intolerance of ambiguity as an emotional and perceptual personality variable. *Journal of Personality, 18*, 108–143.

Frenkel-Brunswik, E. (1951). Personality theory and perception. In R. R. Blake & G. V. Ramsey (Eds.), *Perception. An approach to personality* (pp. 356–419). New York: Ronald Press.

Freud, S. (1967). *Trauer und Melancholie* (S. 427–446). Ges. Werke, Bd. 10, 4. Auflage. Frankfurt/M: S. Fischer.

Fuchs, T. (2000). Psychopathologie von Leib und Raum. Steinkopf Darmstadt 2000.

Fuchs, T. (2005). Corporealized and disembodied minds. A phenomenological view of the body in melancholia and schizophrenia. *Philosophy, Psychiatry, and Psychology, 12*(2), 95–107.

Fuchs, T. (2011). Depression, Leiblichkeit, Zwischenleiblichkeit. In H. Faller, H. Lang (Hrsg.) Depression. *Klinik, Ursachen, Therapie*. Würzburg: Könighausen & Neumann.

Géraud, M. (2011). Anxiety and Its nosographic and psychopathologic place in German psychiatry. In S. Selek (Ed.), *Different views of anxiety disorders*. Rijeka: InTech Europe.

Goffmann, E. (1961). *Encounters*. Indianapolis, New York: Bobbs-Merrill Company.
Hecht, H., van Calker, D., Berger, M., & von Zerssen, D. (1998). Personality in patients with affective disorder and their relatives. *Journal of Affective Disorder, 51*, 33–43.
Heerlein, A., & Richter, P. (1991). Ambiguitätsintoleranz bei affektiven und schizophrenen Störungen. *Nervenarzt, 62*, 269–273.
Heerlein, A., Santander, J., & Richter, P. (1996a). Premorbid personality aspects in mood and schizophrenic disorders. *Comprehensive Psychiatry, 37*(6), 430–434.
Heerlein, A., Santander, J., & Richter, P. (1996b). Ambiguitätsintoleranz bei endogenen Psychosen aus transkultureller Sicht. *Fortschritte der Neurologie-Psychiatrie, 64*, 358–361.
Heerlein, A. et al. (2002). Persönlichkeitsaspekte bei Zwangskranken und endogen Depressiven. In T. Fuchs, & Ch Mundt (Hg) *Affekt und affektive Störungen. Phänomenologische Konzepte und empirische Befunde im Dialog* (S. 215–230). Paderborn: Ferdinand Schönigh.
ICD-10-V(F). (2005). H. Dilling, W. Momour, & M. H. Schmidt (Hg) Göttingen: H. Huber.
Janzarik, W. (1956). Der lebensgeschichtliche und persönlichkeitseigene Hintergrund des cyclothymen Verarmungswahns. *Archiv für Psychiatrie und Neurologie, 195*, 219.
Janzarik, W. (1957a). Die Schuldthematik und das individuelle Wertgefüge. In N. Petrilowitsch (Hrsg) *Das Gewissen als Problem* (S. 428–473). Darmstadt: Wiss Buchgesellschaft 1966.
Janzarik, W. (1957b). Die hypochondrischen Inhalte der cyclothymen Depression in ihren Beziehungen zum Krankheitstyp und zur Persönlichkeit. *Archiv Psychiatrie Zentralblatt gesammte Neurologie, 195*, 351–372.
Janzarik, W. (1966, 1957) Die zyklothyme Schuldthematik. In N. Petrilowitsch (Hrsg) *Das Gewissen als Problem*. Darmstadt: Wiss Buchges.
Jaspers, K. (1997). *General psychology*, Vol. 1 + 2. Transl. J. Hoenig, & M. W Hamilton. Baltimore, London: John Hopkins University Press.
Kaestner, G. (1947). *Das Wertverhalten der zyklothym Depressiven. Arbeiten zur Psychiatrie, Neurologie und ihren Grenzgebieten (Festschrift für Kurt Schneider)* (S. 159–173). Heidelberg: Scherer, Willsbach.
Kasahara, Y. (1976). The premorbid personality of depression. In Y. Kasahara (Ed.), *Psychopathology of manic-depressive illness* (Vol. I, pp. 1–29). Tokyo: Kobundo.
Kraepelin, E. (1913). Psychiatrie 8. Aufl. III *Band Klinische Psychiatrie II Teil*. Leipzig: Barth.
Kraus, A. (1971a) Der Typus melancholicus in östlicher und westlicher Forschung (der japanische Beitrag M. Shimodas zur premorbiden Persönlichkeit Manisch-Depressiver). *Nervenarzt, 42*, 481–483.
Kraus, A. (1971b) Situationstheoretische Aspekte der Auslösung manisch-depressiver Phasen. In: W. Walcher (Hrsg) Probleme der Provokation depressiver Psychosen. International Symposium, Graz. Brüder Hollinek, Wien, 1971, S. 117–123.
Kraus, A. (1977). *Sozialverhalten und Psychose Manisch-Depressiver*. Stuttgart: Enke.
Kraus, A. (1980). Vom Umgang Manisch-Depressiver mit sozialen Normen. *Medizin, Mensch, Gesellschaft, 5*, S250–255.
Kraus, A. (1982). Identity and psychosis of the manic-depressive. In A. De Koning & J. Jenner Fa (Eds.), *Phenomenology and Psychiatry* (pp. 201–216). London: Academic Press.
Kraus, A. (1988). Ambiguitätsintoleranz als Persönlichkeitsvariable und als Strukturmerkmal der Krankheitsphänomene Manisch-Depressiver. In W. Janzarik (Ed.), *Persönlichkeit und Psychose* (pp. 140–149). Stuttgart: Enke.
Kraus, A. (1991). Methodological problems with the classification of personality disorders: The significance of existential types. *Personality Disorders, 5*(1), 82–92.
Kraus, A. (1994). Phenomenological and criteriological diagnosis. Different or complementary? In J. Sadler, O. Wiggins, & M. Schwartz (Eds.), *Philosophical perspectives on psychiatric diagnostic classification* (pp. 148–160). Baltimore and London: The John Hopkins University Press.
Kraus, A. (1995a). Psychotherapy based on identity problems of depressives. *American Journal of Psychotherapy, 49*, 197–212.

Kraus, A. (1995b). *Analyse phénoménologique des troubles de l'éprouvé corporel dans la mé lancolie* (pp. 11–15). Sp VII: L'Encéphale.
Kraus, A. (1996a). Diagnostic phénomenologique and diagnostic symptomatologique-criteriologique. Synapse, no. spécial, mars 1996: 8–16.
Kraus, A. (1996b). Spezifität melancholischer Verstimmung und Angst. In: H. Lang, & H. Faller (Hrsg.) *Das Phänomen Angst. Pathologie, Genese und Therapie* (pp. 103–121). Frankfurt: Suhrkamp.
Kraus, A. (1996c). Role performance, identity structure and psychosis in melancholic and manic-depressive patients. In Ch. Mundt, M. J. Goldstein, K. Hahlweg, & P. Fiedler (eds.) *Interpersonal factors in the origin and course of affective disorders* (pp. 103–121). London: Gaskell.
Kraus, A. (1998). Thérapie de I'identité des melancholiques et de maniaco-depressives. Troubles de I'identité. *Confrontations Psychiatriques, 39*, 275–292.
Kraus, A. (2005). Phänomenologisch-anthropologische Aspekte der Diagnostik und der Klassifikation in der Psychiatrie: In D. Schmoll, & A. Kuhlmann (Hg) *Symptom und Phänomen* (S. 55–71). München: Karl Alber Verlag, Freiburg.
Kraus, A. (2007). Der Typus melancholicus als Normopath. In H. Lang, H. Faller, & M. Schowalter (Hg.) *Struktur, Persönlichkeit, Persönlichkeitsstörung* (pp. S. 193–209). Würzburg: Königshausen & Neumann.
Kraus, A. (2011). Identitätsorientierte Psychotherapie Melancholischer. In H. Faller, & H. Lang (Hg) *Depression, Klinik, Ursachen, Therapie* (S. 149–164). Würzburg: Königshausen & Neumann.
Kraus, A. (2013). Reaction and development of manics and melancholic depressives. In Th. Fuchs, & G. Stanghellini (Eds.) *Hundred years of K. Jaspers "General Psychopathology"*. Oxford: Oxford University Press.
Kraus, A. (2014a). Der Wahn Melancholischer und Manischer aus der Sicht von Veränderung des Selbst. In T. Fuchs, T. Breyer, S. Micali, & B. Wandruszka (Hrsg) *Freiburg*. München: Verlag Karl Alber.
Kraus, A. (2014b). Das Werden des Sebst Melancholischer in der Sicht Kobayashis' und der Identitätstheorie G.H. Mead's und J.P. Sartres' sowie Alfred Kraus. In F. Schäfer, & M. Roth (Hrsg) *Das Zwischen denken: Marx, Freud und Nishida*. Leipzig : Univeritätsverlag.
Kronmüller, K. T., Backenstrass, M., Reck, C., Kraus, A., Fiedler, P., & Mundt, C. (2002). Einfluss von Persönlichkeitsfaktoren und –struktur auf den Verlauf der Major-Depression. *Nervenarzt, 73*, 255–261.
Kronmüller, K. Th., Backenstrass, M., Kocherscheidt, K., Hunt, A., Fiedler, P., & Mundt, Ch. (2005). Dimensions of the typus melancholicus personality type. Original Paper.
Lang, H. (2003). Melancholie in phänomenologisch- antropologischer und struktural-analytischer Perspektive. In A. Michels (Hrsg) *Jahrbuch für Klinischepsychoanalyse Bd V Melancholie und Depression* (S. 235–249). Tübingen
Mead, G. H. (1934). *Mind, self, and society*. Chicago: University of Chicago Press.
Mead, G. H. (1980). *Geist, Identität und Gesellschaft*. Frankfurt/M: Suhrkamp.
Mundt, C. (2002). Psychological perspectives for the development of future diagnostic systems. *Psychopathology, 35*, 145–151.
Mundt, C., Backenstrass, M., Kronmüller, K.-T., Fiedler, P., Kraus, A., & Stanghellini, G. (1997). Personality and endogenous/major depression: An empirical approach to typus melancholicus. 2. Validation of typus melancholicus core-properties by personality inventory scales. *Psychopathology, 30*, 130–139.
Mundt, Ch. (2011). Depression und Altruismus. Zur Sozialpsychologie und Neurobiologie des Gutseins. In H. Faller, & H. Lang (Hrsg) *Depression. Klinik, Ursachen, Therapie* (pp. 29–37). Würzburg: Königshausen und Heumann.
Mundt, C., Schroeder, A., & Backenstraß, M. (2009). Altruism versus self-centeredness in the personality of depressives in the 1950s and 1990s. *Journal of Affective Disorders, 113*, 157–164.

Reck, C. (2001). *Kritische Lebensereignisse und Depression. Life-Event-Froschung im Überblick.* Pabst SCIENCE Publishers.
Saß, H. (1987). Die Krise der psychiatrischen Diagnostik. *Fortschritte der Neurologie und Psychiatrie, 55*, 355–360.
Sato, T., Sakado, K., Uelhara, T., & Sato, S. (1996). Importance of the melancholic type of personality for research into the premorbid personality of depression. In C. Mundt, M. J. Goldstein, K. Hahlweg, & P. Fiedler (Eds.), *Interpersonal factors in the origin and course of affective disorders.* London: Gaskell.
Schmidt-Degenhard, M. (1983). *Melancholie und Depression.* Stuttgart, Berlin, Köln, Mainz: W. Kohlhammer.
Schmidt-Degenhard, M. (2013). Versteinertes Dasein – Von der Schwarzgalligkeit zur depressiven Episode. In K. Brücher & M. Poltrum (Eds.), *Psychiatrische Diagnostik* (pp. 125–145). Berlin: Parados.
Schmitdt-Degenhard, M. (2005). Interpretative Situageneseforschung. In D. Schmoll, & A. Kuhlmann (Hg) *Symptom und Phänomen. Phänomenologische Zugänge zum kranken Menschen.* Freiburg München: Karl Alber.
Schneider, K. (1967). *Klinische Psychopathologie.* (8. Aufl.). Stuttgart: Thieme.
Stanghellini, G. (2004). *Disembodied spirits and deanimated bodies. The psychopathology of common sense.* Oxford: Oxford University Press.
Stanghellini, G., & Mundt, C. (1997). Personality and endogenous/major depression: An empirical approach to Typus melancholicus. *Psychopathology, 30*, 119–129.
Tellenbach, H. (1961). *Melancholie. Zur Problemgeschichte, Typologie, Pathogenese und Klinik.* Berlin, Göttingen, Heidelberg: Springer.
Tellenbach, H. (1980). Typus Melancholicus. In: Die Psychologie des 20. Jahrhunderts, Band X, Kindler, Zürich.
von Zerssen, D., & Pössel, J. (1990). The premorbid personality of patients with different subtypes of an affective illness. *Journal of Affective Disorders, 18*, 39–50.
von Zerssen, D. (1996a). Forschungen zur prämorbiden Persönlichkeit in der Psychiatrie der deutschsprachigen Länder: Die letzten drei Jahrzehnte. *Fortschritte der Neurologie und Psychiatrie, 64*, 168–183.
von Zerssen, D. (1996b). Melancholic and manic types of personality as premorbid structures in affective orders. In C. Mundt, M. J. Goldstein, K. Hahlweg, & P. Fiedler (Eds.), *Interpersonal factors in the origin and course of affective disorders* (pp. 65–88). London: Gaskell.
Zerssen von, D. (1977). Premorbid personality and affective psychoses. In Burrows (ed.) *Handbook of studies of depression* (pp. 79–103). Amsterdam-London-New York: Excerpta Medica.
Zerssen von, D. (2000). Persönlichkeit und affektive Störungen. In C. Mundt et al. (Hg) *Psychiatrie der Gegenwart, Band IV: Schizophrenie und affektive Störungen.* New York Heidelberg Berlin: Springer.
Zerssen von, D. (2001). Personality and affective disorder. In: Contemporary Psychiatry (Vol. 3, 1st ed.). In N. Sartorius et al. (Eds.) *Specific psychiatric disorders* (pp. 279–296). Berlin, Heidelberg: Springer.

The Phenomenological Approach to Patients with Bizarreness

11

Gareth S. Owen

The word "bizarre" in ordinary language simply means odd or very odd. Standard dictionaries define it in this way. Because of that, the word will associate with our ordinary language use of "madness" or whichever words a society uses, at a given time, to point toward behaviours, expressions and experiences considered abnormal or pathological.

But gaining expertise in psychopathology is to learn to go beyond ordinary language characterisations of madness. The apprenticeship involves developing approaches that enable one to (a) see different patterns in odd behaviour and experience (diagnostic types); (b) develop abilities to make sense of, empathise with and not shun mental states that go beyond the reach of common social communication (understanding); and (c) avoid error when attributing pathology (medicalising) or abnormal psychology (psychologising).

This chapter starts with three cases of bizarreness. These are used to discuss some interpretative issues in patients who present with bizarreness. Bizarre delusion in the *Diagnostic and Statistical Manual* (DSM) is critically examined, as is the relationship of bizarreness to the clinical phenomenology of schizophrenia. This chapter touches upon some of the communicative challenges that face clinicians and patients with bizarreness and the role of the lifeworld approach. The chapter ends with a summary of points relevant to the psychopathologist in training.

G.S. Owen (✉)
Department of Psychological Medicine, King's College London, Institute of Psychiatry, Psychology and Neuroscience, London, UK

South London and Maudsley NHS Foundation Trust, London, UK
e-mail: gareth.1.owen@kcl.ac.uk

G. Stanghellini, M. Aragona (eds.), *An Experiential Approach to Psychopathology*,
DOI 10.1007/978-3-319-29945-7_11

11.1 Three Cases of Bizarreness

Case 1

A psychiatrist is called to assess a man being held in police custody. The man called the police after assisting an elderly lady reporting a robbery. The police found the man to be impersonating a police officer and arrested him. The man is a foreigner, is not known to the police and is carrying a UK police identification that is a poor-quality cut-and-paste photocopy. Other than asserting that he is a police officer, he is mute. The police sergeant regards it as implausible that he is a police officer and the category "mad" is in the background.

In a psychiatric interview, the man avoids eye contact or communication, and his comportment expresses distress. The psychiatrist asks to see the confiscated belongings. Amongst his papers is a document from a police station in a small island in the Caribbean Sea. The doctor advises the police sergeant to make an international phone call. In cursory fashion, the sergeant speaks to a counterpart in a small island police station who immediately identifies the man as a long-lost colleague who left the island in a state of distress following an event in which he shot a boy during a police raid that went wrong. The psychiatrist returns to the man and recognises his police background and traumatic past, and the man starts to communicate. There is no evidence of major mental illness. The police officers quite literally put their arms around him.

Case 2

You are on a bus and start talking to the person sitting next to you about the weather. The conversation moves on, and the person recounts, thus:

> I went to Samoa. This has been my life in total. I never went there. I was taken there again. We got on the plane that took off, we were supposed to be flying local, we thought, like in France or something. The plane ended up in Tahiti, but the islands were called something in Samoa, so I can't remember whether it was Tahiti or Samoa we were in. I think we were in Samoa, but my family, someone was saying it was Tahiti. We landed on an Island. In those times they never had airstrips. The plane that brought us down was a cargo plane because they never had passenger planes. My brother got hold of me and there was a great white shark in the water, off a fair bit—it looked like somebody was carrying a door on their back—it was that big the shark, its fin.

You find yourself asking yourself: What does he mean? Am I hearing properly? Did he mean to say that? It sounds, you think to yourself, mad.

Note what is happening here. The ordinary familiarity with another is suddenly displaced or rendered problematic. From passively imbibing the other as someone more or less like yourself—communicating a shared concern with the weather—a gulf opens up between you and the communication becomes problematic. The other is now something "other". The experience of bizarreness here is happening in a social, or intersubjective, space—it is a mismatch between the sociality we expect and the sociality we are experiencing, but it is of a different type to case 1. In case 1, we are motivated from the start to get the story. What has happened? What are the historical facts that could make sense of this bizarreness? In case 2, we are motivated to step back from the encounter altogether—we experience puzzlement with the encounter itself.

Case 3

A psychiatrist is interviewing a patient, and the dialogue goes like this:

Patient: What I thought was he was a bird. And then he went into a midget and then into an ant. But I thought he was going through so much torture—you know what I mean?
Psychiatrist: Your father?
Patient: Yeah.
Psychiatrist: So he'd transformed from being. . .
Patient: A bird.
Psychiatrist: A bird.
Patient: To a midget.
Psychiatrist: You mean a small person?
Patient: No a midget is a little fly.
Psychiatrist: A fly. From a bird to a midget to. . .
Patient: Yeah.
Psychiatrist: To a fly. . .
Patient: To an ant.
Psychiatrist: To an ant. And that was real?
Patient: Yes. Well I don't know whether it was real or not but I could see. The pain was—you know what I mean—why was he going through torture you know what I mean.
Psychiatrist: How is that possible do you think? How do you explain that?
Patient: What?
Psychiatrist: Those transformations.
Patient: I thought somebody in here was torturing him and I couldn't understand why?
Psychiatrist: Were you seeing it or hearing it?
Patient: I saw it and could hear him. . . I watched the bird it was going down on the floor. And he was going through so much pain that he couldn't fly. When he was a bird he couldn't fly. And then when he was a midget flying around and then he went to an ant and I was looking at an ant and he was going through torture you know what I mean.
Psychiatrist: So you were seeing your father in the ant.
Patient: Not seeing him in the ant. He was the ant.

Here, bizarreness is a pervasive feature of the dialogue. The experience of "otherness" in case 2 is given, but the psychiatrist is maintaining the patient in a conversation in which meaning is being clarified. Communication is occurring—the psychiatrist and the patient are, so to speak, getting to know each other, but it is a communication where the meaning of words cannot be taken for granted and where the psychiatrist needs to leave space for the experience of the other to be in a different plane—outside the run of what has been referred to as "the axioms of everyday life" (Straus 1958). This is important in order to avoid the error of psychologising—inappropriately forcing bizarre experience into prior psychological theories—be they folk, cognitive, psychoanalytical or other theories—with the pseudo-understanding that can result.

11.2 DSM and Bizarre Delusions

Bizarreness is a particular feature of the diagnosis we call schizophrenia (see below). DSM operationalises bizarreness by linking the descriptor "bizarre" to a class of delusional beliefs ("bizarre delusions"). A bizarre delusion has particular weight in the criterion set defining schizophrenia in DSM. In DSM-5 (American Psychiatric Association 2013), much like earlier versions, delusions are deemed bizarre if they are clearly implausible and not understandable to same-culture peers and do not derive from ordinary life experiences. The manual goes on to list thought withdrawal, thought insertion and delusions of control as exemplars of bizarre delusions and gives an example of a belief that an outside force has removed internal organs and replaced them with someone else's organs without leaving a wound or scar. That would be a bizarre delusion whereas a belief that one is under surveillance by the police, despite a lack of convincing evidence, would not be.

This pragmatic approach has its place and its uses. Contained within it are some of the interpretative points we have already discussed. But there is a clear need to go further. Firstly, is the issue of reliability. Using the DSM construct, different interviewers assessing the same patient agree on there being a bizarre delusion with reliability estimates that are poor in some studies and good in others (Cermolacce et al. 2010). What enables good agreement between raters? These studies indicate that it is not the DSM construct of bizarre delusion alone. Secondly, is the issue of validity. Bizarreness is not exclusive to one psychological function (belief) nor is it exclusive to schizophrenia. Postures, expressions, sensations and representations of all sorts (e.g. bodily representation, drawings, handwriting) can all be bizarre, but they are not beliefs. Beliefs can also be bizarre in patients who clearly do not have schizophrenia. Take these examples (all likely to induce profound puzzlement in others):

(a) *Bizarre beliefs emerging in the context of delirium and dementia (after (Cutting* 2012*), p66(4)).*

Irish Catholics from Streatham (London suburb) are driving to Brixton (neighbouring suburb) and harming indigenous people by transmitting decomposed matter into their necks.

There is a "phantom boarder" in the house.

(b) *Bizarre beliefs emerging in the context of depression and mania (Owen, unpublished).*

> I am the only person in the hospital; it is empty. There is no one inside or outside the hospital. Everyone has gone.
>
> I never believed in a creator until 1991, and that was only because my daughter said she was Christ when she was 18 months.

So DSM is (a) not giving sufficient guidance to the interviewer to identify bizarre delusions in schizophrenia with much precision and (b) over-restricting the clinical phenomenology of bizarreness to beliefs held by people with schizophrenia.

11.3 Bizarreness and the Clinical Phenomenology of Schizophrenia

As we have seen, bizarreness has been linked to schizophrenia. This predates DSM, and the roots of this are worth the psychopathologist in training knowing about—history lending orientation. In Kraepelin and Bleuler, much of their descriptive work attests to the peculiarity, or oddness, in the patients they grouped under the category schizophrenia (Kraepelin initially calling it "dementia praecox"). Kraepelin's metaphor "the orchestra without a conductor" captures his impression of strangeness (think of the music of an orchestra as it warms up before the arrival of the conductor). Bleuler's emphasis on "autism" as a critical feature of the grouping summarises his impression of oddness.

The European psychiatrists Jaspers, Rümke and Schneider conducted more rigorous phenomenological analysis of bizarreness. Jaspers drew attention to "understandability" or the process by which one grasps a mental state by way of its social or psychological antecedents, for example, understanding the development of a character in a novel. This is the point made by case 1 where the bizarreness melts away when the historical and biographical information becomes known. Jaspers taught that this kind of understanding can experience limits in psychiatry—not limits of time, information or imagination on the part of the interviewer but limits of principle. There are cases of bizarreness, said Jaspers, where, despite considerable effort in gaining personal and contextual information, understanding does not emerge and "ununderstandability" presents as primary. Jaspers taught that these limits of understandability have significance vis a vis the diagnosis of schizophrenia. In other words, when we experience ununderstandability in clinical interviews, the concept "schizophrenia" can be considered.

Rümke drew attention to the intersubjective (social) element discussed in case 2. In interaction, Rümke taught that one can become aware of a characteristic absence of a communication instinct. Rümke thought this could be identified as a feeling in the experienced interviewer and that the psychopathologist needs to learn to identify it in himself/herself. By that he meant that the evidence for this lack of communication instinct was not to be found in what the psychiatrist impersonally observes in the patient but in the feeling that manifests in the interviewer during an interaction. Rümke tried to characterise this feeling as "a stiffness of affect" (calling it the "praecox feeling") (Rumke 2012). He acknowledged the potential problems with reliability, but gave it weight in the diagnosis of schizophrenia.

Schneider tried to render the whole approach more practical. As well as the intersubjective phenomenon that may be present at interview, he thought that there were symptoms that were particularly good indicators of core schizophrenia. Most of these symptoms have an affinity to what other German psychopathologists called "Ich-Storung" or disturbances of the self.

Schneider considered them as indicating "a primary disorder of the consciousness of a subject's own execution of mental functions" (John Cutting, personal correspondence). But ultimately, he simply listed symptoms—all of them odd experiences—and called them "first rank" (i.e. of particular significance, or heuristic value, for a diagnosis of schizophrenia) (Cutting 2012; Schneider 1974; Mellor 1970). They are:

1. Audible thoughts (voices speaking thoughts aloud)
2. Voices arguing (two or more hallucinatory voices discussing the subject in the third person)
3. Voices commenting on ones actions (voices describing subject's activities as they occur)
4. Somatic passivity (the experience of influences playing on the body or the experience of bodily sensations imposed by external agency)
5. Thought withdrawal (thoughts cease and subject simultaneously experiences them as removed by external force)
6. Thought insertion (thoughts have quality of not being mine and are ascribed to external agency)
7. Thought broadcasting (thoughts escape, or diffuse, into the outside world where they are experienced by others)
8. Made feelings (feelings not mine and attributed to external agency)
9. Made impulses (drive or impulse seems to be alien and external)
10. Made volitional acts (actions and movements not experienced as mine and felt to be under outside control)
11. Delusional perception (normal perception which has a private, highly significant, anomalous meaning)

So the clinical phenomenology of bizarreness has been coupled to the clinical phenomenology of a diagnostic entity—schizophrenia. That this linking should be so tight is doubtful. As we have seen, the bizarre features of other major psychiatric illnesses (e.g. organic brain syndromes, affective disorders) can be striking but have received much less phenomenological attention than schizophrenia. The psychopathologist needs to be careful about diagnosing schizophrenia on the basis of finding bizarreness without further qualification. The *quality* of the bizarreness is important as is its pervasiveness in the whole course of the illness.

11.4 Bizarre Lifeworlds

Models of psychosis span neuroscience, cognitive psychology and social science. As scientific models, their primary value lies in the power to predict mental states and to modify them. As it currently stands, the power of existing models to do this is limited. Some models can extend our imaginative grasp of bizarreness somewhat (Kendler and Campbell 2014). With the lifeworld approach to bizarreness, imaginative grasp is the main goal. In distinction to the scientific modelling referred to, the lifeworld approach does not have prediction or intervention as a sine qua non. Instead, the primary value is to *illuminate* the worlds of people with mental disorders a little bit like how an anthropologist illuminates the world of a far off culture and tribe to enable communication with it and distinguish it from other cultures and tribes. The approach aspires to, as it were, *pure understanding*, and its role in improving scientific modelling, whilst to be hoped for, is not a sole motive.

The lifeworld approach cannot be fully accounted for here. It comprises an approach that draws heavily upon philosophy—particularly those parts of philosophy called phenomenology, existentialism, hermeneutics and philosophical anthropology. The approach is not recent although recent guides to old literatures are now available (Broome et al. 2012) and new work continues. The approach looks at bizarreness, as other aspects of psychopathology, in terms of change to categories of human experience such as time, space, self, body, value, etc. Binswanger carried out one of the earliest lifeworld analyses of autism in schizophrenia (Broome et al. 2012). One of his cases involved a 39-year-old married woman with schizophrenia named Ilse who loved her father but wanted to stop his tyrannical behaviour toward her mother. She put her right hand into a burning stove in order to show her father "what love can do". In his analysis, Binswanger tries to focus on the core phenomenological features or this ordeal by fire. He considers them to be (1) a quality of climbing too high ("extravagant"), (2) a kind of tortured logic ("perverse") and (3) a role play-like behaviour ("manneristic"). In more recent lifeworld analyses of bizarreness in patients with schizophrenia, it is seen as constituted by a mode of experiencing characterised by hyperflexivity with respect to self (Sass and Parnas 2003) or, seen from a different perspective, an inability to evaluate pragmatically (Stanghellini 2004; Cutting 1997). Sass has drawn illuminating attention to the affinities this lifeworld has with the cultural zeitgeist of "modernism" (Sass 1992) and Cutting and McGhilchrist to the affinities with the neuropsychology of the left hemisphere of the human brain when working alone (McGhilchrist 2009; Cutting 1997). On these more recent accounts, Ilse's "ordeal by fire" could be seen as an act constituted by logic without common sense and by hyperreflexivity. Her ordeal by fire "role play" (disordered though it seems) could be seen as a modernist performance—and one that the right hemisphere of the brain would disavow.

In general, rather than taking bizarreness, by itself, as pathological or as identical to one diagnosis, the lifeworld approach traces bizarreness to an underpinning alteration, or disproportion, in human experiencing.

11.5 Communication

In the clinical interaction with bizarreness, we can often experience, as in case 3 but also in (a) and (b) above, a refractory struggle to achieve communication. An ongoing dispute that runs through the history of psychiatry/psychology is the extent to which such communication is possible and also what successful communication in this setting is supposed to comprise. Much of the psychopathologist's apprenticeship here will be to learn to accept that there are moments of communicative contact and understanding and moments when it is far off indeed. Taking communication for granted, or over-projecting an imagined lifeworld, needs to be guarded against. In the spirit of phenomenology, we need to go to the things themselves, and if the phenomenon is, at times, a communicative impasse, then that is the phenomenon.

But clinicians also need to guard against retreating to a psychologically safe position whereby communicating with patients with bizarreness is avoided—risking de-humanising both of them. With patients like case 3 the clinician is given a communicative challenge but it is neither frightening nor meaningless.

The clinician taking an interest in the lifeworlds of their patients with bizarreness is going to be more interested in communication and more equipped to put communication at the core of their clinician–patient relationship.

11.6 Summary

We can conclude with the following points:

Bizarre presentations can melt away in the face of careful psychosocial assessment. Competence in that assessment therefore protects against medicalising (case 1).

The sense of the other as "other" within a communication has a distinctive phenomenological structure that can help to correctly identify the patient with bizarreness (case 2).

Bizarreness of belief has been strongly linked to schizophrenia but bizarreness is not specific to belief (expressions, perceptions, etc. can be bizarre) nor to schizophrenia (bizarreness may be seen in organic syndromes and in affective disorders).

The clinical phenomenology of bizarreness in schizophrenia has a specific quality.

Patients with bizarreness can present communicative challenges. The lifeworld approach to bizarreness offers the clinician–patient relationship support.

Acknowledgements This work was supported by the Wellcome Trust.

References

American Psychiatric Association. (2013). DSM-5: Diagnostic and statistical manual of mental disorders (5th Ed.). American Psychiatric Publishing.

Broome, M., Harland, R., Owen, G. S., & Stringaris, A. (Eds.). (2012). *The Maudsley reader in phenomenological psychiatry*. Cambridge: Cambridge University Press.

Cermolacce, M., Sass, L., & Parnas, J. (2010). What is bizarre in bizarre delusions? A critical review. *Schizophrenia Bulletin, 36*, 667–679.

Cutting, J. (1997). *Principles of psychopathology, two worlds - two minds - two hemispheres*. Oxford: Oxford University Press.

Cutting, J. (2012). *A critique of psychopathology*. Berlin: Parados Verlag.

Kendler, K. S., & Campbell, J. (2014). Expanding the domain of the understandable in psychiatric illness: An updating of the Jasperian framework of explanation and understanding. *Psychological Medicine, 44*(1), 1–7.

McGhilchrist, I. (2009). *The Master and his Emissary*. New Haven: Yale University Press.

Mellor, C. S. (1970). First rank symptoms of schizophrenia. *British Journal of Psychiatry, 117*, 15–23.

Rümke, H. (2012). The nuclear symptom of schizophrenia and the praecox feeling. In M. Broome, R. Harland, G. Owen, & A. Stringaris (Eds.), *The Maudsley reader in phenomenological psychiatry*. Cambridge: Cambridge University Press.

Sass, L. (1992). *Madness and modernism*. Cambridge, MA: Harvard University Press.

Sass, L., & Parnas, J. (2003). Schizophrenia, consciousness and the self. *Schizophrenia Bulletin, 29*, 427–444.

Schneider, K. (1974). Primary and secondary symptoms in schizophrenia. In S. R. Hirsch & M. Shepherd (Eds.), *Themes and variations in European psychiatry*. Bristol: Wrights.

Stanghellini, G. (2004). *Disembodied spirits and deanimated bodes: The psychopathology of common sense*. Oxford: Oxford University Press.

Straus, E. W. (1958). Aesthesiology and hallucinations. In R. May, E. Angel, & H. Ellenberger (Eds.), *Existence*. New York: Basic Books.

Capgras Syndrome

12

Femi Oyebode

12.1 Introduction

The Capgras syndrome is perhaps one of the best-known examples of the delusional misidentification syndromes. It is characterized by the firmly held but false belief that an impostor has replaced a familiar person (Abbate et al. 2012; Christodoulou et al. 2009; Ellis et al. 1994; Silva and Leong 1992). The other delusional misidentification syndromes include Frégoli syndrome, syndrome of intermetamorphosis, syndrome of subjective doubles, delusion of inanimate doubles and reduplicative paramnesia (Anderson and Williams 1994; Christodoulou et al. 2009; Ellis et al. 1994). Central to these conditions is the unifying theme of "the double". In Frégoli syndrome the subject believes that an unfamiliar person is really a disguised familiar person, whereas in the syndrome of intermetamorphosis, the subject believes that the unfamiliar and familiar person are identical because of shared physical characteristics such as hair colour or shape of the nose. The syndrome of subjective doubles is characterized by the belief that a double of the self is abroad in the world acting in such a way as to damage the subject's reputation. The delusion of inanimate doubles refers to the belief that inanimate objects have been duplicated and replaced, whereas reduplicative paramnesia refers to the belief that places have been duplicated.

The delusional misidentification syndromes occur in schizophrenia, in affective disorders and in organic brain diseases (Christodoulou et al. 2009; Feinberg and Roane 2005; Förstl et al. 1994; Joseph et al. 1999; Oyebode 2008; Sidoti and Lorusso 2007). There is evidence that the right hemisphere has a role in the pathogenesis of these disorders (Cutting 1991; Ellis 1994; Förstl et al. 1991) and that impairment of face processing including impairment of face recognition

F. Oyebode (✉)
National Centre for Mental Health, University of Birmingham, 25 Vincent Drive, Edgbaston, Birmingham B15 2FG, UK
e-mail: Femi.Oyebode@bsmhft.nhs.uk

G. Stanghellini, M. Aragona (eds.), *An Experiential Approach to Psychopathology*,
DOI 10.1007/978-3-319-29945-7_12

memory is an important underlying anomaly in subjects who present with delusional misidentification syndrome (Breen et al. 2000; Edelstyn et al. 1996, 1998; Oyebode 2008; Paillère-Martinot et al. 1994; Silva and Leong 1995). The fact that delusional misidentification syndromes are associated with neurological, neuropsychological and neurophysiological correlates makes them ideal subjects for further investigation as to the origin and genesis of delusions (Christodoulou et al. 1981; Förstl et al. 1994; Ismail et al. 2012; Munro 1994; Paillère-Martinot et al. 1994; Papageorgiou et al. 2003, 2005).

In this chapter, I will describe a paradigmatic case of Capgras syndrome with a view to analyzing the central, typical and characterizing features emphasizing the first-person account and subjective experience. I will then discuss the phenomenology, diagnosis, classification, pathogenesis, management and outcome of delusional misidentification syndromes.

Case Study

Case History

A female patient first presented at age 56 years in acute emotional distress manifest as total insomnia, motor restlessness, agitation and a profound inability to fully verbally express or explain her problems. This sudden onset had occurred in the setting of her husband discovering, by chance, that she had been having an affair with the same married man for 32 of their 37-year marriage. Her husband had decided to sue for divorce. She had prior history of "depression" at age 26 years that had spontaneously remitted after a few weeks.

She was one of the six children and there was no family history of psychiatric disorder. She had two children of her own. She worked as a cashier and was described as an outgoing and sociable individual who "has a lot of vitality".

This presenting clinical picture improved over a 4-week period, and she made a full recovery without requiring any medical treatment. The diagnosis was adjustment disorder (ICD-10F43). She suffered a relapse after 6 months. The relapse was precipitated by contact with her ex-lover who had by now become involved with another woman. On this occasion, the patient presented with intense anxiety, motor restlessness and marked tension and expressed a multiplicity of delusional beliefs including the belief that she was being followed and watched, that unidentified individuals were gaining entrance into her home whilst she was at work and tampering with her possessions including her bank account. She was socially withdrawn and harboured ideas of guilt and unworthiness. Her condition continued to deteriorate over the following 3 months as she refused to be seen or treated by psychiatrists. Eventually she was compulsorily admitted. On admission she denied feeling low spirited and claimed that her sleep, appetite and weight were all normal. She admitted that she did not "have much energy" but this was only "because we don't eat the right food". On examination she was well kempt, agitated, restless, tremulous and fidgety. She said that she had heard someone say on the TV that she was to telephone her lover. She expressed ideas of worthlessness as follows: "I am a terrible person, I am a devious liar. I never help anyone. I'm so hard". She expressed delusions of poverty believing that her family had no money and that their home might be repossessed. This belief appeared to have some basis in fact as it turned out that her husband was a compulsive gambler and owed £ 4000 in debt. She denied being ill and said "There's nothing wrong with me, it's just domestic doctor". She remained uncooperative with the treatment and was eventually discharged after 2 weeks but followed up at home and outpatients for the following 14 months.

Her third episode occurred after she deteriorated significantly over a 4-week period with features of depressed mood, motor restlessness and agitation and insomnia, and, significantly, she expressed the belief that all her relatives including her husband and her two sons were impostors. She threatened a neighbour who she believed was an impostor. She expressed the belief that the hospital was not the "real" hospital and that the "real" hospital had been closed down and that the hospital staff were not "real" nurses and neither was the doctor responsible for her care a "real" doctor. She said, "You're a bogus doctor". She believed that her granddaughter was "swapped at birth". She expressed the belief that people were talking about her behind her back. She believed that she was ugly and that she "had nothing to be happy about". This deterioration appeared to have occurred in the context of significant stressful life events: Her husband lost his job, her mother had a stroke and her sister had subarachnoid haemorrhage. Her condition improved in response to a combination of trifluoperazine and lofepramine, and she made a full recovery.

She then had five further admissions with the same clinical profile. In addition to the features described above in the last two admissions, she presented with orofacial and appendicular dyskinesia, high-stepping gait and decline in cognitive functions. Furthermore she was also diagnosed with multiple myeloma from which she subsequently died as direct result of anaemia.

Investigations included serial formal Wechsler Adult Intelligence Scale (WAIS) that was reported as follows: 1988, Full Scale IQ 92, Verbal Scale 91, Performance Scale 97, and National Adult Reading Test predicted Full Scale IQ 97; 1992, Full Scale IQ 76. She also had CT scan (1996) that was reported as follows: Appearances do suggest some degree of atrophy, slightly asymmetric, involving the frontal and temporal lobes particularly. The cause for this is uncertain, and the distribution is by no means definite for Alzheimer's disease although such is possible.

Case Analysis

This case is illustrative of the complexity of Capgras syndrome and related conditions. It demonstrates the interrelationships between descriptive psychopathology, pathogenesis, neurology and neuropsychology. I shall take each of these in turn.

12.2 Descriptive Psychopathology

Formally speaking, this patient presented with abnormalities of mood complicated by delusions. She had delusions of persecution, delusions of poverty, delusions of ugliness, delusions of worthlessness and Capgras delusion involving family members, nurses, doctors and the hospital itself. This meant that she met the criteria for recurrent depressive disorder, severe depression with psychotic features on each of her hospital admissions (ICD-10F33.4).

The Capgras syndrome was only one of a number of psychotic symptoms that the patient exhibited. It is rare that Capgras syndrome or any of the other delusional misidentification syndromes occurs on its own. In other words, Capgras syndrome occurs in the setting of a psychiatric disorder such as mood disorder and is usually part of a complex of delusions and/or hallucinations that the patient experiences.

12.3 Pathogenesis, Neurology and Neuropsychology

The initial presentation in this case arose in the context of the discovery of a long-standing adulterous sexual relationship by the patient's spouse. The dynamics of this significant and stressful life event definitely informed the content of the patient's psychotic symptoms, namely, her delusions of worthlessness, reference and persecution. It was understandable that she felt unworthy and that she regarded herself "a devious liar". However, the extent and quality of her beliefs were exaggerated and had the hallmarks of delusional beliefs, namely, incorrigibility and a lack of openness to counter argument and exploration. The fact of the husband's gambling problem also clearly influenced the patient's delusion of poverty despite the fact that she had sufficient funds in the bank. And finally the delusion of ugliness was understandable in the context of the patient's lover's new sexual relationship. The stressful event(s) can be seen to be relevant with respect to precipitating the patient's condition and also lending colour to the content of the patient's psychosis.

There is a well-established link between organic brain disease and delusional misidentification syndromes. This case also exemplifies this recognized relationship. The patient, subsequent to her initial presentation, developed deterioration in her cognitive functions demonstrated on serial neuropsychological testing as described above. This decline in function was also confirmed by fronto-temporal atrophy on CT scan making the diagnosis of fronto-temporal dementia very likely.

Whether or not the patient's recurrent depression and fronto-temporal dementia are independent conditions is a moot point. It is also difficult to comment on what the relationship of the patient's multiple myeloma is to her psychiatric disorder(s).

The patient's treatment and response to treatment were that of the primary underlying condition, namely, psychotic depression.

12.4 Phenomenology

It is important to examine the subjective experience of an individual who presents with delusional misidentification syndrome and in this instance with Capgras syndrome. This is to draw a distinction between descriptive psychopathology and phenomenology. It is a truism to say that descriptive psychopathology relies on phenomenology; the emphasis in descriptive psychopathology is in the selection and delineation of abnormal phenomena, the description of abnormal subjective experience and the accurate use of terminology, whereas the emphasis in phenomenology is in the structure of subjective experience with a view to determining what a sense of reality consists of Ratcliffe (2008a), and of course this approach is not restricted to abnormal phenomena.

In Capgras syndrome, an individual is making a claim that a familiar person (in the case described above involving spouse and children, the treating doctor and even the hospital) is not what they seem. The question is how to understand this subjective experience and the erroneous conclusion from the patient's perspective. The empirical literature (see discussion below) has shown that in prosopagnosia (inability to recognize familiar faces), there is covert recognition of familiar faces as demonstrated by skin conductance studies (Bauer 1984). This finding laid the foundation for the proposal that there are at least two face recognition pathways, one dealing with iconic face recognition and the other with autonomic recognition. The application of this finding to Capgras syndrome suggested that the two-stage process demonstrated in prosopagnosia was also relevant in Capgras syndrome, but in Capgras syndrome, the fault lay in an absent or attenuated autonomic recognition pathway resulting in the iconic image of a familiar person not evoking the usual, accompanying autonomic arousal and recognition, thereby resulting in the delusional belief that a familiar person had been replaced by an impostor. Phenomenological accounts of the world we live in and experience point to the role of value and purposes in transforming a lifeless and empty world into the world that solicits and motivates us to action (Ratcliffe 2008a; Solomon 1993). It is easy to see how this relates to Capgras syndrome. Familiar others are imbued with the valence of our emotions and are recognizable as who they are, not merely by the accuracy of iconic face recognition, but also by the appropriate and congruent autonomic arousal. As Ratcliffe says when we encounter the world, "people sometimes talk of feeling alive, dead, distant, detached, dislodged, estranged..." (Page 68) (2008a). These feelings refer to the manner in which our emotions supplement the world we encounter with value. It is the absence or attenuation of these feelings that underpins the declaration by the patient that impostors have replaced a familiar other. If this were merely a matter of distortion of normal feelings, then there would be many more cases of Capgras syndrome. In other words, even though "a loss of all or many of those subtle affective responses that ordinarily constitute a background of relatedness between a person and her spouse, without any precipitating events or pronounced negative emotions...", amounts to a different experience even if still constitutive of recognition (Ratcliffe 2008b), it would not normally result in Capgras syndrome.

The emphasis is that face recognition does not take place in a void but is always contextual. As Ratcliffe argues "If the perceived person did not fall into place within a framework of expectation or if a characteristic field of possibilities did not form around that person, even though her actual appearance were exactly like that of a spouse, then the result would be an experience of her as identical in actual appearance to the spouse but somehow very different" (2008b). This is to say in

Ratcliffe's terms that affective interconnectedness is involved in recognition of others. This account is elegant and probably true to a degree but is yet problematic. Capgras syndrome and the other delusional misidentification syndromes do not only affect recognition of persons but also objects and places. Indeed all sensory modalities can be affected including audition, gustation and touch. More remarkably, as distinct from prosopagnosia where the inability to recognize familiar faces involves recognition of all familiar faces, in delusional misidentification syndromes, the delusions are transitory and affect only a select few familiar others, objects or places. Furthermore, the demonstrated impairments in face recognition memory and face processing are traits not state markers. In other words even when the patient is no longer expressing delusional beliefs, the underlying abnormalities persist. Finally, the impairments are not restricted to face processing but to all visual processing of complex objects (Oyebode 2008). The demonstrated abnormalities in delusional misidentification syndromes inform our understanding of face recognition in general but there is more to delusional misidentification syndromes than mere alterations in affective connectedness.

12.5 Diagnosis and Classification of Delusional Misidentification Syndromes

Delusional misidentification syndromes are, strictly speaking, not syndromes at all. They are different but related phenomena that centre on the theme of "the double". The aim, when any of these phenomena is noted to be present in a patient, is firstly to describe the phenomenon, name it and then establish what the underlying psychiatric disorder is, whether this be schizophrenia, mood disorder, delusional disorder or an organic disorder such as Alzheimer's dementia (Oyebode and Sargeant 1996). It is important to be aware of the range of other neurological and physical disorders that have been described in association with delusional misidentification syndromes such as multiple sclerosis (Sidoti and Lorusso 2007), urinary tract infection (Salviati et al. 2013), parkinsonism (Roane et al. 1998), Parkinson's disease (Cercy and Marasia 2012; Pagonabarraga et al. 2008), cortical atrophy (Joseph et al. 1999) Alzheimer's dementia (Ismail et al. 2012; Jedidi et al. 2013), dementia with Lewy bodies (Thaipisuttikul et al. 2013), subarachnoid haemorrhage (Bouckoms et al. 1986) and cerebral infarction (Jocic and Staton 1993; de Pauw et al. 1987).

The delusional misidentification syndromes most commonly include Capgras syndrome, Frégoli syndrome, syndrome of intermetamorphosis, syndrome of subjective doubles and reduplicative paramnesia. There has been repeated call for consensus regarding terminology, definition and classification of these conditions (de Pauw 1994). Several authors have proposed differing classifications (Roessner and Rössner 2002; Silva and Leong 1994; Silva et al. 1990; Weinstein 1994). Silva's recommended classification that includes "subjective" Frégoli, "reverse" intermetamorphosis and other new phenomena is likely to unnecessarily widen the boundaries of delusional misidentification syndromes. Furthermore, other authors have included misidentification of mirror images and TV images and the so-called phantom boarder syndrome as part of the delusional misidentification syndromes (Förstl et al. 1991). Again, this approach seeks to widen the reach of these syndromes by including phenomena that do not have at their centre notions of "the double". Misidentification of TV and mirror images as real points to the loss of capacity to distinguish between objects and their images. Some of the misidentification of mirror images of the self relates more to prosopagnosia for familiar faces than to delusional misidentification syndromes. More recently, clonal pluralization of self, relatives or others has been proposed as a variant of delusional misidentification syndromes in which an individual believes that there are many physical and psychological copies of a given original (Ranjan et al. 2007).

Weinstein has argued for a classification system that regards the delusional misidentification disorders as determined by a belief in duplicates, and hence a classification according to whether the duplication is expressed in the modalities of person, place, time and event, objects, parts of the body or self might reduce complexity (Weinstein 1994). However, this classification is likely to lose sight of the commonalities between Capgras phenomenon, for example, that involves coexisting duplication of person, place, time and events, etc., as these would all be classified differently. There is little doubt that delusional misidentification syndromes occur as a continuum from a positive pole consisting of minor forms of déjà vu experience to reduplicative paramnesia and a negative pole from depersonalization to nihilistic delusions (Sno 1994). What is significant is that there is at present no fully satisfactory classification of delusional misidentification syndromes. Derealization and depersonalization can occur in the prodromal phase of delusional misidentification syndromes, and hence there is some case for depersonalization having an intrinsic role in the process that produces delusional misidentification syndromes (Todd et al. 1981). This at least means that the argument for regarding delusional misidentification syndromes as being part of a continuum as proposed by Sno is promising as a basis for further inquiry (Sno 1994).

Delusional misidentification syndromes are commonly regarded as rare conditions. Estimates of the prevalence range from 0.001 to 4.1 % (Joseph 1994; Kirov et al. 1994; Moselhy and Oyebode 1997). Early reports suggested that these disorders occur exclusively in females but it is now clearly established that males are afflicted as well (1997).

12.6 Pathogenesis

12.6.1 Psychodynamic Explanations

Coleman argued for ambivalence as an essential psychodynamic mechanism in delusional misidentification syndromes, namely, that the misidentified individual is one with whom the patient has an ambivalent relationship (Coleman 1933). This view is shared by several other authors who also emphasize the fact that only a small number of specific individuals are misidentified, and this confirms that ambivalence is important and central (Dally and Gomez 1979; Enoch 1963; Enoch et al. 1967; Moskowitz 1972; Vogel 1974). The problem with this approach is simply that it is not always obvious that the emotional relationship is marked either by ambivalence or a negative attitude. And in any case delusional misidentification for objects and places for which ambivalence is far from obvious widely occurs (Moselhy and Oyebode 1997).

Other authors have emphasized the role of "splitting" of internalized object representation (Berson 1983), and regression to a phase in childhood before object constancy was established (Jackson et al. 1992) or of regression to archaic forms of thinking that occurs in psychosis (Todd et al. 1981) as the basic anomaly in delusional misidentification syndromes. What is clear is that these explanatory hypotheses cannot account for the range of cases seen nor can they account for the associations with neurological lesions or impairments in face processing that have been demonstrated in delusional misidentification syndromes.

12.6.2 Neurological Explanations

Delusional misidentification syndromes have been associated with a number of neurological lesions (Moselhy and Oyebode 1997). In a series of 29 cases, diffuse cortical atrophy, posterior fossa or subcortical abnormalities were demonstrated on CT scans, and cortical dysrhythmia and focal epileptiform discharges on EEG were reported (Joseph 1985). There is also substantial evidence of the role of the right (non-dominant) hemisphere in delusional misidentification syndromes (Cutting 1991; Madoz-Gúrpide and Hillers-Rodríguez 2010) including findings of significantly enlarged right anterior horn region in patients with delusional misidentification syndrome in the context of Alzheimer's disease (Förstl et al. 1991) and the development of delusional misidentification syndromes following right temporoparietal infarction (de Pauw et al. 1987). In addition, in reduplicative paramnesia, there is evidence of bilateral anterior cortical atrophy, subcortical atrophy and involvement of the cerebellar vermis atrophy (Joseph et al. 1999). But perhaps the most important findings are the reports of Capgras syndrome in association with inter-ictal psychosis and infarction of the occipitotemporal junction thereby drawing attention to the role of the occipital cortex in delusional misidentification syndromes (Lewis 1987) and of involvement directly of the fusiform gyrus therefore pointing to a role for the same brain areas in both delusional misidentification syndromes and prosopagnosia (Hudson and Grace 2000). Other investigators have shown that in Alzheimer's disease presenting with Capgras syndrome, there is significant hypometabolism in orbitofrontal and cingulate regions bilaterally and in left median areas and relative hypermetabolism in bilateral superior temporal and inferior parietal regions (Mentis et al. 1995). It is probably true to say that an integrative model is required that relates the differing roles of the various cortical regions to the production of delusional beliefs, for example, identifying lesions in the right frontal regions as important in releasing left-sided hyperinferential states that are liable to cause delusion formation (Ismail et al. 2012).

Christodoulou and colleagues (1981) initially proposed psychophysiological changes and anomalies in delusional misidentification syndromes. More recently there is emerging evidence of abnormal P300 in association with working memory in delusional misidentification syndromes suggesting failure to allocate sufficient attentional resources to sensory stimulus (Papageorgiou et al. 2002, 2003, 2005).

12.6.3 Neuropsychological Explanations

There is growing evidence of impairment of face recognition memory in the absence of impairment of verbal recognition memory in delusional misidentification syndromes (Bidault et al. 1986; Edelstyn et al. 1996, 1998; Ellis 1998; Ellis et al. 1994; Oyebode 2008). These reported impairments are at least as severe as those in individuals with acquired right-sided brain injury. This is important and interesting precisely because it points to the same underlying mechanisms as in prosopagnosia. In prosopagnosia, it is now established that covert face recognition takes place via the intact ventral pathway linking the occipital cortex with medial temporal structures, thereby bypassing the damaged dorsal pathway that links occipital cortex via longitudinal fasciculus with the parietal cortex (Bauer 1984). It is hypothesized that in Capgras syndrome, the dorsal pathway is impaired with a sparing of the ventral pathway (the opposite of what happens in prosopagnosia) with the result that face recognition is intact but the sense of familiarity is disrupted, thereby producing the belief that a familiar person is an impostor (Ellis et al. 1992). This is an elegant and testable hypothesis that has now been confirmed (Ellis et al. 1997; Hirstein and Ramachandran 1997), with the proviso that the putative dorsal pathway is yet to be demonstrated (Breen et al. 2000) and that the dissociation between overt and covert recognition is not as clear-cut as once thought (Fiacconi et al. 2014), thus making room for further elaborations and refinements to the original hypothesis. There is also evidence that in addition to the markedly reduced magnitude of skin conductance responses to familiar faces compared to normal samples, patients with Capgras syndrome also demonstrated impairment in judging gaze directions and concluded that models looking in different directions were different individuals (Hirstein and Ramachandran 1997). It is also relevant that there may be differences in the demonstrable face processing impairments between Capgras and Frégoli syndromes, respectively (Walther et al. 2010). There are other proposals including the notion of disconnection between various cortico-visuo-limbic pathways that result in the lack of resolution of the differing representations of personal experience including face representations (Joseph 1985), the role of preconscious perceptual processing (Fleminger 1992, 1994), a form of agnosia of identification (Luauté and Bidault 1994), impairment of the attribution of uniqueness to self, others and objects (Margariti and Kontaxakis 2006) and the place of "mindreading" in delusional misidentification syndromes (Hirstein 2010). These additional hypotheses have yet to be confirmed by further empirical study.

12.6.4 Forensic Aspects

Violence in patients with delusional misidentification syndromes, particularly Capgras syndrome, has been reported in the literature (Crane 1976; Silva et al. 1992, 1993, 1994a, b; Thompson and Swan 1993; Woytassek and Atwal 1985). It is now clear that violence occurs not only in Capgras syndrome but also in syndrome of subjective doubles (Christodoulou 1978) and syndrome of intermetamorphosis (Barton and Barton 1986). The original case of Frégoli syndrome by Courbon and Fail involved a female patient who was admitted following an assault on a former employer whom the patient accused of being in disguise (Moselhy and Oyebode 1997). But patients presenting with delusional misidentification syndrome can themselves be victims of violence as well as being perpetrators of violence (De Pauw and Szulecka 1988). There is some evidence that individuals with delusional misidentification who are violent are less likely to use weapons than other patients who express delusional beliefs and that grandiose beliefs, thought disorder, generalized hostility and a previous history of violence are predictors of violence in individuals who present with delusional misidentification syndromes (Silva et al. 1995).

12.7 Management, Course and Outcome

The treatment of delusional misidentification syndrome is the treatment of the primary, underlying psychiatric disorder. It is important to rule out a primary organic brain disease as the cause and the investigation ought to include MRI or CT scan and neuropsychological tests in order to exclude intracranial pathology including the various causes of dementia.

There are no studies of the long-term outcome of delusional misidentification syndromes. However, there is no reason to believe that response to treatment is likely to be any different from that of the underlying condition.

12.8 Conclusions

Delusional misidentification syndromes are natural experiments that allow a focused approach to investigating the neural and neuropsychological substrate of delusions. It is already well established that the same brain regions that subserve the function of face recognition are involved in delusional misidentification syndromes. It is also true that both the right (non-dominant hemisphere) and the frontal lobes are implicated. These conditions are also revealing the processes and mechanisms that underlie face recognition, attribution of identity and the relationship between delusional misidentification syndromes and the impairments that are present in other psychiatric disorders such as schizophrenia in the absence of delusional misidentification syndromes. Finally, despite the growing body of knowledge about the neural mechanisms, delusional misidentification syndromes continue to demonstrate that a holistic approach that involves the integration of descriptive psychopathology, the patient's subjective experience, the social and cultural context and the biology of psychiatric disorders is required for a thorough understanding of any psychiatric phenomena.

References

Abbate, C., Trimarchi, P. D., Salvi, G. P., Quarenghi, A. M., Vergani, C., & Luzzatti, C. (2012). Delusion of inanimate doubles: Description of a case of focal retrograde amnesia. *Neurocase, 18*(6), 457–477. doi:10.1080/13554794.2011.627344.

Anderson, D. N., & Williams, E. (1994). The delusion of inanimate doubles. *Psychopathology, 27* (3–5), 220–225.

Barton, J. L., & Barton, E. S. (1986). Misidentification syndromes and sexuality. *Bibliotheca Psychiatrica, 164*, 105–120.

Bauer, R. M. (1984). Autonomic recognition of names and faces in prosopagnosia: A neuropsychological application of the guilty knowledge test. *Neuropsychologia, 22*(4), 457–469. Retrieved from Google Scholar.

Berson, R. J. (1983). Capgras' syndrome. *The American Journal of Psychiatry, 140*(8), 969–978.

Bidault, E., Luauté, J. P., & Tzavaras, A. (1986). Prosopagnosia and the delusional misidentification syndromes. *Bibliotheca Psychiatrica, 164*, 80–91.

Bouckoms, A., Martuza, R., & Henderson, M. (1986). Capgras syndrome with subarachnoid hemorrhage. *The Journal of Nervous and Mental Disease, 174*(8), 484–488.

Breen, N., Caine, D., & Coltheart, M. (2000). Models of face recognition and delusional misidentification: A critical review. *Cognitive Neuropsychology, 17*(1), 55–71. doi:10.1080/026432900380481.

Cercy, S. P., & Marasia, J. C. (2012). *Journal of Neuropsychiatry and Clinical Neurosciences, 24,* E3–4). United States. doi:10.1176/appi.neuropsych.11010016

Christodoulou, G. N. (1978). Syndrome of subjective doubles. *The American Journal of Psychiatry, 135*, 249–251.

Christodoulou, G. N., & Malliara-Loulakaki, S. (1981). Delusional misidentification syndromes and cerebral 'dysrhythmia'. *Psychiatria Clinica, 14*(4), 245–251.

Christodoulou, G. N., Margariti, M., Kontaxakis, V. P., & Christodoulou, N. G. (2009). The delusional misidentification syndromes: Strange, fascinating, and instructive. *Current Psychiatry Reports, 11*(3), 185–189.

Coleman, S. M. (1933). Misidentification and non-recognition. *Journal of Mental Science, 79,* 42–51.

Crane, D. L. (1976). More violent capgras. *The American Journal of Psychiatry, 133*(11), 1350.

Cutting, J. (1991). Delusional misidentification and the role of the right hemisphere in the appreciation of identity. *The British Journal of Psychiatry. Supplement*, (14), 70–5.

Dally, P., & Gomez, J. (1979). Capgras: Case study and reappraisal of psychopathology. *The British Journal of Medical Psychology, 52*(3), 291–295.

de Pauw, K. W. (1994). Delusional misidentification: A plea for an agreed terminology and classification. *Psychopathology, 27*(3–5), 123–129.

De Pauw, K. W., & Szulecka, T. K. (1988). Dangerous delusions. Violence and the misidentification syndromes. *The British Journal of Psychiatry, 152*, 91–96.

de Pauw, K. W., Szulecka, T. K., & Poltock, T. L. (1987). Frégoli syndrome after cerebral infarction. *The Journal of Nervous and Mental Disease, 175*(7), 433–438.

Edelstyn, N. M. J., Oyebode, F., & Barrett, K. (1998). Delusional misidentification: A neuropsychological case study in dementia associated with parkinson's disease. *Neurocase, 4*(3), 181–188.

Edelstyn, N. M., Riddoch, M. J., Oyebode, F., Humphreys, G. W., & Forde, E. (1996). Visual processing in patients with frégoli syndrome. *Cognitive Neuropsychiatry, 1*(2), 103–124. doi:10.1080/135468096396587.

Ellis, H. D. (1994). The role of the right hemisphere in the capgras delusion. *Psychopathology, 27* (3–5), 177–185.
Ellis, H. D. (1998). *Cognitive Neuropsychiatry, 3*: 81–89. England. doi:10.1080/135468098396170
Ellis, H., De Pauw, K., Christodoulou, G. N., Luaute, J. P., Bidault, E., & Szulecka, K. (1992). Recognition memory in psychotic patients. *Behavioural Neurology, 5*(1), 23–26. doi:10.3233/BEN-1992-5104.
Ellis, H. D., Luauté, J. P., & Retterstøl, N. (1994). Delusional misidentification syndromes. *Psychopathology, 27*(3-5), 117–120.
Ellis, H. D., Young, A. W., Quayle, A. H., & De Pauw, K. W. (1997). Reduced autonomic responses to faces in capgras delusion. *Proceedings. Biological Sciences/The Royal Society, 264*(1384), 1085–1092. doi:10.1098/rspb.1997.0150.
Enoch, M. D. (1963). The capgras syndrome. *Acta Psychiatrica Scandinavica, 39*(3), 437–462.
Enoch, M. D., Trethowan, W. H., & Barker, J. C. (1967). *Some uncommon psychiatric syndromes.* Bristol: John Wright.
Feinberg, T. E., & Roane, D. M. (2005). Delusional misidentification. *The Psychiatric Clinics of North America, 28*(3), 665–683. doi:10.1016/j.psc.2005.05.002. 678–679.
Fiacconi, C. M., Barkley, V., Finger, E. C., Carson, N., Duke, D., Rosenbaum, R. S., et al. (2014). Nature and extent of person recognition impairments associated with capgras syndrome in lewy body dementia. *Frontiers in Human Neuroscience, 8*, 726. doi:10.3389/fnhum.2014.00726.
Fleminger, S. (1992). Seeing is believing: The role of 'preconscious' perceptual processing in delusional misidentification. *The British Journal of Psychiatry, 160*, 293–303.
Fleminger, S. (1994). Delusional misidentification: An exemplary symptom illustrating an interaction between organic brain disease and psychological processes. *Psychopathology, 27*(3–5), 161–167.
Förstl, H., Besthorn, C., Burns, A., Geiger-Kabisch, C., Levy, R., & Sattel, A. (1994). Delusional misidentification in alzheimer's disease: A summary of clinical and biological aspects. *Psychopathology, 27*(3–5), 194–199.
Förstl, H., Burns, A., Jacoby, R., & Levy, R. (1991). Neuroanatomical correlates of clinical misidentification and misperception in senile dementia of the Alzheimer type. *The Journal of Clinical Psychiatry, 52*(6), 268–271.
Hirstein, W. (2010). The misidentification syndromes as mindreading disorders. *Cognitive Neuropsychiatry, 15*(1), 233–260. doi:10.1080/13546800903414891.
Hirstein, W., & Ramachandran, V. S. (1997). Capgras syndrome: A novel probe for understanding the neural representation of the identity and familiarity of persons. *Proceedings. Biological Sciences/the Royal Society, 264*(1380), 437–444. doi:10.1098/rspb.1997.0062.
Hudson, A. J., & Grace, G. M. (2000). Misidentification syndromes related to face specific area in the fusiform gyrus. *Journal of Neurology, Neurosurgery, and Psychiatry, 69*(5), 645–648.
Ismail, Z., Nguyen, M.-Q., Fischer, C. E., Schweizer, T. A., & Mulsant, B. H. (2012). Neuroimaging of delusions in Alzheimer's disease. *Psychiatry Research, 202*(2), 89–95. doi:10.1016/j.pscychresns.2012.01.008.
Jackson, R. S., Naylor, M. W., Shain, B. N., & King, C. A. (1992). Capgras syndrome in adolescence. *Journal of the American Academy of Child and Adolescent Psychiatry, 31*(5), 977–983.
Jedidi, H., Daury, N., Capa, R., Bahri, M. A., Collette, F., Feyers, D., et al. (2013). Brain metabolic dysfunction in capgras delusion during alzheimer's disease: A positron emission tomography study. *American Journal of Alzheimer's Disease and Other Dementias.* doi:10.1177/1533317513495105.
Jocic, Z., & Staton, R. D. (1993). Reduplication after right middle cerebral artery infarction. *Brain and Cognition, 23*(2), 222–230. doi:10.1006/brcg.1993.1056.
Joseph, A. B. (1985). Focal central nervous system abnormalities in patients with misidentification syndromes. *Bibliotheca Psychiatrica, 164*, 68–79.
Joseph, A. B. (1994). Observations on the epidemiology of the delusional misidentification syndromes in the Boston metropolitan area: April 1983-june 1984. *Psychopathology, 27* (3–5), 150–153.

Joseph, A. B., O'Leary, D. H., Kurland, R., & Ellis, H. D. (1999). Bilateral anterior cortical atrophy and subcortical atrophy in reduplicative paramnesia: A case-control study of computed tomography in 10 patients. *Canadian Journal of Psychiatry. Revue Canadienne De Psychiatrie, 44*(7), 685–689.
Kirov, G., Jones, P., & Lewis, S. W. (1994). Prevalence of delusional misidentification syndromes. *Psychopathology, 27*(3–5), 148–149.
Lewis, S. W. (1987). Brain imaging in a case of capgras' syndrome. *The British Journal of Psychiatry, 150*(1), 117–121.
Luauté, J. P., & Bidault, E. (1994). Capgras syndrome: Agnosia of identification and delusion of reduplication. *Psychopathology, 27*(3-5), 186–193.
Madoz-Gúrpide, A., & Hillers-Rodríguez, R. (2010). Capgras delusion: A review of aetiological theories. *Revista De Neurologia, 50*(7), 420–430.
Margariti, M. M., & Kontaxakis, V. P. (2006). Approaching delusional misidentification syndromes as a disorder of the sense of uniqueness. *Psychopathology, 39*(6), 261–268. doi:10.1159/000095730.
Mentis, M. J., Weinstein, E. A., Horwitz, B., McIntosh, A. R., Pietrini, P., Alexander, G. E., et al. (1995). Abnormal brain glucose metabolism in the delusional misidentification syndromes: A positron emission tomography study in Alzheimer disease. *Biological Psychiatry, 38*(7), 438–449.
Moselhy, H., & Oyebode, F. (1997). Delusional misidentification syndromes: A review of the Anglophone literature. *Neurology Psychiatry and Brain Research, 5*(1), 21–26.
Moskowitz, J. A. (1972). Capgras' symptom in modern dress. *International Journal of Child Psychotherapy, 1*, 45–64.
Munro, A. (1994). Delusional disorders are a naturally occurring 'experimental psychosis'. *Psychopathology, 27*(3–5), 247–250.
Oyebode, F. (2008). The neurology of psychosis. *Medical Principles and Practice, 17*(4), 263–269. doi:10.1159/000129603.
Oyebode, F., & Sargeant, R. (1996). Delusional misidentification syndromes: A descriptive study. *Psychopathology, 29*(4), 209–214.
Pagonabarraga, J., Llebaria, G., García-Sánchez, C., Pascual-Sedano, B., Gironell, A., & Kulisevsky, J. (2008). A prospective study of delusional misidentification syndromes in Parkinson's disease with dementia. *Movement Disorders, 23*(3), 443–448. doi:10.1002/mds.21864.
Paillère-Martinot, M. L., Dao-Castellana, M. H., Masure, M. C., Pillon, B., & Martinot, J. L. (1994). Delusional misidentification: A clinical, neuropsychological and brain imaging case study. *Psychopathology, 27*(3–5), 200–210.
Papageorgiou, C., Lykouras, L., Alevizos, B., Ventouras, E., Mourtzouchou, P., Uzunoglu, N., et al. (2005). Psychophysiological differences in schizophrenics with and without delusional misidentification syndromes: A P300 study. *Progress in Neuro-Psychopharmacology and Biological Psychiatry, 29*(4), 593–601. doi:10.1016/j.pnpbp.2005.01.016.
Papageorgiou, C., Lykouras, L., Ventouras, E., Uzunoglu, N., & Christodoulou, G. N. (2002). Abnormal P300 in a case of delusional misidentification with coinciding capgras and frégoli symptoms. *Progress in Neuro-Psychopharmacology and Biological Psychiatry, 26*(4), 805–810.
Papageorgiou, C., Ventouras, E., Lykouras, L., Uzunoglu, N., & Christodoulou, G. N. (2003). Psychophysiological evidence for altered information processing in delusional misidentification syndromes. *Progress in Neuro-Psychopharmacology and Biological Psychiatry, 27*(3), 365–372. doi:10.1016/S0278-5846(02)00353-6.
Ranjan, S., Chandra, P. S., Gupta, A. K., & Prabhu, S. (2007). Clonal pluralization of self, relatives and others. *Psychopathology, 40*(6), 465–467. doi:10.1159/000108126.
Ratcliffe, M. (2008a). *Feelings of being: Phenomenology, psychiatry and the sense of reality*. Oxford: Oxford University Press. Retrieved from Library of Congress or OCLC Worldcat.
Ratcliffe, M. (2008b). The phenomenological role of affect in the capgras delusion. *Continental Philosophy Review, 41*(2), 195–216. doi:10.1007/s11007-008-9078-5.

Roane, D. M., Rogers, J. D., Robinson, J. H., & Feinberg, T. E. (1998). Delusional misidentification in association with parkinsonism. *The Journal of Neuropsychiatry and Clinical Neurosciences, 10*(2), 194–198.
Roessner, V., & Rössner, V. (2002). A new classification of the delusional misidentification syndromes. *Psychopathology, 35*(1), 3–7.
Salviati, M., Bersani, F. S., Macrì, F., Fojanesi, M., Minichino, A., Gallo, M., et al. (2013). Capgras-like syndrome in a patient with an acute urinary tract infection. *Neuropsychiatric Disease and Treatment, 9*, 139–142. doi:10.2147/NDT.S39077.
Sidoti, V., & Lorusso, L. (2007). Multiple sclerosis and capgras' syndrome. *Clinical Neurology and Neurosurgery, 109*(9), 786–787. doi:10.1016/j.clineuro.2007.05.022.
Silva, J. A., & Leong, G. B. (1992). The capgras syndrome in paranoid schizophrenia. *Psychopathology, 25*(3), 147–153.
Silva, J. A., & Leong, G. B. (1994). *Comprehensive Psychiatry, 35*, 244. United States.
Silva, J. A., & Leong, G. B. (1995). Visual-perceptual abnormalities in delusional misidentification. *Canadian Journal of Psychiatry. Revue Canadienne De Psychiatrie, 40*(1), 6–8.
Silva, J. A., Leong, G. B., Garza-Treviño, E. S., Le Grand, J., Oliva, D., Weinstock, R., & Bowden, C. L. (1994a). A cognitive model of dangerous delusional misidentification syndromes. *Journal of Forensic Sciences, 39*(6), 1455–1467.
Silva, J. A., Leong, G. B., Weinstock, R., Sharma, K. K., & Klein, R. L. (1994b). Delusional misidentification syndromes and dangerousness. *Psychopathology, 27*(3-5), 215–219.
Silva, J. A., Leong, G. B., Weinstock, R., & Klein, R. L. (1995). Psychiatric factors associated with dangerous misidentification delusions. *The Bulletin of the American Academy of Psychiatry and the Law, 23*(1), 53–61.
Silva, J. A., Leong, G. B., Weinstock, R., & Wine, D. B. (1993). Delusional misidentification and dangerousness: A neurobiologic hypothesis. *Journal of Forensic Sciences, 38*(4), 904–913.
Silva, J. A., Leong, G. B., & Shaner, A. L. (1990). A classification system for misidentification syndromes. *Psychopathology, 23*(1), 27–32.
Silva, J. A., Leong, G. B., & Weinstock, R. (1992). The dangerousness of persons with misidentification syndromes. *The Bulletin of the American Academy of Psychiatry and the Law, 20*(1), 77–86.
Sno, H. N. (1994). A continuum of misidentification symptoms. *Psychopathology, 27*(3-5), 144–147.
Solomon, R. C. (1993). *The passions: Emotions and the meaning of life*. Indianapolis: Hackett Publishing. Retrieved from Google Scholar.
Thaipisuttikul, P., Lobach, I., Zweig, Y., Gurnani, A., & Galvin, J. E. (2013). Capgras syndrome in dementia with lewy bodies. *International Psychogeriatrics/IPA, 25*(5), 843–849. doi:10.1017/S1041610212002189.
Thompson, A. E., & Swan, M. (1993). Capgras' syndrome presenting with violence following heavy drinking. *The British Journal of Psychiatry, 162*, 692–694.
Todd, J., Dewhurst, K., & Wallis, G. (1981). The syndrome of capgras. *The British Journal of Psychiatry, 139*, 319–327.
Vogel, B. F. (1974). The capgras syndrome and its psychopathology. *The American Journal of Psychiatry, 131*(8), 922–924.
Walther, S., Federspiel, A., Horn, H., Wirth, M., Bianchi, P., Strik, W., & Müller, T. J. (2010). Performance during face processing differentiates schizophrenia patients with delusional misidentifications. *Psychopathology, 43*(2), 127–136. doi:10.1159/000277002.
Weinstein, E. A. (1994). The classification of delusional misidentification syndromes. *Psychopathology, 27*(3-5), 130–135.
Woytassek, L. E., & Atwal, S. S. (1985). Capgras syndrome in court. *The Nebraska Medical Journal, 70*(11), 392–394.

Perplexity

13

Clara S. Humpston and Matthew R. Broome

13.1 Introduction

In this chapter we aim to examine the phenomenon of perplexity in the context of delusional mood/atmosphere, two terms which are often used interchangeably (however, some argue delusional mood is a consequence of delusional atmosphere and that the latter term should be used; see Berner 1991): despite its relative absence in the current diagnostic manuals, perplexity is considered a common observation in the psychosis prodrome (Nelson et al. 2012) and one of the key disturbances of self-world awareness, alongside others such as hyper-reflexivity (Sass and Parnas 2003). In the *Schedules for Clinical Assessment in Neuropsychiatry* (SCAN, Wing et al. 1990), there is a specific item on delusional mood and perplexity (item 18.001, in Chap. 18 'Experiences of Thought Disorder and Replacement of Will', p. 152) which is defined as:

> Respondents feel that familiar surroundings have changed in a way that may be difficult to describe but that is charged with significance and self-reference and, above all, puzzling. Something odd seems to be going on and the atmosphere may rapidly seem to become ominous and threatening. Respondent seeks for an explanation, which may be based on misinterpretations of ordinary observations or on perceptual abnormalities. This part of the episode often ends abruptly, with the formation of hallucinations or delusions.

An alternative definition for perplexity is 'a sense of lacking immersion in the world, lack of spontaneous grasping of commonsensical meanings, puzzlement, and alienation' (Parnas et al. 2011, p. 200); perhaps unsurprisingly, perplexity deprives the prodromal individual of the ability to find everyday taken-for-granted

C.S. Humpston (✉)
School of Psychology, Cardiff University, Cardiff CF24 4HQ, UK
e-mail: HumpstonCS@cardiff.ac.uk

M.R. Broome
Department of Psychiatry, University of Oxford, Oxford OX3 7JX, UK

G. Stanghellini, M. Aragona (eds.), *An Experiential Approach to Psychopathology*,
DOI 10.1007/978-3-319-29945-7_13

meaning in the world as well as the basis upon which he perceives himself as an integrated and self-governing being. By using a detailed account of a clinical case ('Laurie'), our goal is to immerse the readers directly into the patient's first-person perspective. Then we will discuss Laurie's experiences against a background of contemporary literature in both philosophy and psychiatry and explore the clinical presentation of perplexity in terms of phenomenology, before offering some suggestions for the assessment, diagnosis and treatment of early psychosis. One focus of our discussion will be Klaus Conrad's stage model of beginning schizophrenia, in particular his concepts of 'Trema' preceding an 'Apophany' in the onset of psychosis (Mishara 2010; Broome et al. 2012), which will be explored in greater detail in the forthcoming sections. We would like the readers to bear in mind that there is no such thing as a 'typical' textbook case; the complexity and heterogeneity of psychosis, especially during its prodrome where many non-specific disturbances are present, preclude the possibility of a case study which can account for all the different manifestations a clinician might encounter. However, we do hope to shed some light on our understanding of this highly puzzling and very often deeply distressing experience by putting the patient's perspective on the centre stage.

The Case of Laurie[1]

It took over 3 years before Laurie received an accurate diagnosis of psychosis. Even after being diagnosed within the psychotic disorder spectrum, the actual labels had varied between schizophrenia, schizoaffective disorder and persistent delusional disorder depending on the responsible clinician. As a result of the delay in diagnosis, she was never referred to the early intervention for psychosis service, and effective treatment with antipsychotics was severely delayed, although this is rather atypical in terms of wider clinical practice and service models in the UK. The first signs that something was 'different' about her could be traced back to her childhood. Being an only child, Laurie had always tended to isolate herself from other children of her age and had practically no playmates until primary school where she was forced to mingle with others, something she never really got used to doing. She reported that it was not necessarily because she was worried others would not like her; instead, she did not care what other children or adults thought about her—rather than making friends with real people, she much preferred the company of her own imagination. She would draw little storyboards on the walls of her room (much to the annoyance of her grandparents who were her caregivers), for example, a series of stick figures which had no strict or logical rules for a storyline. Still she enjoyed her imaginary world very much; social interaction seemed a small and worthwhile price to pay in exchange. Laurie said that she could not grasp the 'hidden rules' of how to deal with others—indeed, throughout her life experiences, people were something she had to *deal with* unwillingly, albeit with a handful of exceptions. She could not understand how or even why her peers held birthday parties: what was there to celebrate? Perhaps more importantly, even when she was

[1] Patient name and identifiable factors have been changed to protect anonymity.

a child, she wondered what the meaning and purpose of such activities were. She was the kind of child who loved asking 'why?' When she learnt to read she would wonder why words had meaning and significance, why each letter was in the shape it was and why they were arranged in predefined ways to make sense.

By the time Laurie became a teenager, this sort of constant doubt and questioning had not ceased. She still had a very active imagination and very few friends at secondary school. Her grades were amongst the top of her year group and she had received much praise from the teachers, but she did not seem to be bothered by exams and classes although she did enjoy learning new things, partly because she wanted to have the knowledge to answer the questions she always had in mind. Yet some of these questions were becoming distracting. This perpetual mental question mark was turning into a hindrance, and her imagination was gaining a foreign quality—almost a kind of autonomy—she would find thoughts and images in her mind which she did not remember creating even though they were not unpleasant at the beginning. They were just random thoughts and images of everyday chores. Even colours of the objects in her surroundings seemed distorted sometimes: they would appear brighter and more vivid. Sounds in the external world started to get louder; occasionally, this would occur simultaneously when the images and thoughts popped into her mind. These experiences continued rather 'peacefully' until she was 17, when she first began to turn the question mark inwards and doubt whether the subtle changes in her thinking and perception were from her own imagination or from *something else*, something she could not control. This 'something else' became the new focus of her intense questioning and ruminations, and an initially confusing but harmless world was starting to gain a sinister feeling, a sense of unexplainable and impending threat.

Why do I have to question? Why do I have to question this questioning itself? Gradually then suddenly, Laurie came to the conclusion that she did not *want to* question after all. She simply *had to* question because this doubt—this constant, persistent and unforgiving sense of unidentifiable uneasiness intensifying day by day—was not a part of her imagination. Something major in the real world was about to happen or was already happening, and she was the only one who could detect it. The world and its inhabitants were stranger than ever; their hidden rules turned against her and her only. Yet still, she was almost fascinated by the promise of danger because she just *knew* she had to continue questioning; otherwise, her enemies would win. 'I don't understand anything anymore', Laurie explained. 'It's as if everything has a new meaning and at the same time entirely meaningless. Everything is a cipher, a signal sent by my unseen enemies. No, in fact it is not just an as if feeling. I know everything has changed for certain'. It was a very insidious process; soon before everything started crashing down, she felt extremely anxious, a kind of unpredictable yet inescapable doom about to engulf her entire existence. Indeed, her whole being, her life, everything she had was in grave danger. Although she still could not pinpoint who or where the enemies were, by this point she was absolutely certain that she was being hunted down. She would lose everything, including her autonomy as a person and freedom of thought. In fact, her enemies had already begun the operation in order to fully control her every thought, emotion and behaviour. Yet at the same time, she felt unreal and dead inside, almost as a direct proof that her enemies were taking over her mind. 'I was not anxious or depressed because I was feeling sad or panicky. I was *forced* to think and feel things I didn't want to think or feel'. Such ideas had persisted until this day. For Laurie, the loss of her autonomy was only the beginning. Thoughts that were not hers were penetrating and infiltrating her mind from without, accumulating in an amorphous mental space until there was nothing of hers left. 'I actually have a good analogy', she said. 'My brain is nothing but a remotely accessible virtual storage device. Anyone can view, change or modify the data inside without leaving a single trace of evidence behind, and those people are my real enemies'. She became even more withdrawn and depressed, and it was the depression that brought her to the attention of her general practitioner. Nevertheless, nobody had ever asked her why she was so depressed, and she did not confide in medical professionals just in case they were one of *them* as well. Indeed, for Laurie the eventual onset of her psychosis was almost an unpreventable consequence of what was happening to her *externally*. Like many sufferers of psychosis, she did not and could not realise it was an internal shift of perception, an entire reorientation of existence and reality. The thoughts started to vocalise in the air. 'To me the voices are not the biggest problem. The biggest problem is the thought interference, all the messages coming and going'. There had to be something behind all this. Her enemies were planning something. *Yes, this was it. They were monitoring me via a device in my head.*

When this seemingly sequential and perfectly logical conclusion dawned on Laurie, it was such a revelation that she almost felt at ease for the first time in months. How else could anyone know her thoughts and interfere with them if they did not have direct access to her brain? She regretted her 'stupidity' for not having realised this sooner. It was not her who had changed, of course. In fact, she was the only one that had *not* changed. It was the world and most people (if not everyone else) in this distant, unfamiliar yet so intimately intimidating world who had turned against her. She never found out the answer why she was the target; it seemed that she never would.

13.2 The Phenomenology of Early Psychosis

The case of Laurie above illustrates in detail the subjective experiences of the transition from the psychosis prodrome or at-risk mental state to the onset of bizarre delusions of control and persecution. The initially benign imaginations in everyday life have slowly turned into something much more sinister, to the extent that the distinction between such imaginations and external reality is severely blurred. Disturbances of ego boundaries or the demarcation between the internal and the external have been noted as some of the key symptoms of schizophrenia (Schneiderian first-rank symptoms), and more recently this type of self-disturbances has been the focus of prodromal research as well and is viewed as fundamental markers of psychosis vulnerability by some authors (Nelson et al. 2008). The level of selfhood in this type of disturbance is the very basic, minimal, pre-reflexive sense of self at the core of all other layers of self-knowledge (e.g. personal identity) and is the background against which all the taken for grantedness of experience is constructed (Cermolacce et al. 2007). As a result, any disruption in this level of selfhood will likely lead to significant consequences in one's relationships to the world and to himself and in extreme cases, a sense of psychological annihilation due to the loss of 'mineness' in thinking, perception and behaviour. However, the psychosis prodrome does not usually start with such extreme states of self-disturbance. Instead, as with Laurie's case, the onset of psychosis is often insidious and gradual, beginning with a sense of estrangement of the individual from the world and other people. In Laurie's case, this started very early in her childhood and continued into adolescence, yet this is not always an indication that the actual prodrome started then. It is unfortunate that early warning signs are often only found retrospectively, although the presence of such signs is not always a trigger for later transition to psychosis. In fact the term 'prodrome' is debatable as it necessarily implies transition to a psychotic episode, and some have suggested that it should be reserved as a solely retrospective concept (Yung and McGorry 1996) as the at-risk mental state only predicts transition in around 30 % of individuals (Fusar-Poli et al. 2012). Nevertheless, in individuals who do transition to frank psychosis, impairments in social functioning are apparent (Niendam et al. 2007; Addington et al. 2008), yet there is hardly any research on the connection between a damaged self-world relationship and, say, social withdrawal. Curiously in Laurie's case, she did not simply withdraw from social life due to anxiety or discomfort in situations with others; instead, she 'did not care what others thought of her'. Her preference towards a rich imaginary life seems to be the reason why she was willing to 'exchange' social interaction with her own internal world which is almost equivalent to Bleuler's concept of 'schizophrenic autism' or 'withdrawal to inner life' (Parnas et al. 2002). There is some evidence that fantasy proneness and imaginative absorption are associated with dissociative experiences and hallucination proneness (Levin et al. 2004; Perona-Garcelán et al. 2008; Humpston et al. 2016) in healthy volunteers and established schizophrenia patients with hallucinations, although their roles in the psychosis prodrome remain inconclusive. However, this is not an indication that a highly active imagination *causes* psychosis or even that psychotic symptoms are simply 'imagined'. As Laurie describes, the imagination component of her experience only became problematic when it gained a foreign quality and deviated from her control. The ability of voluntary control is a useful differentiator between internally and externally generated stimuli or events: in terms of phenomenology, for example, one's own thoughts will only become alien when one loses the sense of agency of ownership of these thoughts such as in the case of thought insertion. Laurie did indeed report 'thoughts and images she did not remember creating' even though they lacked a delusional elaboration to begin with. The concept of 'mental automatism' proposed by de Clérambault ('an automatic ideation that has become strange in a stream of thought processes without any definite sensorial or perceptional change'; Kim et al. 1994, p. 435) is also reflected here in Laurie's spontaneous thoughts 'popping into' her mind without her attributing them to an external source. Still, we have argued previously that delusional elaboration is not a prerequisite for phenomena such as thought insertion (Humpston and Broome 2015) and the key lies within the loss of ownership and agency of thoughts regardless of how one explains them. This 'primordial' form of thought interference persisted for Laurie before the attachment of any personal meaning or significance, creating an 'ideal' environment for subsequent delusions to form.

One of the most influential theories for this stage of psychosis is that of aberrant salience (Kapur 2003) which does have some overlap with phenomenological accounts of delusional mood and atmosphere. In Karl Jaspers' seminal work *General Psychopathology* (Jaspers 1962), delusional atmosphere is viewed as the very first stage of disordered subjective experience contributing to the formation of fully fledged delusions, as reflected by our case study ('something major in the real world was about to happen or was already happening') signifying an external attribution of salience. The subtle perceptual changes ('sounds in the external world started to get louder') in Kapur's account of salience and the attribution of personal significance and meaning can also be applied to internal events which contribute to the sense of perplexity and bafflement. The affective component ('a sense of unexplainable and impending threat') in delusional atmosphere which is emphasised in Jaspers' approach could be an epiphenomenon arising from aberrant salience attribution or being overwhelmed by the constant bombardment of sensory input (Broome et al. 2005b). All three forms of disturbance (personal significance, altered perception and heightened affective reactivity) are reported in Laurie's case, and it is extremely difficult if not impossible to establish causal relationships between them. Even the basic nature of delusional atmosphere, the 'psychologically irreducible and phenomenologically final' assumption of primary delusions has been brought under question (Maj 2013) as the consequence and not the cause of a disturbed self-world awareness. Even the very idea that delusions are always beliefs is debatable, and even non-delusional beliefs can be overtly irrational (Gerrans 2001; Berrios 1991; Bortolotti 2010): delusions could simply be expressions of anomalous perceptual experiences which carry metaphorical and not literal meanings to the individual. In a sense, this account is useful in the understanding of delusions—if they are not simply incorrigible and unintelligible beliefs, they might be more understandable—what Jaspers himself considered 'alien' and 'incomprehensible' as expressed by the delusional patient may in fact be representations of experiences so bizarre and indescribable that the only way to attach any meaning and explanation to them is by an elaboration equally bizarre to everyone else except the person himself who is gripped by such experiences. In addition, is it always the case that delusional mood and atmosphere are specific to the genesis of 'primary delusions' in psychosis, and if so, why are such phenomena so closely related to psychosis onset? To date, there is no consensus regarding what is actually pathognomonic of schizophrenia, and as a result such issues remain open to research. In the following sections, we will explore why the sense of perplexity could indeed be a diagnostic marker for the beginning of psychosis and argue that delusions, whether they are beliefs or not, arise as the 'natural' consequences of extreme and often irreversible alterations in an individual's self-world relationships and not just as a result of distortions in external sensory experiences.

13.3 Sense of Perplexity in Delusional Mood

As mentioned in the Introduction, we will now discuss in detail Klaus Conrad's stage model of 'beginning schizophrenia', which is viewed as an evolutionary process suggestive of eventual progression (Berner 1991). Relatively little of Conrad's work has been translated into English until recently (Mishara 2010; Broome et al. 2012), allowing us to gain a better insight into his understanding of, and approach to, the psychosis prodrome. Although Conrad was not the one who coined the terms 'delusional mood/atmosphere' (Jaspers first used the term delusional atmosphere based on the construct of delusional mood by F. W. Hagen), he was one of the first to expand these concepts and provided new foundations for descriptive psychopathology research. He observed that the duration of the psychosis prodrome could vary between days, months or even years, where the patient experiences 'an increasingly oppressive tension, a feeling of nonfinality or expectation' (Mishara 2010). The sense of perplexity arises in the first stage of Conrad's model for the prodrome, namely, 'Trema' ('stage fright' from Greek), during which 'everything that lies in the periphery to one's attention, what is behind or not part of the current thematic focus becomes a potential threat' and the sense of threat 'spreads to the entire perceptual field...nevertheless, the subject does not attribute the changes to his own state but externalises them to some yet to be understood process in the world' (Mishara 2010, p. 10). It is very interesting how Conrad chose the colloquial name for 'stage fright' as the first stage of the prodrome as if the patient was suddenly put on a 'stage', under the spotlight and observation of an unseen audience. This kind of stage fright is not the same as that where the 'performance' has been 'rehearsed' beforehand; instead, it is an unexpected, unpredictable and unexplainable focus of attention directed at the patient and the patient alone, with the whole world watching him (which is akin to the more recent concept of the 'Truman Show' delusion; see Mishara and Fusar-Poli 2013). In our case study, Laurie clearly reports this kind of 'Trema': 'the world and its inhabitants were stranger than ever, their hidden rules turned against her and her only'. It would naturally be an extremely frightening experience for anyone fighting a battle against a 'strange' world and its 'hidden' rules. Such words carry a sinister feeling to say the least; by using these words, Laurie conveys the fear, the 'promise of danger' she had experienced during the 'Trema' period—and the source of this fear is exactly the sense of perplexity towards the world and its inhabitants, something she had felt since early childhood ('she could not grasp the "hidden rules" of how to deal with others'). In a world where only she cannot understand the 'why' and 'how' of the behaviour of other people, it should be no surprise that she feels fearful and threatened. As a response to a threatening world, of course one will gather as much information as possible in order to counteract the threat and fight against her 'unseen enemies'. Therefore, every little detail in the environment comes to the forefront of attention; a perceptual gestalt according to Conrad 'takes on saliency even before the patient orients to it'. What this generates is a perpetual dilemma, a paradox which leads to even more perplexity because the patient is forced to pay more attention to the surroundings as the result of the sheer incoming flow of stimuli overloading the senses, but at the same time, it does not solve the original problem of the threat, hence creating a vicious circle. In Laurie's case, this takes the form of her constant, almost obsessional questioning: 'she just knew she had to continue questioning, otherwise her enemies would win'. Her saying that 'everything has a new meaning and at the same time entirely meaningless' captures the nature of this paradox precisely. However, she also expresses a great degree of certainty and conviction ('I *know* everything has changed *for certain*') which is again paradoxical—how can anyone be so convinced about something that is 'entirely meaningless'? She did not know who her enemies were at this time, yet she was 'absolutely certain that she was being hunted down'; she was forced to question everything, yet she accepted the existence of, and the threat posed by, her enemies without questioning. It is an irreconcilable case that she questions because she has to win against her enemies whose malign force which causes her to question in the first place is beyond questioning. The net result is an even stronger sense of perplexity which feeds into itself and the loop continues. Interestingly, the consequence of Laurie's potentially losing to her enemies is psychological annihilation, and the biggest threat is not physical harm or death ('she would lose everything, including her autonomy as a person and freedom of thought') which may well be a worse outcome than anything physical for her as she had always treasured her imaginary life even when it became exhausting and distracting. Of course, she could not realise that it was her imagination that tormented her: consistent with Conrad's theory, it was the external world and most people in the world that turned against her ('she was the only one that had *not* changed').

However, the perplexity associated with 'Trema' cannot possibly continue forever. Just as Laurie reports, the moment at which a delusion forms and surfaces to the forefront of experience is a 'gradual then sudden' process followed by an intense feeling of revelation or, as Conrad calls it, an 'Apophany' (derived from 'revelation' in Greek). This second stage of the beginning of schizophrenia is termed an 'aha experience' (*Aha-Erlebnis*) not dissimilar to a 'eureka moment' which quite literally offers unprecedented explanations to everything the patient has been experiencing right up until this 'Apophany'. Unlike the highly disturbing and distressing perplexity in the 'Trema' stage, the realisation (no matter how 'out of touch with reality' it may sound) that there is a reason, in Laurie's case her unseen enemies trying to monitor her mind via a device planted in her brain, a malevolent plot behind all this brings a tremendous sense of relief ('she almost felt at ease for the first time in months') adding to the regret or the 'gutted' feeling that she should have realised sooner. From her own words, she was almost disappointed in herself that her 'stupidity' had led her to ignore something so logical, so obvious that should have been self-evident all along. According to Conrad, the 'aha experience' signifies a loss of the patient's ability 'to distance from the experience, to achieve an exchange of reference frames or perspectives, to consider the situation- even temporarily- with the eyes of the others' (Broome et al. 2012, p. 178). In other words, there is a kind of solipsism involved, a fundamental failure to adopt someone else's perspective and a full immersion in one's own internal world. For

Laurie, however, this is nothing new as she had always preferred solitude and imagination to external reality. To cite another example, the storyboards and stick figures she drew which did not follow a logical storyline could probably be seen as an indication of the solipsism and a desire to create her own rules in order to deal with the perplexity caused by the 'social world'. Indeed, the formation of Laurie's delusions follows exactly the same pattern except this time she was not aware that she created the delusions herself. Just like the feeling of fulfilment after the completion of a storyboard, the delusion offered her a solution upon which she could formulate new strategies to continue the fight with her enemies. She had finally found meaning and significance which were deeply connected to the very essence of her being. This leads to the third stage in Conrad's model, 'Anastrophe' (derived from Greek, 'turning back'), which has direct relevance to the sense of solipsism mentioned above. Conrad explains 'Anastrophe' as 'a reflexive turning back on the self in which the universe is experienced as revolving around the self as middle point', and the delusions are a 'reorganisation' of the patient's subjective experiences. The patient's self appears to be a *passive* middle point of all perceptions and events occurring in the world where everything is intimately self-referential. Nevertheless, once again this gives rise to a paradox. Although the sense of perplexity during the 'Trema' stage is temporarily alleviated by the delusional 'Apophany', the 'Anastrophe' stage may bring back the perplexity because the self is again a passive entity at the mercy of all the confusion caused by a fragmented self-world relationship. At least in Laurie's account, her worst fear was the loss of autonomy of thought; her self was only momentarily 'in charge' (even if she might not realise it) when the delusion was created, yet the content of such delusion had plunged her deeper in the perplexity for the very reason that she had lost autonomy ('my brain is nothing but a remotely accessible virtual storage device').

In our opinion, there is a more basic change taking place during the three stages of Conrad's model of beginning schizophrenia, which is the loss of 'common sense' at the root of the perplexity interwoven within the prodromal experience. The loss of autonomy and control described by Laurie can be viewed as a reflection of one's alienation from common sense; this could be due to a secondary (i.e. metacognitive) deficit in social processing (e.g. likely to be that in theory of mind) rendering common sense inaccessible or due to a more primary problem in how one *experiences* the world and its inhabitants which prevents the formation of a firm grasp on the basic understanding of self and other at a level even before theory of mind could take place. In other words, the kind of loss of common sense we propose, which is the focus of the next section, is an unavailability rather than inaccessibility deeply rooted in a disturbed and unstable self-world awareness.

13.4 Loss of 'Common Sense'

Considering that common sense (or its deficit) is central to the definition of perplexity as mentioned in the Introduction (a 'lack of spontaneous grasping of commonsensical meanings', Parnas et al. 2011), it would be useful to explore how this contributes to the patient's experience and why it might have arisen in a given individual. Indeed, Stanghellini (2000) also links the lack of common sense in psychosis with perplexity in acute cases and with autism in chronic schizophrenia, drawing from ideas of Blankenburg's (Broome et al. 2012, p. 159). However, because common sense seems such an intrinsic construct in our society, it is actually difficult to find an accurate definition for something most of us easily take for granted. Here we will adopt a Wittgensteinian definition as outlined in Stanghellini's abovementioned paper that common sense is a 'set of rules of the game that discipline human behaviours' (p. 778). This has direct relevance to our clinical case: in Laurie's account, she mentioned more than once about the 'hidden rules' governing the behaviours of others which she could never decipher. These hidden rules might well be the exact set of rules of the game by which Wittgenstein defines common sense. The continuous questioning of 'why?' (and the self-perpetuating question of 'why do I ask why?') since Laurie's childhood is an example not only of perplexity itself but also of a disturbed self-world awareness that prevents her from relating to others and understanding external reality. This disruption in one's core relationship to self and world separates what should be inseparable and reciprocal, namely, the connection between one's sense of immersion in the immediate world and the world's enveloping of the basic self; such disruption has been proposed as the essential feature of self-disturbances in prodromal psychosis (Nelson et al. 2009).

To a certain degree, Laurie's questioning did not result in a *total* alienation from reality; after all, there were a handful of exceptions in her life to which she could relate. Instead, it is the instability of this self-world relationship that led to the loss of common sense. It is worth noting that we are suggesting a loss (and not just a lack) of common sense here and this loss occurs at the very basic level of awareness without one's employing of any secondary or metacognitive processes. In other words, as we argued at the end of the previous section, a highly unstable yet still somewhat functional (as opposed to a completely blocked or impermeable self-world relationship) has made common sense unavailable and not just inaccessible. The sequence of events is that this instability leads to the loss of common sense which in turn leads to the feelings of perplexity. All three stages can occur without any active deliberation; again we think they are more akin to an automatic chain reaction than processes which involve volitional control. Laurie simply could not understand the rules of the game—whether she wanted to or not was irrelevant. Although she *preferred* her own company which might suggest that she *chose* to isolate herself (we will come back to this later), the end result would have remained the same. Common sense as a summation of 'social knowledge' which constitutes the implicit rules of the human world is, or at least should be, an automatic and pre-reflexive inferential process, and the attribution of which is effortless.

On the other hand, common sense as 'intuitive attunement' enables members of a society to successfully utilise these rules in order to understand and explain the *meaning* of social situations including other people's intentions. The givenness of common sense in any society is a prerequisite for the attunement of an individual in that society; as a consequence, a loss of common sense will almost naturally place the affected individual outside of what the social rules can regulate and therefore dramatically impair his ability to identify with that society. Stanghellini (2000) suggests that in psychosis, the damage to common sense can be at the conceptualisation level or the attitudinal level. In the former, an individual's social knowledge network is either deficient (atrophy) or overly expansive (hypertrophy). For example, in a hypertrophic state of knowledge, a single stimulus can trigger an infinite stream of free associations ('automatic consciousness') which could lead to the thought disorders seen in schizophrenia. Alternatively, the loss of common sense can be resulted from a sense of distrust and scepticism against intuition or an obsessional emphasis on rationality (for a fascinating study on logic and psychosis, see Owen et al. 2007). The latter approach implies the pathological process is actively willed by the patient ('an active and voluntary bracketing of common sense'), and this may indeed seem to be the case in Laurie's account, at least during the very first stage of her psychosis. The extreme scepticism towards everyday experience is a top-down process which destroys the intuitive nature of common sense and shifts more towards a 'morbid rationalism' or even an 'apoplexia philosophica' (interestingly, the word 'apoplexy' is also used in medicine as a term for internal bleeding) which quite literally paralyses the patient into a catatonic state because what is originally a coping strategy against the perplexity of reality by creating new rules (rather similar to Laurie's storyboards) has turned into a distorted, purely intellectualistic nihilism where the world is made of thoughts alone, and thus life in this world can no longer be lived within corporeality.

Despite debates about rationality and will aside, however, we think that the loss of common sense in Laurie's case is not simply a personal choice, and neither is it an active nor voluntary process. For Laurie, the mere idea of common sense was unfamiliar from the very beginning, and therefore she was compelled to make the 'choice' to establish her own rules in order to cope with everything else in the world. Perhaps this is why her delusions manifested as those of control and persecution—she had very little autonomy in deciding how she could navigate through the perplexity, and the only solution seemed to be that she had to let go of volition all together even though she was not aware of making this choice. Earnshaw (2011) argues that 'the discounting of the common sense world-picture is possible because of a breakdown in the atmosphere of trust' (p. 145), which is deeply engrained in our social knowledge and skills. Once this trust has been compromised or even destroyed, the world becomes a terrifying place where nothing can be understood naturally or intuitively, and this is where persecutory delusions ensue. If the breakdown of trust lies at the root of the loss of common sense, is it possible that the psychotic process has already started much earlier which renders the patient paranoid and mistrustful? Again it would be extremely naïve to assume a causal relationship in any case; however, in our opinion, the actual delusion itself forms *after* the breakdown of trust and the loss of common sense, but the feeling of uncanniness (without a delusional elaboration) and perplexity in delusional mood as a prerequisite for the 'Apophany' would have been present for a long time beforehand. Once the delusions have formed, they drive the mistrust even deeper into the patient's cognitive structure which then turns into yet another vicious circle. Delusions by nature are not the 'real' solutions or explanations for the external world, even though they might appear to be much more concrete and 'rational' than common sense and intuition. A third and more fundamental dimension of the disorder of common sense in psychosis is that of perception (see Uhlhaas and Mishara 2007): the perceptual field is thought to be directly connected to the pre-reflexive sense of being in the world and is therefore the basis of any continuity in a person's existence and self-consciousness. In psychosis, the self and the world in which the self resides are no longer a harmonious entity; the patient's embeddedness in the world and the embodiment within his self are drastically altered. The self becomes a distant object of observation and constant scrutiny, to the point that the entire self-experience diminishes. Further, the distance between experience and observation applies to the patient's relationship to the world as well, a sense of detachment from the social norms (which we argue again is not a willed action) and hence a loss of common sense. Indeed to us, the loss of common sense underlying feelings of perplexity on both perceptual and cognitive levels is the most subtle yet most significant indicator of a severely disturbed self which lies at the core of the phenomenology of psychosis and which signals the start of the prodromal stage (in other words, an even earlier stage before 'Trema'). In the next section, we will move on to a later stage and consider the actual formation of delusions. Why is it that of all the potential explanations for perplexity, including the feeling of uncanniness and loss of common sense and trust, those of a delusional nature always come to the forefront of experience? Previously, we have mentioned the bizarreness of such experience and delusions as metaphorical representations; here we will offer a more detailed discussion of another intrinsic process for humans—the need for understanding and the search for meaning.

13.5 Delusional Elaboration and the Search for Meaning

In our clinical case, it is apparent that Laurie had had pervasive difficulties grasping the meaning and significance of everyday events since early childhood (wondering why letters were arranged in certain ways to 'make sense' and the purpose of birthday parties); it seems that she knew there was a meaning—in fact, everything *had to* have a meaning—but one which was beyond her understanding. When her delusions 'dawned on her', all the constant doubt and questioning dissipated, and she took in this new meaning without asking the usual 'why' at all. Laurie's perspective is reflected in another previously published first-person account in *Schizophrenia Bulletin* (Hawkes 2012) explicitly titled 'Making Meaning', in which the author calls her delusions 'deep meaning' where she 'makes meaning where there is none' before concluding that it is in essence 'the result of random but coordinated activity in the brain'. Indeed, this propensity to attribute significance and draw connections between perceived events when there is none, in particular against others in social situations, is called 'Apophenia' (Fyfe et al. 2008) which has direct relevance (and is not only linguistically similar) to the stage of

'Apophany' coined by Conrad. Let us consider the point when Laurie concluded 'this constant, persistent and unforgiving sense of unidentifiable uneasiness intensifying day by day was not a part of her imagination'. Undoubtedly, this was the moment when she finally found (or at least started to find) meaning 'in the real world' for the very reason that everything that had been puzzling her really did happen. Even when she was a child, her questioning about the meaning of ordinary daily activities seemed a parallel process with her rich internal life. As we have argued previously, psychosis is not simply 'imagined' because the act of imagining is no longer a willed action: her imaginative processes have gained autonomy, simultaneous with a loss of autonomy of her own thoughts (Parnas and Sass 2001). Her imagination was no longer private and under her volitional control; however, delusions may still be viewed as *imaginings* even though they are not wilfully imagined. Currie (2000) suggests there are two stages of delusion formation from imagination: first, a misidentification of imaginings as reality and, second, a propensity for imaginings to become beliefs. The fact that one's imagination is not directly accessible to the external world or others unless he explicitly makes the imagined content available ('epistemic asymmetry') is no longer true with Laurie, even though she still maintained a kind of knowledge that the perceived events occurred in her subjective psychological space *in the first instance* ('epistemic primacy') before diffusing outwards. The perceptual properties of these seemingly internal mental events, whether they were unconsciously assigned at a later stage or automatically acquired, created an experiential distance (and disturbance) between herself and what should be an intimately accessible awareness. This perceptualisation of imagination (Rasmussen and Parnas 2015) significantly accentuates the salience and reality of internally generated events, and the contrast between the 'realness' of this externalisation and the original perplexity is not something anyone could easily ignore. As a consequence, a (delusional) meaning is attached to the external nature of the experience, and this meaning is reinforced as long as the experience itself maintains externality, and this particular meaning is often resistant to contrary evidence, perhaps due to some kind of memory consolidation (the moment of 'Apophany' is so strongly imprinted that it is extremely difficult to take on a different perspective). However, this approach implies that the prodromal individual, after experiencing a long period of perplexity, is not 'searching' for meaning but simply takes on the most salient meaning available and discards all the other alternative meanings without any consideration. If this is always the case, why is it that perplexity leads to drastically different conclusions for different individuals, especially when there is supposedly no conscious or willed guidance of thought (or imagination)?

We think that perhaps the answer lies in the structure of consciousness, in particular the 'fringe' component (alongside the 'nucleus') of consciousness as proposed by William James (James 1950) and discussed by Carr (2010): the fringe is not the focus of overt and explicit attention and is often nonsensory and in the periphery of awareness. Feelings of knowing, familiarity and expectation are example characteristics of the fringe component, together with feelings of intention, agency and ownership of thought and action. They are denoted as 'feelings' for the very reasons that they are 'diaphanous and translucent', something that is not solid or graspable. The fringe component of conscious experience also involves a sense of 'rightness', of 'harmony', of fit and, most importantly, of *meaningfulness* manifested as 'a signal of tight fit, coherence, or compatibility between the nucleus and the fringe' (Carr 2010, p. 196). This feeling of rightness is key to making sense of a thought, perception or an external event: according to James himself, when something makes sense, there is a 'subjective feeling of rationality' (even if it is objectively irrational or plain wrong), and when the sense of rightness is hindered, we will be inevitably 'dissatisfied and perplexed'. Carr (2010) argues that delusions arise because of the same kind of rightness feeling with the proto-psychotic anomalous experiences and that delusions serve the purpose of eliminating the discord or dissonance between what is in the core field of awareness in the nucleus of consciousness and what is felt in the fringe. He posits that 'the delusional explanation thereby creates harmony between the contents of consciousness in the nucleus and the patient's associative network and in doing so induces a feeling of rightness or good fit in the fringe'. As a result of the intense and pervasive feeling of rightness brought about by the delusional elaboration, the patient may even find aesthetic value in the delusions which validates the original (albeit abnormal) experience via a coherent context between experience and explanation. The consequence is the persistence and maintenance of delusions in the face of contradictory objective evidence because the subjective 'goodness of fit' is so overwhelmingly powerful (which is also reflected in Wittgenstein's approach to aesthetics, in that 'the attraction of certain kinds of explanation is greater than you can conceive'). We believe that the 'charm' of a delusional elaboration is not necessarily always the result of 'anything that clicks': although the concept of the Jamesian 'fringe' is already very compelling, we would like to add that the fringe experience is different to each individual and the definition of the 'feeling of rightness' is extremely variable both between and within individuals. The prodromal individual did not simply 'decide' on a delusion after searching through all the alternative meanings, at least not consciously or even willingly—instead, the delusional elaboration is something that 'dawns on' them regardless of whether there has been an internal searching process or not. Perhaps the sense of perplexity before 'Apophany' is already an index of 'searching for meaning', and the delusion is the meaning itself. When there is questioning, there needs to be a corresponding answer; when there is perplexity, there also needs to be an attribution of meaning. When such meaning evades conscious scrutiny, it will appear particularly persuasive and logical, no matter how one reaches the conclusion in the first place. Therefore, the delusional elaboration is the fruition of a mutually (in terms of both the nucleus and the fringe of consciousness) well-fitted resolution of perplexity and not of an action-guiding, deliberative inference or personal choice.

13.6 Clinical Implications

We opened Laurie's account with the observation that both her diagnosis and treatment of psychosis were severely delayed; in fact, the reasons for this were manifold, and in this section, we would like to elaborate further in order to offer some suggestions for clinical practice. Perhaps in many ways Laurie was not a 'typical' case of psychosis in her teenage years, and the length of the prodromal period (over 3 years) in addition to the lack of functional impairment, at least in the beginning, were somewhat puzzling to the clinician who was treating her for her depressive symptoms which were what brought her to the attention to her GP in the first place. Unfortunately, due to both Laurie's unwillingness to confide in the GP and the GP's own inattentiveness to the *nature* of Laurie's depression, nobody came to the realisation that the affective symptoms manifested as a secondary reaction to an underlying psychosis. Nevertheless, even her psychotic symptoms were vague and ambiguous at the time which further complicated her receiving an accurate diagnosis. We therefore suggest that in terms of early assessment, the clinician might need to enquire further into *why* the patient has a certain complaint, is it masking something deeper, and why is the patient reluctant to talk about it? Help-seeking behaviour by the individual himself is not always prevalent in psychosis at least during the acute phase due to a lack of insight, yet the unspecific mental health symptoms in a prodromal patient may still encourage him to seek help not for the psychosis itself but for the sheer distress and confusion he is experiencing even though he does not easily volunteer this information (Addington et al. 2002; Rietdijk et al. 2011). We think that when a primary care clinician faces complaints of depression and anxiety (as the GP is usually the first point of contact), it might be useful to also screen for basic psychotic symptoms—not necessarily frank psychosis such as delusional ideation and hallucinations, but more about very subtle changes in thought and perception both of the patient's self and of the external world. One example would be 'Do things appear changed somehow in a way you cannot easily describe?' or 'Do you feel something strange is happening to you?' Of course these are very general questions and may not carry any diagnostic specificity in the long term, but at least they could serve as very tentative early warning signs that the patient might be at risk for psychotic *symptoms* (note not necessarily a *diagnosis* of psychosis) and might require a follow-up clinical interview. Although a detailed assessment using questionnaires for basic symptoms or even self-disturbances (Nelson et al. 2012; Parnas et al. 2005) may be practically difficult to implement (usually a GP appointment only lasts 10 min) in a primary care setting, asking a few simple questions about the patient's subjective experience takes just as long as deciding which antidepressant to use and writing a prescription.

Although there is currently no recognised diagnostic label for attenuated psychosis (as mentioned before, some argue that the prodrome is only a retrospective concept) and even if there was, the predictions made about the progression to actual psychosis would remain very much unreliable. As a result, we do not think a diagnostic label at this stage is very useful for the clinician or the suffering individual because although accurate diagnoses can lead to effective treatment, they should never replace a clinician's duty to treat distressing symptoms no matter what the diagnosis might be in the end. This is why the early intervention for psychosis (EIP) services can play a major role in alleviating the patient's suffering by embracing diagnostic uncertainty and target individual complaints. However, on occasion, referral to the EIP services has an additional step in that access to EIP requires a responsible clinician from secondary care (i.e. a psychiatrist) who will decide whether it is necessary or appropriate for a certain patient to receive input from the EIP services. In contrast, ideally patients displaying very early psychotic symptoms should be triaged by EIP services straight away and directly from primary care, as such teams typically have greater experience in eliciting subtle psychotic psychopathology than general mental health teams (Broome et al. 2005a). In Laurie's case, her consultant psychiatrist did not even consider the possibility for psychosis at all because at the time Laurie was referred to him by her GP, she was not frankly delusional or hallucinating even though severe depression is less common in teenagers and should have rung alarm bells. When it became apparent that Laurie did indeed suffer from a psychotic disorder, the consultant still never made the referral to the EIP services because she had been under the community mental health team 'for too long'. In our opinion, both GPs and psychiatrists need to be better educated about the very early signs of psychosis and stop insisting on equating 'psychosis' with 'a severe break from reality and zero insight' or even a sudden drop in levels of functioning. Instead, perhaps clinicians should spend more time *listening* to the patient: what has he been experiencing and what might this potentially *mean*? Perhaps just as the patient himself needs a meaning and an explanation for his experiences, the clinicians also need to find out the 'why' and the 'how' of the symptoms presented to them and to enquire about subtle and nebulous experiences. Psychiatric diagnoses unlike their counterparts in general medicine are based on judgements and not test results; consequently, a wrong judgement or even a right judgement made at the wrong time can be extremely detrimental. In the psychosis prodrome, if a diagnosis of schizophrenia, for example, is made too early or too late, this will affect the patient's prognosis because in the former case, it will likely make the patient even more distressed due to the stigma associated with psychotic illnesses and in the latter case (such as with Laurie), it may cause delay in both pharmacological and psychological treatments. It may sound somewhat idealistic but a diagnosis can only serve its purpose and do more good than harm when it is made timely and when it is necessary. Accuracy comes secondary to necessity—sometimes it is simply not necessary to label someone's *personal experiences* into a medical category. The potential presence of an underlying (psycho-)pathology does not always mean we should further pathologise his experiences.

We strongly believe that treatment (medication and/or talking therapy) should commence as soon as it is necessary based on the level of distress caused to the sufferer and not just on the scores of a diagnostic tool or questionnaire. Whether the patient has 'insight' or not, the decisions made on treatment options should closely involve the patient and his carers. The use of antipsychotic medications in the psychosis prodrome is still very much controversial, but if possible, the decision should be on a case-to-case basis according to the level of distress and risk whilst minimising potential ethical issues (Cornblatt et al. 2001). Again this might be unrealistic due to a shortage of experienced medical staff or funding for mental health services (especially with psychological therapies); we do think that in some cases, the use of (very) low-dose antipsychotic drugs can be immensely beneficial at an early stage even if used to dampen down the overwhelming feelings of uneasiness and anxiety. Psychological therapies, on the other hand, should perhaps aim at equipping the patient with adaptive coping strategies in order to deal with the distress caused by his experiences in the first instance instead of solely focusing on reorganising the patient's thinking patterns or beliefs. Although the sense of perplexity and confusion in early psychosis as discussed in this chapter can be extremely resistant to intervention and change, if detected early enough, the individual might be able to learn the skills necessary to reorient himself and re-establish his self-world relationship with the right kinds of help which are determined on an individual basis. Fortunately for Laurie, she did eventually manage to switch to a psychiatrist with whom she could establish a good rapport and who immediately identified her treatment needs. Laurie still experiences thoughts that are not hers and hears that odd voice from time to time, and she is still highly imaginative even today; she never considers herself 'recovered', but perhaps it is never her ultimate goal whatever the definition of 'recovery' might be. In her own words, she has finally learnt to accept that there will always be things she cannot comprehend in this world and the sense of perplexity may never fully diminish; however, she now views her psychosis as a kind of parallel process that stays with her but does not interfere with her life as much as it once did. This understanding is also a 'revelation' which will stay with her, but one for which she is grateful.

13.7 Conclusion

Through the experiences of 'Laurie', we have presented a clinical scenario of the psychosis prodrome with the sense of perplexity and delusional mood/atmosphere as its focus. Using Laurie as a paradigmatic case study, we have emphasised on the roles a disturbed self-world awareness plays in the pathogenesis of perplexity and argued that factors and processes such as a loss of common sense are at the centre of the prodrome by providing evidence in the context of contemporary medical and philosophical literature. We have discussed the importance of self-disturbances in the phenomenology of psychosis in general before offering some suggestions for clinicians. Indeed, the 'first impression' a clinician presents to a highly distressed prodromal patient can never be underestimated in terms of establishing a valuable therapeutic relationship and helping the patient regain his sense of self and clarity of thought, and this process cannot happen easily by simply writing a prescription for antipsychotics. Biological psychiatry and phenomenological psychopathology should work together and not against each other as there is a large degree of synergism, not antagonism, between the two disciplines. The study of the subjective experiences and biological investigations are both invaluable tools with the aim of alleviating the patient's suffering, as we can only achieve this goal when we accept that such suffering originates from deep within a person's own self and not just a malfunctioning brain. Perhaps when clinicians begin to adopt this attitude more often and acknowledge that subjective experience is just as valid as objective observation, it will also help the patient realise that although the world can indeed be a perplexing place for his self, there is always the prospect of integration and reconciliation between the external and internal 'realities'.

References

Addington, J., Penn, D., Woods, S. W., Addington, D., & Perkins, D. O. (2008). Social functioning in individuals at clinical high risk for psychosis. *Schizophrenia Research, 99*(1), 119–124.

Addington, J., Van Mastrigt, S., Hutchinson, J., & Addington, D. (2002). Pathways to care: help seeking behaviour in first episode psychosis. *Acta Psychiatrica Scandinavica, 106*(5), 358–364.

Berner, P. (1991). Delusional atmosphere. *British Journal of Psychiatry, 159*, 88–93.

Berrios, G. (1991). Delusions as wrong beliefs: A conceptual history. *British Journal of Psychiatry, 159*, 6–13.

Bortolotti, L. (2010). *Delusions and other irrational beliefs*. Oxford: Oxford University Press.

Broome, M. R., Harland, R., Owen, G. S., & Stringaris, A. (Eds.). (2012). *The Maudsley reader in phenomenological psychiatry*. Cambridge: Cambridge University Press.

Broome, M. R., Woolley, J. B., Johns, L. C., Valmaggia, L. R., Tabraham, P., Gafoor, R., et al. (2005a). Outreach and support in south London (OASIS): Implementation of a clinical service for prodromal psychosis and the at risk mental state. *European Psychiatry, 20*(5), 372–378.

Broome, M. R., Woolley, J. B., Tabraham, P., Johns, L. C., Bramon, E., Murray, G. K., et al. (2005b). What causes the onset of psychosis? *Schizophrenia Research, 79*(1), 23–34.

Carr, V. J. (2010). Beauty and belief: William James and the aesthetics of delusions in schizophrenia. *Cognitive Neuropsychiatry, 15*(1-3), 181–201.

Cermolacce, M., Naudin, J., & Parnas, J. (2007). The "minimal self" in psychopathology: re-examining the self-disorders in the schizophrenia spectrum. *Consciousness and Cognition, 16*(3), 703–714.

Cornblatt, B. A., Lencz, T., & Kane, J. M. (2001). Treatment of the schizophrenia prodrome: Is it presently ethical? *Schizophrenia Research, 51*(1), 31–38.

Currie, G. (2000). Imagination, delusion and hallucinations. *Mind & Language, 15*(1), 168–183.

Earnshaw, O. (2011). Losing anchoring in the everyday: The role of trust in commonsense and its breakdown in delusions. PhD Thesis.

Fusar-Poli, P., Bonoldi, I., Yung, A. R., Borgwardt, S., Kempton, M. J., Valmaggia, L., et al. (2012). Predicting psychosis: Meta-analysis of transition outcomes in individuals at high clinical risk. *Archives of General Psychiatry, 69*(3), 220–229.

Fyfe, S., Williams, C., Mason, O. J., & Pickup, G. J. (2008). Apophenia, theory of mind and schizotypy: Perceiving meaning and intentionality in randomness. *Cortex, 44*(10), 1316–1325.

Gerrans, P. (2001). Delusions as performance failures. *Cognitive Neuropsychiatry, 6*(3), 161–173.

Hawkes, E. (2012). Making meaning. *Schizophrenia Bulletin, 38*(6), 1109–1110.

Humpston, C. S., & Broome, M. R. (2015). The spectra of soundless voices and audible thoughts: Towards an integrative model of auditory verbal hallucinations and thought insertion. *Review of Philosophy and Psychology*, 1–19.

Humpston, C. S., Walsh, E., Oakley, D. A., Mehta, M. A., Bell, V., & Deeley, Q. (2016). The relationship between different types of dissociation and psychosis-like experiences in a non-clinical sample. *Consciousness and Cognition, 41*, 83–92.

James, W. (1950). *The principles of psychology* (Vol. 1). New York: Dover Publications.

Jaspers, K. (1962). *General Psychopathology* (J. Hoenig & M. W. Hamilton, Trans.). Manchester, UK: Manchester University Press.

Kapur, S. (2003). Psychosis as a state of aberrant salience: A framework linking biology, phenomenology, and pharmacology in schizophrenia. *American Journal of Psychiatry, 160* (1), 13–23.

Kim, Y., Takemoto, K., Mayahara, K., Sumida, K., & Shiba, S. (1994). An analysis of the subjective experience of schizophrenia. *Comprehensive Psychiatry, 35*(6), 430–436.

Levin, R., Sirof, B., Simeon, D., & Guralnick, O. (2004). Role of fantasy proneness, imaginative involvement, and psychological absorption in depersonalisation disorder. *The Journal of Nervous and Mental Disease, 192*(1), 69–71.

Maj, M. (2013). Karl Jaspers and the genesis of delusions in schizophrenia. *Schizophrenia Bulletin, 39*(2), 242–243.

Mishara, A. L. (2010). Klaus Conrad (1905–1961): Delusional mood, psychosis, and beginning schizophrenia. *Schizophrenia Bulletin, 36*(1), 9–13.

Mishara, A. L., & Fusar-Poli, P. (2013). The phenomenology and neurobiology of delusion formation during psychosis onset: Jaspers, Truman symptoms, and aberrant salience. *Schizophrenia Bulletin, 39*(2), 278–286.

Nelson, B., Fornito, A., Harrison, B. J., Yücel, M., Sass, L. A., Yung, A. R., et al. (2009). A disturbed sense of self in the psychosis prodrome: Linking phenomenology and neurobiology. *Neuroscience and Biobehavioural Reviews, 33*(6), 807–817.

Nelson, B., Thompson, A., & Yung, A. R. (2012). Basic self-disturbance predicts psychosis onset in the ultra high risk for psychosis "prodromal" population. *Schizophrenia Bulletin, 38*(6), 1277–1287.

Nelson, B., Yung, A. R., Bechdolf, A., & McGorry, P. D. (2008). The phenomenological critique and self-disturbance: Implications for ultra-high risk ("prodrome") research. *Schizophrenia Bulletin, 34*(2), 381–392.

Niendam, T. A., Bearden, C. E., Zinberg, J., Johnson, J. K., O'Brien, M., & Cannon, T. D. (2007). The course of neurocognition and social functioning in individuals at ultra high risk for psychosis. *Schizophrenia Bulletin, 33*(3), 772–781.

Owen, G. S., Cutting, J., & David, A. S. (2007). Are people with schizophrenia more logical than healthy volunteers? *The British Journal of Psychiatry, 191*(5), 453–454.

Parnas, J., Bovet, P., & Zahavi, D. (2002). Schizophrenic autism: clinical phenomenology and pathogenetic implications. *World Psychiatry, 1*(3), 131.

Parnas, J., Møller, P., Kircher, T., Thalbitzer, J., Jansson, L., Handest, P., & Zahavi, D. (2005). EASE. Examination of anomalous self-experience. *Psychopathology, 38*(5), 236–258.

Parnas, J., Raballo, A., Handest, P., Jansson, L., Vollmer-Larsen, A., & Saebye, D. (2011). Self-experience in the early phases of schizophrenia: 5-year follow-up of the Copenhagen Prodromal Study. *World Psychiatry, 10*(3), 200–204.

Parnas, J., & Sass, L. A. (2001). Self, solipsism, and schizophrenic delusions. *Philosophy, Psychiatry, and Psychology, 8*(2), 101–120.

Perona-Garcelán, S., Cuevas-Yust, C., García-Montes, J. M., Pérez-Álvarez, M., Ductor-Recuerda, M. J., Salas-Azcona, R., et al. (2008). Relationship between self-focused attention and dissociation in patients with and without auditory hallucinations. *The Journal of Nervous and Mental Disease, 196*(3), 190–197.

Rasmussen, A. R., & Parnas, J. (2015). Pathologies of imagination in schizophrenia spectrum disorders. *Acta Psychiatrica Scandinavica, 131*(3), 157–161.

Rietdijk, J., Hogerzeil, S. J., van Hemert, A. M., Cuijpers, P., Linszen, D. H., & van der Gaag, M. (2011). Pathways to psychosis: Help-seeking behavior in the prodromal phase. *Schizophrenia Research, 132*(2), 213–219.

Sass, L. A., & Parnas, J. (2003). Schizophrenia, consciousness, and the self. *Schizophrenia Bulletin, 29*(3), 427–444.
Stanghellini, G. (2000). Vulnerability to schizophrenia and lack of common sense. *Schizophrenia Bulletin, 26*(4), 775–787.
Uhlhaas, P. J., & Mishara, A. L. (2007). Perceptual anomalies in schizophrenia: Integrating phenomenology and cognitive neuroscience. *Schizophrenia Bulletin, 33*(1), 142–156.
Wing, J. K., Babor, T., Brugha, T., Burke, J., Cooper, J. E., Giel, R., et al. (1990). SCAN: Schedules for clinical assessment in neuropsychiatry. *Archives of General Psychiatry, 47*(6), 589–593.
Yung, A. R., & McGorry, P. D. (1996). The prodromal phase of first-episode psychosis: Past and current conceptualizations. *Schizophrenia Bulletin, 22*(2), 353–370.

Self-Disorders in Schizophrenia

14

Mads Gram Henriksen and Julie Nordgaard

14.1 Introduction

The aim of this chapter is to elicit and discuss certain anomalies of self-experience (i.e., self-disorders), which empirical studies consistently have found to aggregate significantly in schizophrenia spectrum disorders but not in other mental disorders (Parnas and Henriksen 2014). From the outset, it is important to stress that self-disorders are *nonpsychotic* experiential phenomena. Thus, accounting for the experience of delusion or hallucination is principally beyond the scope of this chapter (for some considerations on these issues, see, e.g., Sass 1994, 2014; Henriksen 2013; Henriksen and Parnas 2014; Henriksen et al. 2015).

One of the first things you realize when interviewing patients about their self-disorders is that these experiential anomalies typically have been present from childhood or early adolescence, i.e., they appear to be mainly trait-like features, persisting prior to psychosis but, from our experience, usually also after remission has been established. In this chapter, we focus on a single patient, who offers rich descriptions of some of the most typical and frequently reported self-disorders in schizophrenia. Today, self-disorders are best assessed with the *Examination of*

M.G. Henriksen (✉)
Center for Subjectivity Research, University of Copenhagen, Njalsgade 140-142, Building 25, 5th floor, 2300 Copenhagen, Denmark

Psychiatric Center Glostrup, University Hospital, University of Copenhagen, Copenhagen, Denmark

Faculty of Health and Medical Sciences, Institute of Clinical Medicine, University of Copenhagen, Copenhagen, Denmark
e-mail: mgh@hum.ku.dk

J. Nordgaard
Faculty of Health and Medical Sciences, Institute of Clinical Medicine, University of Copenhagen, Copenhagen, Denmark

Psychiatric Research Unit, Region Zealand, University Hospital, Copenhagen, Denmark

G. Stanghellini, M. Aragona (eds.), *An Experiential Approach to Psychopathology*,
DOI 10.1007/978-3-319-29945-7_14

Anomalous Self-Experience scale (Parnas et al. 2005a), viz., the EASE scale. For the sake of clarity, we refer to items and item numbers found in the EASE scale in our analysis of the patient's experiences (Sect. 14.2).

We have structured the chapter in the following way: first, we introduce the patient and offer a quite lengthy vignette, illuminating a selection of some of her most central self-disorders and touching upon the core of her suffering. Second, we analyze the patient's experiences in the light of contemporary phenomenological research, and we address the psychopathological core that appears to underlie the various manifestations of self-disorders. Third, we offer a brief overview of the results from empirical studies on self-disorders. Finally, we discuss the format of the psychiatric interview that explores these psychopathological phenomena and the appropriate approach to the interview.

A Case Story

The patient "K" is a 25-year-old female. At the age of 23, she was hospitalized for the first time due to severe suicidal ideation, and she was diagnosed with paranoid schizophrenia (ICD-10/DSM-IV). In the last couple of years, she has regularly been in contact with an outpatient clinic, and she has taken antipsychotic medication from time to time. "K" is studying at the university and lives alone in an apartment. She has friends and is in touch with her family but the contact is fairly unstable. When we meet her, she is hospitalized for the second time, again due to suicidal ideation.

Sense of self. Already from early childhood, she felt very different from others: "I feel like I'm not a natural human being or a proper human being or something like that. I have always tried so much to be a real human being, but I have the feeling that I'm not." In school, she says, "I was a total pushover, very manageable, extremely pleasing. At home, I could be very selfish, greedy, and very dictatorial—all the things that were forbidden for me to be in school. There, I always pretended to take it easy, but when I got home it felt as if I had being holding my breath the entire day. I would go into my room and cry for hours. It was a very peculiar grief. I don't know where it came from. It was not that I was sad about something specific. It was everything. I think it has something to do with the fact that I don't feel like I have a core or a substance... Increasingly, I began to feel that I sort of fused with the surroundings... And I had a hard time recognizing myself from hour to hour, day to day." She elaborates on her feeling of not being a natural human being. "I had this idea that I didn't look human and that everybody was sort of being nice to me and played along. Seriously, when I passed others in the street, they were polite and didn't stare too much, but they would think "what was that?" That is, I really thought that I wasn't recognizable as a human being." She describes the first time she had the experience of looking inhuman. "I remember it very precisely. I must have been 4 or 5 years old. I was starting dance class and I was looking in the mirror. I was standing next to the other kids and I remember that I looked alien. I felt like I sort of stuck out from that large wall mirror. As if I wasn't a real child. This feeling has been very persistent from very early on."

Others and common sense. She reports that she often ponders on the big questions in life. "I have always taken things, you know, a little heavier than others. I was sort of more thin skinned or something. I have always struggled to understand why people didn't take life more seriously. I mean, "How can you just walk around, be named 'Angie,' buy butter, and take riding lessons?" Every morning, when I wake up, I realize like for the first time that this is the real reality, that we are all going to die, that we don't know why we are here, that nothing makes sense... This is one of the reasons why I feel different from others. They walk around and talk on their phone, plan what they want to do... It puzzles me that I haven't gotten used to it. Everyday I realize that the sky is just above us, right... infinity is so near, we don't know why we are here, and we will all die...It hurts me that it is so easy and natural for the rest of the world. They don't even think about it." This also makes social behavior difficult for her. "I always feel that it is like enormously feigned when I have some social interaction. It feels false, like I can't react naturally or sincerely like everyone else...I have the experience that there are two of me: the one that interacts with someone and then there is the real me, who sits there behind. For example, 'I sense that the one I'm talking to finds my statement a little transgressive, so I add a little humor here to establish an ironic distance. That may perhaps... yes, that worked well...' And I do it, like, simultaneously. I don't feel present at all." It is not only in relation to the big questions or sociality that she finds herself different from others. "For others, simple everyday things are incredibly easy. When we are hungry, we eat; when we are thirsty, we drink. It's elementary... But for me it's not like that. I feel like I don't have that natural balance, because I can get so lost in my own thoughts... If I, say, think or read, I can sit for 10 h and sort of forget my body and the physical world, and then suddenly realize, I really need to pee or my bones are aching from sitting in this chair... When I had roommates, I would adopt their daily rhythm. For example, when they ate, I would eat something; when they showered, I would take a shower, etc. It's not that I don't know these things. When I am alone, I must have a plant or pet in my room. You know, like a physical watermark, reminding me that the world is still spinning, that time passes. Like, "well, I see the flower needs water. I too am a living organism, so I also need water." It has always been like that. If there wasn't a world to remind me that time passes and that I am not in some sort of time vacuum, I could sit with a book until I starved to death."

Stream of consciousness. "I have a lot of problems with my memory. I can get completely alienated from my own memories. It's like the distinction between what you hear, see, and read dissolves and everything floats. For example, I can be extremely sad about something tragic that has happened to me and then suddenly realize, oh no, it was just that movie yesterday that ended badly. It's as if the context is cast away but the feeling remains intact... When that distinction dissolves, my trains of thought just race so fast that I can't keep up. I can't make heads or tails of the thoughts. It's like your brain talks faster than you can listen. I know these trains of thought come from within me, but I can get very insecure because their acoustic quality is identical with the quality of a voice of someone standing next to me... It feels as if these trains of thought aren't really my own."

The body. "I have always had a difficult relation to my body. Sometimes, while lying down, I have had the experience that my shoulders were dislocated or dismantled, and then I couldn't move... I have a very hard time feeling my body and the demarcation of my body. Then I have to do like this [she repeatedly puts pressure on her left arm with her right hand] just to feel something... to sort of merge my thoughts and my body... to have a leash on the kite so it doesn't fly away... It's as if there is a distance between my body and my mind. It's like my mind is a little puppeteer, sitting far away, controlling my body. It's not like I see myself from above or something. But it's like I'm not in my body or not attached to it. It's like my body is an appendix that hangs below me. My body feels alien to me and I get annoyed that it demands stuff. I wish I could be free of it. My relation to my body is as if I got a dog without realizing how bothersome it would be, and I just want to send it away." She also has a problematic relation to her own specular image: "For 10 years of my life, I couldn't stand looking at myself in the mirror, and I still have a very hard time doing it. It was not like 'no, I don't like it that much,' but more like 'turn off the light, turn the mirror around, smash it, avoid it completely.' I couldn't stand it at all. It wasn't that I didn't think I looked pretty. It was because I felt I didn't look human. I would be happy, if I just looked human."

14.2 Analysis of Self-Disorders

In a remarkably lucid manner, "K" describes a variety of self-disorders, whose distinctness we now will elicit. Subsequently, we will briefly address the assumed core underlying this panoply of experiential anomalies in schizophrenia. For the sake of clarity, we discuss clusters of self-disorders, following the four divisions in the case story. Yet, it is noteworthy that all these anomalous self-experiences are intrinsically interrelated.

"K's" enduring feeling of not being a natural, proper or real human being is at the very core of her suffering. She reports that this feeling dates back to early childhood. Patients with schizophrenia often report feelings of being profoundly different from others (*Anderssein*) or just "wrong." While the more precise quality of this feeling can remain ineffable for some patients, other patients, like "K," can clearly describe it. When exploring the nature of this feeling, it typically becomes evident that it cannot be exhaustively accounted for by any concrete, mundane, or *ontic* property (e.g., being too clever or feeling stupid, being too slim or fat, having other interests or hobbies than one's peers, coming from another cultural or familial background, etc.). Rather, what usually looms up is a pervasive sense of being *ontologically* different, i.e., a feeling of being different in which one's very humanity is at stake (e.g., feeling inhuman, alien, or perhaps another category of human). For "K," as for many other patients, the feeling of not being a real human is a constant source of solitude, isolation, and suffering. This particular feeling has also been aptly described by Prof. Elyn Saks, who lives with schizophrenia. In her autobiography, she writes, "[one] of the worst aspects of schizophrenia is the profound isolation—the constant awareness that you're different, some sort of alien, not really human" (2007, 193f.). For "K," this feeling is intertwined with an experience of lacking a "core" or "substance," which compromises her most intimate feeling of identity (i.e., she reports difficulties in recognizing herself from hour to hour, etc.). In connection to her description of not having a core, she reports that she felt that she "sort of fused with the surroundings." This is a conspicuous statement, perhaps indicative of a transitivistic experience, but we would need more information about the quality of the actually lived experience to be sure that what "K" reports here is in fact a self-disorder in the area of transitivism (e.g., 4.5). Moreover, her pervasive lack of self-identity seems also to be operative in her social behavior, where she, in school, describes herself as "a total pushover, very manageable, extremely pleasing." This description seems to be indicative of a hyper-adaptive attitude, reflecting a great need to accommodate to others' opinions, which, in this context, often revolves around a persistent feeling of not having an opinion of one's own (*Haltlosigkeit*). In the EASE scale, the feelings of being radically different from others, of lacking core, and of *Haltlosigkeit* are all manifestations of a single self-disorder, viz., "diminished sense of basic self" (2.1).

Another key aspect of her feeling of being different is expressed in her description of others. In her view, she perpetually ponders on the big questions in life, whereas others do not really take live seriously and tend to be occupied with trivialities or superficialities (e.g., "How can you just walk around, be named 'Angie', buy butter, and take riding lessons?"). She observes others talking on the phone and planning their activities, whereas she everyday realizes anew, as she put it, "that the sky is just above us, right... infinity is so near, we don't know why we are here, and we will all die." It puzzles her that she has not gotten "used to it," and it hurts her that "it is so easy and natural for the rest of the world." "They don't even think about it," she says. This cluster of experiences entails quite a few self-disorders, which we will now address from the vantage point of three of them, i.e., "loss of common sense" (2.12), "solipsistic grandiosity" (5.8), and "hyper-reflectivity" (2.6).

First, loss of common sense has for a long time been considered one of the essential features of schizophrenia (e.g., Blankenburg 1971, 2001; Stanghellini 2004). As in the case of "K," loss of common sense is frequently related to feelings of *Anderssein*, and it typically manifests as an inability to simply take for granted what is a matter of fact for nearly everybody, e.g., reflected in questions such as "why do people say 'hello' to each other?", "why is the sky blue?", or "why is a knife called a knife?". The point is of course not that "K" raises questions that others usually do not raise (if that was the point, most scientists and philosophers would also suffer from loss of common sense). Rather, the point is that these questions perpetually articulate themselves and require explicit attention and reflection on her behalf, because she cannot rest content with assumption. But what does this mean? Ordinarily, we navigate in life on the basis of a multiplicity of assumptions that lure in the tacit background of our awareness (e.g., when walking, my behavior manifests that I am committed to the assumption that "the ground is solid" even though I have formed no such assumption). These fundamental assumptions or, as Thornton put it, "certainties expressed by our actions" (Thornton

2008, 164) belong to an intersubjectively constituted and shared horizon of acting and knowing within which all knowledge and action take place. In other words, this horizon is not a matter of knowledge but is prior to knowledge. Therefore, it is also not something we simply can acquire by means of reasoning or logic—as one of Blankenburg's patients put it, "[it] is the kind of thing you just get naturally" (2001, 308) or, as "K" said at one point, "[it's] not that I don't know these things." Emphasis must therefore be on the fact that she still, after more than two decades, cannot get "used to" the ordinary, everyday life with all its trivialities and unquestioned assumptions, and consequently she finds herself deprived of the sense of "naturalness" she perceives in others. This horizon forms what Blankenburg called "common sense," which appear to have the same foundational, epistemological status as Wittgenstein's "framework propositions" or Searle's "background capacities" (Henriksen 2013). Against this backdrop, it should be evident that loss of common sense in schizophrenia is not a matter of having insufficient knowledge but reflects instead an instability in the basic, immediate attunement and resonance with the world, which usually involves an impaired pre-reflective grasp of the meaning of everyday objects, events, and social interactions. Typical manifestations of loss of common sense in schizophrenia include being occupied with questions that others take for granted, difficulties in telling what is situationally appropriate and contextually relevant from what is not, an idiosyncratic sense of taste and tact, etc.

Second, solipsistic grandiosity refers to a sense of superiority, exhibited either in speech or behavior, over one's fellow humans, leaving others to be seen as ignorant fools, occupied predominantly by superficial or trivial aspects of existence. This sense of grandiosity has a different coloring that the kind of grandiosity one may find in, say, narcissism, where others' appraisal, and admiration play a far more significant role. "K" exhibits solipsistic grandiosity, when she said, "How can you just walk around, be named 'Angie', buy butter, and take riding lessons?" Often, solipsistic grandiosity is associated with another self-disorder, i.e., a feeling of having extraordinary insights into hidden dimensions of reality. There is a fairly strong indication that "K" also has the experience of "extraordinary insight" (5.4), e.g., she said several times that everyday she realizes anew "that the sky is just above us, right. . . infinity is so near" etc., but we would need further a description of the quality of her experience to potentially be able to rate this self-disorder as present.

Third, hyper-reflectivity refers to exaggerated and self-alienating forms of self-consciousness that is characterized by a recurring and excessive tendency to take aspects of the environment or oneself as objects of intense reflection (Sass and Parnas 2003). As in the case of "K," hyper-reflectivity is very often coupled with loss of common sense. Some patients report that they constantly reflect upon everyday events or objects in an attempt to decode their meaning. The objects of hyper-reflectivity may, however, also be aspects of oneself that normally only lurk in the background of our awareness, e.g., the *way* one thinks, listens, speaks, or interacts with others. In this case, hyper-reflectivity can take the form of self-monitoring, which may be operative alongside the patient's interactions with others and the world. This is also vividly described by "K," when she said, e.g., "I have the experience that there are two of me: the one that interacts with someone and then there is the real me, who sits there behind..." In the EASE scale, this form of self-monitoring is rated as a subtype of "distorted first-person perspective" (2.2.2). Moreover, her excessive tendency to hyper-reflect and self-monitor compromises her feeling of being present in social interactions ("I don't feel present at all"), which should be rated in the EASE scale as a form of "diminished presence" (2.4). This self-disorder usually involves a feeling of distance to the world or a sense of barrier between oneself and the world (e.g., as if being in a cheese dome) or a decreased ability to become affected, touched, drawn, motived, etc., by others, objects or events, and often patients complain about not being fully present or participating in the world. Finally, "K" indicates the presence of another self-disorder, viz., "I-split" (2.7.1), which refers to an experience of one's self being divided into semi-independent parts ("there are two me...").

"K's" feeling of being alienated from her own memories appears to be founded mainly on her experience of the dissolving or, at least, unstable distinction between "what you hear, see, and read." She reports that she can be "extremely sad about something tragic" that has happened to her and then suddenly realize that this tragic event did in fact not happen to her; it was something that happened to someone else, e.g., a character in a movie. "K's" experience is a typical example of a self-disorder, which in the EASE scale is termed 'inability to discriminate modalities of intentionality" (1.10), referring to an experience of being uncertain about whether or not one's experience, occurring or recalled, is, say, a perception, a memory, or a phantasy. For example, some patients, like "K," can be unsure or, at times, entirely unable to tell whether or not they themselves experienced something or if they merely read or heard about it or saw it in a movie. Other patients report that they can be uncertain about whether or not they have just thought something or spoken aloud. When this distinction dissolves, she said, "my trains of thought just race so fast that I can't keep up. I can't make heads or tails of the thoughts. It's like your brain talks faster than you can listen. I know these trains of thought come from within me, but I can get very insecure because their acoustic quality is identical with the quality of a voice of someone standing next to me... It feels as if these trains of thought aren't really my own." Here, "K" describes three additional self-disorders. First, she describes "thought pressure" (1.3), i.e., an experience of having many thematically *unrelated* thoughts or trains of thought occurring simultaneously or immediately after each other and with a clear loss of meaning. Often, the semantic content of these thoughts is neutral to the patient. Another patient described thought pressure with the analogy of "rockets shooting in all directions at once. It's one big chaos" (Henriksen and Nordgaard 2014, 437). Second, she describes "perceptualization of inner speech or thought" (1.7.1), i.e., her thoughts have an acoustic or auditory quality, allowing her to listen to her own thoughts spoken aloud internally. It is noteworthy that she does not believe that others can hear her thoughts or have access to them; if that was the case, then it would amount to a Schneiderian first-rank symptom of schizophrenia. In our experience, patients, who have thoughts aloud, usually report that it always has been like this, making it very ego-syntonic, and usually this particular self-disorder does not seem to involve a great deal of suffering. Third, "K" describes "loss of thought ipseity" (1.2), i.e., a feeling that some thoughts are deprived of the sense of mine-ness, e.g., appearing somehow alien, anonymous or as if they were not generated by the patient, yet the patient has no doubt that these thoughts are in fact generated by her. It is important to note that this feeling does not primarily pertain to the content of the thought.

Finally, "K" reports a complicated relationship with her own body, which feels alien to her—e.g., "[it's] as if there is a distance between my body and my mind. It's like my mind is a little puppeteer, sitting far away, controlling my body. It's not like I see myself from above or something. But it's like I'm not in my body or not attached to it. It's like my body is an appendix that hangs below me." Here, she vividly describes experiences of both "psychophysical split" (3.4) and "somatic depersonalization" (3.3)—she also rules out the possibility of understanding her experience as an "out-of-the-body" experience or, in EASE terms, as "dissociative depersonalization" (2.8). First, "psychophysical split" refers to a feeling as if the body and mind do not really fit together or are somehow disconnected—this is well described in the example above but also when she described how she tries to "merge my thoughts and my body... to have a leash on the kite so it doesn't fly away." In a seminal paper, Fuchs (2005) has described how disturbances of the lived body's transparency (i.e., its "mediated immediacy") can be altered in psychopathological conditions—e.g., patients with schizophrenia can become detached from the mediating processes and experience that they do not *inhabit* their body in the normal, unproblematic way ("disembodiment of the self"), whereas patients with melancholia rather tend to experience themselves as *imprisoned* in their own body, collapsed into its spatial-material boundaries, and unable to transcend their body and reach the world ("corporealization of the self"). Fuchs's description of disembodiment seems to us to capture a key aspect of "K's" experience of psychophysical split (e.g., "I'm not in my body..."). Second, "somatic depersonalization" refers to an experience of perceiving one's own body or parts of it as strange, alien, disconnected from each other, etc.—this is reflected, e.g., in "K's" description of her body as an "an appendix" that hangs below or in her comparison of her body to a demanding "dog," she would to give away if she could. In the same vein, she said that her body feels alien to her. She also reports that she is annoyed be the fact that her body demands stuff from her (e.g., to eat, drink, move, pee, etc.). Stanghellini has used the expression of "deanimated bodies" to articulate a kind of mechanization or objectification of the lived body in schizophrenia (2004, 127ff., 153ff.). In our view, this notion also captures important aspects of "K's" experiences of somatic depersonalization. Furthermore, "K" reports an experience of her shoulders sometimes becoming "dislocated or dismantled," and in such situations, she is, though fully conscious, unable to move. Again, she offers a description of somatic depersonalization. The experience of not being able to move may, however, also be an instance of "motor disturbance" (3.8.3), i.e., partial or complete blockage of intended motor actions (e.g., moving or speaking), but we would need her to further elaborate on this experience to feel confident that this particular self-disorder is present. Additionally, she describes "mirror phenomena" (3.2), "I couldn't stand looking at myself in the mirror (. . .) It was not like 'no, I don't like it that much', but more like 'turn off the light, turn the mirror around, smash it, avoid it completely'." Mirror phenomena refer to experiences of either unusually frequent, intense looking in the mirror, or entirely avoiding mirrors. Typically, patients look for or perceive changes in their face, and some patients may become surprised or even frightened by what they see, which regularly prompt them to avoid mirrors. The latter was the case for "K"; she explicitly said, "I felt I didn't look human."

It seems that we are back where we started, trying to understand a core feature of her suffering, namely, her enduring feeling of being radically different from others and of looking inhuman. The latter merits a few observations. How are we to understand the complaint of "looking inhuman?" When describing mirror phenomena, she said, "I *felt* I didn't look human," which seems to suggest that it is a *feeling*, a disturbing feeling obviously, but nonetheless just a feeling. When she described the onset of this experience, occurring in dance class, she said, "I was standing next to the other kids and I remember that I looked alien. I felt like I sort of stuck out from that large wall mirror. As if I wasn't a real child." Here, it is less obvious that it is just a feeling. She said that she *looked* alien and that she *felt* like she stuck out from the mirror (which in itself is a peculiar way of describing the feeling). Note also that she did not say that she felt like she stood out from the other kids but that she "sort of stuck out from that large wall mirror," which might be indicative of spatial-visual alterations in her perceptual field. At the very least, we should here consider the possibility that when looking in the mirror, she might perceive perceptual changes of her face or body, which can be rated as mirror phenomena, subtype 2 (3.2.2), in the EASE scale. Finally, she also described the experience of looking inhuman in the context of others perceiving her in the street, "[seriously], when I passed others in the street, they were polite and didn't stare too much, but they would think 'what was that?' That is, I really thought that I wasn't recognizable as a human being." This experience is obviously closely intertwined with her profound feeling of *Anderssein* and her experience of looking inhuman (mirror phenomena). Given the persistency of this disturbing experience and the manner in which she phrases it (e.g., "I really thought that I wasn't recognizable as a human being"), it seems to us to almost approach the level of delusion. However, we would need further examples and descriptions from her to confidently evaluate the quality of these perhaps different experiences of looking inhuman.

We have discussed "K's" experiences through the prism of self-disorders, and it is our hope that the reader now has a fairly good grasp of her experiential life, psychopathology, suffering, and of some of the core problems she face in life. Through this kind of active, mutual, phenomenological exploration of her experiences (see Sect. 14.4), we found unity and meaningful coherences in her experiences (symptoms) and behaviors (signs) that otherwise might appear fragmented, enigmatic, or perhaps incomprehensible. In other words, exploring self-disorders may increase the understanding of our patients and their lifeworlds. This kind of understanding relies on a reconstruction of the patients' altered experiential life and lifeworld and on imagining the impact these alterations can have on their self-understanding, emotions, expressivity, behavior, language use, etc. We also suggest that this kind of understanding enables a form of empathy by allowing us to understand something of what it might be like to experience the world as patients with schizophrenia sometimes do (Henriksen 2013). Using Ratcliffe's term, this kind of "radical empathy" requires, as he aptly has pointed out (2012), a suspension of ordinary, taken-for-granted assumptions about the world and how we usually experience it and a willingness and commitment to contemplate the possibility of structurally different ways of being-in-the-world. It is, however, not just the psychiatrist who gains a better understanding of the patient. In our experience, exploring self-disorders with patients may also facilitate a more individual and biographically coherent self-understanding on their part—this seemed also to be the case with "K."

Finally, the case story and the analysis both illustrate that self-disorders are not sharply delimited, independent symptoms but rather mutually implicative, interdependent aspects of a more comprehensive psychopathological Gestalt. So far, we have not addressed the core of this Gestalt, and it is beyond the scope of this chapter to do so in full detail (see instead Sass and Parnas 2003; Parnas 2011; Henriksen and Parnas 2012). Yet, three observations merit attention. First, the "self," which we suggest is "disordered" in schizophrenia (when we speak of "self-disorders"), does not refer to complex aspects of selfhood (e.g., reflected in notions such as "personality" or "social identity") but to a very basic experience of being a self, which signifies that we live our life in the first-person perspective, as a self-present, single, temporally persistent, bodily, and bounded subject of experience and action (Henriksen and Parnas 2014)—it follows from our analysis of "K's" experiences that nearly all of these "dimensions," which jointly facilitate the basic experience of being a self, are threatened in her case. Moreover, these "dimensions" are not of our making; descriptions of problems along these "dimensions" have a long history in psychiatry and can be traced back to Pick's work (1904/1996) on pathologies of self-consciousness and possibly even further back. In short, the basic experience of being a self refers to the first-personal givenness of experience, which immediately and implicitly facilitates a sense of "mine-ness" that transpires through the flux of time and changing modalities of consciousness. It is this very basic experience of being a self that appears to be fragile or unstable in schizophrenia, prompting, as in the case of "K," disturbing experiences of a profoundly diminished sense of "mine-ness" of one's own thoughts, actions, body, etc. Second, this basic experience of being a self is not something like a core or substance that operates behind our manifold experiences, somehow tying them together, but a feature or product of the very givenness of consciousness—e.g., when I speak, listen, see, or move, these experiences are given to me in such a way that I am always already pre-reflectively aware that *I am the one who speaks*, *listens*, *sees*, *moves*, etc., i.e., I have no need for self-reflection or self-perception to assure myself of being myself. Following Henry (1973), we may say that this basic experience of being a self arises from the "auto-affectivity" of consciousness. By implication, the pathogenetic core of the Gestalt of schizophrenia may be an instability or disturbance of the "auto-affectivity" of consciousness. Third, the very idea that the central disturbance in schizophrenia is a disorder of the self is not novel. It was ventilated more or less explicitly in most foundational texts on the concept of schizophrenia (e.g., Bleuler 1950; Kraepelin 1913; Minkowski 1927; Schneider 1950; Jaspers 1997), but until recently, systematic and empirical corroboration of this fundamental, clinical intuition was lacking.

14.3 Empirical Results

In 2005, the EASE scale was published (Parnas et al. 2005a). The EASE scale is a semi-structured psychometric instrument for a qualitative and quantitative assessment of self-disorders. Today, it has been translated into ten languages (see www.easenet.dkfor details). The scale comprises 57 main items, aggregated into five domains: (1) cognition and stream of consciousness, (2) self-awareness and presence, (3) bodily experiences, (4) demarcation/transitivism, and (5) existential reorientation/solipsism. The EASE scale has a monofactorial structure (Raballo and Parnas 2012; Nordgaard and Parnas 2014) and exhibits a very high internal consistency (Cronbach's alpha > 0.900; Nordgaard and Parnas 2014) and good-to-excellent inter-rater reliability among trained and experienced psychiatrists or clinical psychologists (Parnas et al. 2005a; Møller et al. 2011; Nelson et al. 2012; Nordgaard and Parnas 2012).

Jointly, the empirical studies using the EASE scale or pre-EASE analog scales demonstrate the following results: (1) self-disorders aggregate selectively in schizophrenia and schizotypal disorders but not in disorders outside the schizophrenia spectrum (Parnas et al. 2005b; Raballo et al. 2011; Nordgaard and Parnas 2014); (2) patients with schizophrenia and patients with schizotypal disorder score statistically similar on the EASE scale (Raballo and Parnas 2012; Nordgaard and Parnas 2014); (3) self-disorders discriminate first-admission cases with bipolar psychosis from schizophrenia, even after adjusting for the differences in the scores on the PANNS-derived positive and negative symptom scales (Haug et al. 2012a), and self-disorders occur more frequently in residual schizophrenia than in remitted bipolar psychosis (Parnas et al. 2003); (4) self-disorders have been found to occur in individuals who are biologically related to probands with schizophrenia (Raballo and Parnas 2011); (5) prospective studies have shown the following results: self-disorders are identifiable among nonpsychotic help-seeking adolescents (Koren et al. 2013); self-disorders predict transition to psychosis in an ultrahigh risk sample (Nelson et al. 2012); and high baseline scores of self-disorders were predictive of a subsequent diagnostic transition to the schizophrenia spectrum in a 5-year follow-up study of first-admitted non-schizophrenia spectrum patients (Parnas et al. 2011); (6) correlational studies have found the following results: self-disorders correlate with social dysfunction (Haug et al. 2014) and suicidality (Skodlar and Parnas 2010; Haug et al. 2012b) in schizophrenia, respectively; self-disorders correlate positively with positive and negative symptoms, formal thought disorders, and perceptual disturbances, respectively (Nordgaard and Parnas 2014); no correlations have been found between self-disorders and IQ (Nordgaard and Parnas 2014) or neurocognitive measures (Nordgaard et al. 2015), except for impaired verbal memory (Haug et al. 2012c). For a detailed review of empirical pre-EASE and EASE-based studies on self-disorders, see Parnas and Henriksen (2014).

14.4 The Phenomenological Interview in Psychiatry

We obtain information about our patients' psychopathological experiences mainly by talking with the patients, observing their behavior, and by talking with their relatives. Prior to the psychopathological interview, it is necessary to consider the object of inquiry and the appropriate way of examining the object. The object of a psychopathological interview is of course symptoms and signs (Berrios 2002; Markova and Berrios 2009). In contrast to somatic medicine, psychiatric symptoms and signs are not something close to third-person data, which would render them publicly accessible and mutually independent entities, devoid of subtle or complex forms of meaning and suitable for context-independent definition and measurement. In somatic medicine, symptoms and signs have no intrinsic meaning, and they merely guide us toward the underlying physiological substrates. In psychiatry, we do, with only a very few exceptions, not know the causal referents in any diagnostically relevant sense. Thus, a psychiatrist finds herself in a quite different situation than, say, a surgeon or cardiologist (Jaspers 1997; Spitzer 1988). The psychiatrist is not confronting an organ or body part but another *person*, i.e., another embodied consciousness with its realm of meaning. It is important to stress again that patients do not manifest a series of independent symptoms or signs. Rather, their symptoms and signs are usually interdependent and mutually implicative, forming certain meaningful wholes that are interpenetrated by experiences, feelings, expressions, beliefs, and actions—all permeated by biographical detail.

Interviewing patients about their self-disorders is not an easy task. It requires considerable clinical experience, a certain level of psychopathological scholarship, and inter-rater reliability training in the phenomenological use of the EASE scale. Some self-disorders may be fleeting or elusive, perhaps even verging on something ineffable. There are several reasons for this. First, many self-disorders, targeted by the EASE scale, possess a pre-reflective quality, i.e., they are usually lived as *modes* rather than *objects* of the patients' experience. In other words, self-disorders affect more the structure than the content of experience, i.e., self-disorders are often not in the explicit focus of attention but tend to lurk or operate in the background of our awareness. Second, given that the structure of experiencing typically has been altered for years before contact with psychiatric services, many self-disorders have usually become quite ego-syntonic—this aspect may offer a new framework for understanding poor insight into illness in schizophrenia (Henriksen and Parnas 2014). Third, several self-disorders may even undermine the patient's capacity for self-expression. Fourth, many patients seem to consider this kind or level of experience as uniquely private (in contrast to, say, auditory verbal hallucinations, which tend to be regarded more as a common knowledge), and therefore the patients may view these experiences as embarrassing, "inhuman," or deeply disturbing (Parnas et al. 2005a; Nordgaard et al. 2013).

Evidently, for the patient to convey to the psychiatrist the type of experiences, we are exploring here, a certain intimacy and trust between the interviewer and the patient are required. It is therefore mandatory to try to establish a neutral, yet caring rapport with the patient, and ideally to provide the patient with a possibility to act as a partner in a shared, mutually interactive exploration. The patient must be willing to make an effort to explore his own experience and experiencing. Most importantly, no matter how uncommon or bizarre the reported experiences may seem to the interviewer, she must remain neutral, calm, yet with a restrained interested-caring attitude, and tacitly convey to the patient that she is familiar with the sort of psychopathology that is being expressed. The interviewer should never adopt a curious or voyeuristic posture or a judgmental or valuing attitude. What is being explored is how the patient experiences herself and her world and not an objectively or medically prescribed "reality" or "morbidity" of these experiences. From the patient's perspective, these experiences and the way he experiences simply amount to his being-in-the-world ("It's just who I am").

All psychopathological interviews should be performed in a semi-structured way—as Willig (2008) put it, "[the] semi-structured interview provides an opportunity for the interviewer to hear the patient talk about particular aspects of their life or experience. The questions function as triggers that encourage the patient to talk. Through his or her comments, the interviewer steers the interview to obtain the relevant data." Performing such an interview requires that the interviewer is intimately familiar with the relevant psychopathology. The patient should be encouraged to speak freely, rarely be interrupted, and given time for reflection and recollection. It can be helpful to propose examples of pathological experiences to the patient. To verify the presence of a given self-disorder, the patient must always describe, often upon request, in detail and by his own words at least one concrete example of an experience, and only on this ground may the interviewer score the relevant self-disorder as present, if the concrete example fulfills the relevant item definition. In other words, a simple, affirmative answer ("yes") to a question about a given self-disorder is never enough to rate this item as present. In the ideal situation, the interview consists of a patient-doctor mutually interactive reflection—e.g., the interviewer poses a question, the patient tries to respond, then the interviewer perhaps reformulates the answer by proposing an example, and becomes corrected by the patient, who provides another example of his own experience and in his own words.

Moreover, the interviewer must try to capture essential features of the experience in question through a further probing and using imaginative (or eidetic) variation, meaning that the interviewer, in her inquiry and attempts to represent the patient's experience, may change some aspects of the experience and retain others in order to strip the experience of its accidental and contingent features. The purpose is to grasp the features that are constitutive or essential for this type of experience, e.g., the essential differences between thought pressure and rumination, between pseudo-obsessions and true obsessions, etc. Yet, it is also important to recognize the limits to this process; it might not be possible for the patient to give a clear description, and if pressured, the patient might change the subject or become frustrated. Additionally, asking questions about one symptom after the other is not an adequate way of obtaining psychopathological information.

Finally, it is highly recommendable to open the psychopathological interview by asking for a detailed social history, which is fairly easy, because it's factual, usually "safe," and because most people actually like to talk about themselves and their lives. Allow the patient to speak freely, but within certain limits. This part of the interview serves to establish rapport and trust, but it always provides an initial picture of the patient and of her potential psychopathology, e.g., reflected in patterns of interpersonal functioning (e.g., behavior patterns across different ages, isolation, insecurity, suspiciousness, sexuality), educational achievements, work stability, tenacity, flexibility, ability to make choices, professional inclinations, spare time interests, etc. Finally and most importantly, the social history provides information of the *context* on the basis of which the patient's experiences are to be understood (e.g., are certain self-disorders bound to specific situations or do they occur in virtually any situation, etc.).

14.5 Conclusion

In this chapter, we illuminated and discussed self-disorders on the basis of a single case story. The notion of disordered self as the core disturbances in schizophrenia is as old as the schizophrenia concept itself (Parnas 2011), and it is, as we have shown, consistent with recent empirical studies. In short, self-disorders seem to constitute a crucial schizophrenia spectrum vulnerability phenotype. In our view, self-disorders hold great value for increasing the understanding our patients and their experiences, for early intervention efforts, for differential diagnosis, and self-disorders have potentially important nosological implications (e.g., they may help sharpen the diagnostic boundaries between schizophrenia and psychotic affective illness).

Finally, it is noteworthy that many of our patients, during an EASE interview, express feelings of relief when realizing that the interviewer is familiar with the nature of their experiences or that others suffer from similar experiences; this may to some extent counterbalance, though perhaps only transiently, the patients' feeling of ontological dissimilarity and existential loneliness. Therefore, discussing self-disorders in group sessions may have a psychotherapeutic value. In our view, a psychotherapeutic approach that is better informed about the core of the patients' suffering, vulnerability, and experiential life is likely to improve its efficacy (Skodlar et al. 2013).

Funding and Conflicts of Interest

Funding M.G.H. was funded partly by the Carlsberg Foundation (#2012010195).

Conflicts of Interest None.

References

Berrios, G. E. (2002). Conceptual issues. In J. A. den Boer, P. Willner, & H. D'haenen (Eds.), *Biological psychiatry* (pp. 3–24). New York: Wiley.

Blankenburg, W. (1971). *Der Verlust der natürlichenSelbstverständlichkeit. EinBeitragzurPsychopathologie symptomarmer Schizophrenien*. Stuttgart: Enke.

Blankenburg, W. (2001). First steps toward a psychopathology of "commonsense", trans. Mishara, A. L. *Philosophy, Psychiatry, and Psychology, 8*, 303–315.

Bleuler. E. (1950). *Dementia praecox or the group of schizophrenias*, trans. Zinkin, J. New York: International Universities Press.

Fuchs, T. (2005). Corporealized and disembodied minds. A phenomenological view of the body in melancholia and schizophrenia. *Philosophy, Psychiatry, and Psychology, 12*, 95–107.

Haug, E., Lien, L., Raballo, A., et al. (2012a). Selective aggregation of self-disorders in first-treatment DSM-IV schizophrenia spectrum disorders. *Journa of Nervous and Mental Disease, 200*, 632–636.

Haug, E., Melle, I., Andreassen, O. A., et al. (2012b). The association between anomalous self-experience and suicidality in first-episode schizophrenia seems mediated by depression. *Comprehensive Psychiatry, 53*, 456–460.

Haug, E., Øie, M., Andreassen, O. A., et al. (2014). Anomalous self-experiences contribute independently to social dysfunction in the early phases of schizophrenia and psychotic bipolar disorder. *Comprehensive Psychiatry, 55*, 475–482.

Haug, E., Øie, M., Melle, I., et al. (2012c). The association between self-disorders and neurocognitive dysfunction in schizophrenia. *Schizophrenia Research, 135*, 79–83.

Henriksen, M. G. (2013). On incomprehensibility in schizophrenia. *Phenomenology Cognitive Sciences, 12*, 105–129.

Henriksen, M. G., & Nordgaard, J. (2014). Schizophrenia as a disorder of the self. *Journal of Psychopathology, 20*, 435–441.

Henriksen, M. G., & Parnas, J. (2012). Clinical manifestations of self-disorders and the Gestalt of schizophrenia. *Schizophrenia Bulletin, 38*, 657–660.

Henriksen, M. G., & Parnas, J. (2014). Self-disorders and Schizophrenia: A phenomenological reappraisal of poor insight and noncompliance. *Schizophrenia Bulletin, 40*, 542–547.

Henriksen, M. G., Raballo, A., & Parnas, J. (2015) The pathogenesis of auditory verbal hallucinations in schizophrenia: a clinical-phenomenological account. *Philosophy, Psychiatry, and Psychology, 22*, 165–181.

Henry, M. (1973). *The essence of manifestation*, trans. Etzkorn, G. The Hague: Martinus Nijhoff.

Jaspers, K. (1997). *General psychopathology*, trans. Hoenig, J., & Hamilton, M. W. London: The John Hopkins University Press.

Koren, D., Reznik, N., Adres, M., et al. (2013). Disturbances of basic self and prodromal symptoms among non-psychotic help-seeking adolescents. *Psychological Medicine, 43*, 1365–1376.

Kraepelin, E. (1913). Psychiatrie. Ein Lehrbuch für Studierende und Ärzte. Auflage 8, vollständig umgearbeitet. Leipzig: Johann Ambrosius Barth.

Markova, I. S., & Berrios, G. E. (2009). Epistemology of mental symptoms. *Psychopathology, 42*, 343–349.

Minkowski, E. (1927). *La schizophrénie. Psychopathologie des schizoïdeset des schizophrènes*. Paris: Payot.

Møller, P., Haug, E., Raballo, A., et al. (2011). Examination of anomalous self-experience in first-episode psychosis: inter-rater reliability. *Psychopathology, 44*, 386–390.

Nelson, B., Thompson, A., & Yung, A. R. (2012). Basic self-disturbance predicts psychosis onset in the ultra high risk for psychosis 'prodromal' population. *Schizophrenia Bulletin, 38*, 1277–1287.

Nordgaard, J., & Parnas, J. (2012). A semi-structured, phenomenologically oriented psychiatric interview: Descriptive congruence in assessing anomalous subjective experience and mental status. *Clinical Neuropsychiatry, 9*, 123–128.
Nordgaard, J., & Parnas, J. (2014). Self-disorders and schizophrenia-spectrum: A study of 100 first hospital admissions. *Schizophrenia Bulletin, 40*, 1300–1307.
Nordgaard, J., Revsbech, R., & Henriksen, M. G. (2015). Self-disorders, neurocognition, and rationality in schizophrenia: A preliminary study. *Psychopathology, 48*, 310–316.
Nordgaard, J., Sass, L. A., & Parnas, J. (2013). The psychiatric interview: Validity, structure, and subjectivity. *European Archives of Psychiatry and Clinical Neuroscience, 263*, 353–364.
Parnas, J. (2011). A disappearing heritage: The clinical core of schizophrenia. *Schizophrenia Bulletin, 37*, 1121–1130.
Parnas, J., Handest, P., Jansson, L., et al. (2005a). Anomalous subjective experience among first-admitted schizophrenia spectrum patients: Empirical investigation. *Psychopathology, 38*, 259–267.
Parnas, J., Handest, P., Saebye, D., et al. (2003). Anomalies of subjective experience in schizophrenia and psychotic bipolar illness. *Acta Psychiatrica Scandinavica, 108*, 126–133.
Parnas, J., & Henriksen, M. G. (2014). Disordered self in the schizophrenia spectrum: A clinical and research perspective. *Harvard Review of Psychiatry, 22*, 251–265.
Parnas, J., Møller, P., Kircher, T., et al. (2005b). EASE: Examination of anomalous self-experiences. *Psychopathology, 38*, 236–258.
Parnas, J., Raballo, A., Handest, P., et al. (2011). Self-experience in the early phases of schizophrenia: 5-year follow-up of the Copenhagen prodromal study. *World Psychiatry, 10*, 200–204.
Pick, A. (1996). On the pathology of the consciousness of the self, trans. Viviani, R., & Berrios, G. E. *History of Psychiatry, 7*, 324–332.
Raballo, A., & Parnas, J. (2011). The silent side of the spectrum: Schizotypy and the schizotaxic self. *Schizophrenia Bulletin, 37*, 1017–1026.
Raballo, A., & Parnas, J. (2012). Examination of anomalous self-experience: Initial study of the structure of self-disorders in schizophrenia spectrum. *Journal of Nervous and Mental Disease, 200*, 577–583.
Raballo, A., Saebye, D., & Parnas, J. (2011). Looking at the schizophrenia spectrum through the prism of self-disorders: An empirical study. *Schizophrenia Bulletin, 37*, 344–351.
Ratcliffe, M. (2012). Phenomenology as a form of empathy. *Inquiry, 55*, 473–495.
Saks, E. R. (2007). *The center cannot hold*. New York: Hyperion.
Sass, L. A. (1994). *The paradoxes of delusion: Wittgenstein, Schreber, and the Schizophrenic mind*. Ithaca, NY: Cornell University Press.
Sass, L. A. (2014). Delusion and double book-keeping. In T. Fuchs, T. Breyer, & C. Mundt (Eds.), *Karl Jaspers' philosophy and psychopathology* (pp. 125–147). New York: Springer.
Sass, L. A., & Parnas, J. (2003). Schizophrenia, consciousness, and the self. *Schizophrenia Bulletin, 29*, 427–444.
Schneider, K. (1950). *Klinische Psychopathologie*. Stuttgart: Thieme.
Skodlar, B., Henriksen, M. G., Sass, L. A., et al. (2013). Cognitive-behavioral therapy for schizophrenia: A critical evaluation of its theoretical framework from a clinical-phenomenological perspective. *Psychopathology, 46*, 249–265.
Skodlar, B., & Parnas, J. (2010). Self-disorder and subjective dimensions of suicidality in schizophrenia. *Comprehensive Psychiatry, 51*, 363–366.
Spitzer, M. (1988). Psychiatry, philosophy and the problem of description. In M. Spitzer, F. A. Uehlein, & G. Oepen (Eds.), *Psychopathology and philosophy* (pp. 3–18). Berlin: Springer.
Stanghellini, G. (2004). *Disembodied spirits and deanimated bodies. The psychopathology of common sense*. Oxford: Oxford University Press.
Thornton, T. (2008). Why the idea of framework propositions cannot contribute to an understanding of delusions. *Phenomonology and the Cognitive Sciences, 7*, 157–175.
Willig, C. (2008). *Introducing qualitative research in psychology*. Berkshire: Open University Press.

Autism in Schizophrenia: A Phenomenological Study

15

Massimo Ballerini

15.1 The Little *Syd Barrett* of Heavy Metal

Let me call him E. I was not the first psychiatrist to have taken care of him. At that time he lived with his parents, being the major sister away from home. The mother was disappointed with him; she said that her son woke up late in the morning and he was at home all day long; in the evening he remained awake until late staying in his room "mumbling who knows what." The room was his shelter, but few things had remained there: horror comics, books concerning fantasy sagas and occultism, some old music magazines, and his old electric guitar, a sort of mute witness of a time gone forever. In the evening sometimes he left the house and, lonely wanderer, he went around the city streets; he stopped in bars where he would drink heavy and sometimes he took illegal substances. The mother claimed the son told her almost nothing: he appeared detached and shut-in. At least, his mother said, he had not displayed aggressive behavior toward his parents.

During his childhood, he was shy; during adolescence, he was in turmoil. He was hardly in touch with his sister, who was much older than him. He had no real friends and was sometimes aggressive with his peers. He began to cultivate an increasing interest toward the *heavy metal* world: not only for the music but also for the connected mythology—strange creatures, horror themes, satanism, and the occult. He learned to play guitar and joined a heavy metal band. For some time, it seemed to summarize the stereotypes of the genre, both in clothing and in provocative behavior. He had a few brief relationships with girls. At 17 he became more and more withdrawn, and he developed impatience toward other peers. Firstly he quitted the band and then the high school. The onset of psychosis occurred when he was 19 years old. For over a year, he was locked in the house. He was submitted to compulsory admission for assaulting his parents; he had told them that they were

M. Ballerini (✉)
Mental Health Department, Azienda Sanitaria di Firenze, Florence, Italy
e-mail: baller@virgilio.it

G. Stanghellini, M. Aragona (eds.), *An Experiential Approach to Psychopathology*,
DOI 10.1007/978-3-319-29945-7_15

not his parents and admitted to hearing invisible voices. After being discharged, he spent a few months in a residence for psychiatric rehabilitation without appreciable results. Subsequently, there were numerous hospitalizations. During this period, he did not take drugs regularly. The family climate was tense since he tried to attack his parents more than once. Finally after an admission motivated by inappropriate behavior, he was given long-acting antipsychotic treatment, and the aggressive behavior toward his parents regressed. He always refused to take part in psychosocial rehabilitation activities.

The consultations with him were difficult; there was a sense of a barrier, coolness, distance, and impenetrability. The main topics were essentially the news about his everyday life; but it really never happened something effectively new; he did few reports about psychotic symptomatology: he discussed his invisible voices without speaking about their content; he never talked about the delusion of genealogy that seemed to be the root of the aggressive behavior toward his parents. Nonetheless something transpired. Sometimes he spoke about his unquiet adolescence: he remembered his disdainful refusal of his peers, including his past bandmates: "they were really common people; they only liked playing music. If I stayed with them I would lose all my personal ideas." He recalled his fascination with the paranormal: "the reality is not as it seems. I wanted to understand what is behind the appearances." Sometimes he described some disturbances, especially a sort of panic attack: "I have panic attacks. I feel . . . I am going away from myself . . . No, I don't feel myself. . . It is a crisis. No, it is something stable. Yes, but sometime it's harder." He felt distressed when engaged with others: "It's an old story. People seem empty and distant. I do not understand what they want. When I go somewhere I feel unable to take part to things and situations as the others do." Referring to his erratic wanderings, he said: "I am curious; I go to see people . . . what they do and how they perform . . . ." One time I asked him if he was invested by a mission; the answer was sudden and astonishing: "I have a mission, yeah. I have to kill Astaroth . . . I am waiting for him . . . But I have to be on guard. It is . . .. It is . . . They have told me. . . I was E.T. Oh . . . I don't know If I am E.T. A lot of things happened to me. This is my predestination. I was taken by Batman. His son, Robin, took too much extasy . . .. He threatened to implode because he recalled the Sabbath. A bloody Sabbath. I came from planet Megadeath and then I stood with Robins. He is the evil. Perhaps then in my second life I met him. Then I was reborn on a tree on planet Jellystone. I talk with the ranger. He talked to me through the walls. He put me thoughts directly in my head. I met Mr. Magoo in the streets.. I talk with him with the brain. Then in my 4th life I was carried in a laboratory and I was transformed into a cyborg. Oh . . .I received so much surgery on my brain. They enter in my head. Then was made the shake of the galaxy. Now I have the mission to kill the devil. It is very important. It is a prophecy. I have to wait for him. The fate of the human race depends on me." What I believed to be an almost empty fortress with only a few morbid experiences emerging from the inside was effectively a private world animated by an efflorescent imaginative inner life, detached completely by the universally shared symbolism and causalities.

15.1.1 Not Psychopathology But Psychopathologies

There is a plurality (Stanghellini 2009a) of psychopathologies: *descriptive psychopathology* is a detailed description and categorization of morbid experiences and behaviors [see, i.e., the *Allgemeine Psychopathologie* (Jaspers 1913)]; *clinical psychopathology* is voted to delineate reliable diagnostic criteria [see, i.e., the *Klinische Psychopathologie* (Schneider 1950)]. In our case we encounter no difficulty to make a DSM-5 (American Psychiatric Association 2013) diagnosis of schizophrenia: the long lasting of the disorder; the presence of positive, disorganized, negative symptoms with a marked level of social dysfunction and the low relevance of substance abuse are all in touch with the requested diagnostic criteria. Addressing the analysis of the patient's declarations, we can appreciate a series of subtler morbid experiences: though they are still neglected in main diagnostic criteria, they should not be considered merely fringe phenomena as they enrich the clinical picture, delineate the patient's existential standpoint, and contribute to a fine characterization of the schizophrenic phenotype (Sass 1992; Sass and Parnas 2003; Sass and Pienkos 2013; Parnas et al. 2002; Parnas 2011; Stanghellini 2004a; Stanghellini and Ballerini 2007a, 2011a; Stanghellini et al. 2012, 2014a; Fuchs 2007, 2010).

15.1.2 The Phenomenological Way: Hermeneutical or Structural Psychopathology

Phenomenological psychopathology is essentially a hermeneutical approach to morbid subjectivity [see, i.e., *Schizophrenie* (Binswanger 1957)]. It is grounded on patients' subjective accounts of their (morbid) lived experiences, including their contents, their *what-is-like-to-be*, and their phenomenal aspects (Stanghellini 2004b; Fuchs 2010; Nordgaard et al. 2013). The features of a pathological condition emerge from personal subjective experiences articulated in *personal narratives* as *typical invariant constructs* (Stanghellini and Ballerini 2008). These are synthetic schemes of comprehension of a given group of personal narratives and they have to be valid and generalizable to a class of individuals, i.e., people suffering by schizophrenia (Stanghellini and Ballerini 2008). Psychiatric disorders, such as schizophrenia, are not considered a simple collection or a mere checklist of isolated symptoms but as a *structure*, that is, a *Gestalt*, a *meaningful whole* (Stanghellini 2004b; Nordgaard et al. 2013): a *structure* or a *Gestalt* is a web of signs and symptoms—each one is *interconnected* with others according to *internal links*. A *structure* possesses a proper coherent order but paradoxical as in the case of schizophrenia; unitary meaning and global value are disclosed by the internal links between all the single parts [Hjelmslev (1971) quoted in Stanghellini (2009a)]. How can we grasp the meaning of the structure? Psychiatric disorders such as schizophrenia are peculiar existential stances (Binswanger 1957) whose morbid feature is endowed, besides the subjective trouble, in the impossibility (or difficulty) to transcend the *diktat* of the experience; in other words, the morbid experiences impose themselves to patients, overwhelming the capability to cope, resulting in forms of derailment, corrosion, or alienation of the individual's presence in the world (Binswanger 1956). These peculiar forms of existence display an invariant structure residing in the corrosion of the basic organizers of a *person's being in the world*, denominated following Heidegger (Heidegger 1963), *existentialia*: these are the basic features of our presence in the world, the way we live and experience time, space, the body and the self, the others; in the course of clinical settings, *existentialia* are reconstructed through the analysis of personal narratives (Stanghellini 2009a). Corrosion of *existentialia* may account for the morbid arrangement of patients' subjectivity.

Phenomenology assumes that the *lived-body* is the root of the *basic structures of subjectivity* (Merleau-Ponty 1945). Phenomenology operates a distinction between the body-object (the anatomical body or my own body as perceived in a reflective stance) and the body-subject, the pre-reflective, experience of the body. The foundational role of the lived-body or body-subject is referred—following the seminal work of Merleau-Ponty (Merleau-Ponty 1945)—to as *embodiment*; as of today *embodiment* has become a main topic in neuroscience (Varela et al. 1991), including cognitive science (Gallese and Sinigaglia 2011). The body is the medium to live the world (Merleau-Ponty 1945), since it structures the primordial sense of self, named *basic-self or ipseity* (Henry 1990; Damasio 2000; Parnas and Sass 2001; Sass and Parnas 2003; Zahavi 2005; Stanghellini 2004a; Fuchs 2010; Gallagher 2013a); it organizes the *immediate experience of others* and the *self/other demarcation*; finally, it consents our natural *immersion in the world*. The basic structures of subjectivity are precognitive, pre-reflective, and prelinguistic; nonetheless, they possess a certain affective taint: vitality for the basic-self, naturality for endowment in the world, and spontaneity for attunement with others (Parnas et al. 2002; Sass and Parnas 2003). Higher-order, more cognitive, propositional, structures of subjectivity enfold, i.e., the *extended or narrative self or identity, higher-order strategies of intersubjectivity, symbolization processes, values, the temporal arrangement of memories. Existentialia* are all inclusive of the basic, pre-reflective and the higher-order propositional structures of subjectivity. Pre-reflective structures of subjectivity are normally transparent; they become evident when distorted in morbid experiences (Sass and Parnas 2003; Fuchs 2010). Sometimes the patients experience their distortions directly, and other times they reflect themselves in the *quality* of the clinical picture including the psychotic symptoms (see Fig. 15.1).

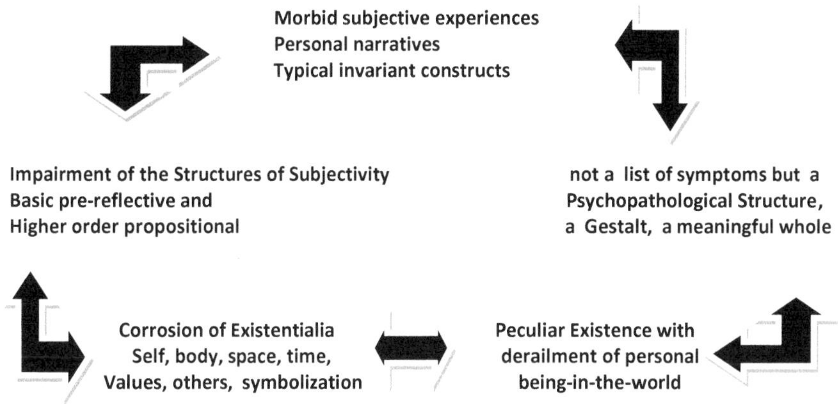

Fig. 15.1 The cycle of phenomenological psychopathology

15.2 Comment

Kretschmer (1921) would have any surprise by the existential arrangement of patient E. What he wrote about schizoid patients retains its full validity if addressed to patients with schizophrenia: "Behind an ever silent facade, which twitches uncertainly with every expiring whim nothing but broken pieces, black rubbish heaps, yawning emotional emptiness, or the cold breath of an arctic soullessness. But from the facade we cannot see what lurks behind [. . .] (Patients) are like Roman houses and villas, which have closed their shutters before the rays of the burning sun; perhaps in the subdued interior light, there are festivities." I was probably the first person admitted *inside the villa* of E. What is the global meaning of this complex and somewhat elusive morbid arrangement of existence? My analysis will be focused on the patient's declarations. My comment will be necessarily tentative, underpinning some crucial points. I will refer to the constructs elaborated by recent empirical research in phenomenology integrating with the classical phenomenological literature.

15.2.1 The Private World

Firstly, I shall provide a global vision of the clinical picture. Patients with schizophrenia, such as E, display an increasingly *marked tendency toward the constitution of a private world detached from attunement, harmony, and vital contact with the social world. A private world filled by an efflorescent imaginative inner life or emptied in a cold rarefaction that leaves only odd and aloof simulacra. The social world, as the horizon of one's own proper presence and life-project, disappears or undergoes a grotesque and paradoxical distortion* (Stanghellini and Ballerini

2011b). This construct is clearly rooted on the notion of *autism*, as depicted by continental psychopathology. Bleuler (1911) introduced the term to depict the *detachment from reality with dominance of inner life;* Kretschmer considered autism, rooted in a paradoxical affective arrangement (comprehensive of coolness and sensitivity), the psychopathological organizer of schizophrenia spectrum (Kretschmer 1921). Minkowsky described *a poor form of autism*, displaying the loss of social attunement, and *a rich form of autism*, where the loss of attunement is replaced with an efflorescent imaginative inner life; autism was considered the *psycho-patho-genetic* mechanism of schizophrenia (Minkowski 1927; Minkowsky 1933). In the following years, despite the contribution of Binswanger (autism as a peculiar arrangement of existence) and Blankenburg (autism as a loss of common sense) (Binswanger 1956; Blankenburg 1971), the construct has progressively vanished from the horizon of mainstream psychiatry since it did not match the standards of modern empirical research (Stanghellini and Ballerini 2011b). In the last decades, the psychopathological literature has renewed its interest for this concept (Gundell and Rudolf 1993; Ballerini 2002). Autism, the expression of the inner core of schizophrenia, has been addressed to the anomaly of the structure *self-others-world* (Parnas et al. 2002) or to *dis-sociality,* a specific disruption of the basic structure of sociality (Stanghellini and Ballerini 2002). Social dysfunction in people with schizophrenia is often restricted to social performance, that is, what patients are unable to do. On the contrary, *dis-sociality* is the "the qualitative disturbance of spontaneous and intuitive participation in social life" (Stanghellini and Ballerini 2002): it encompasses negative features (social roles impairment as job, friends, housekeeping, leisure; lack of common sense and attunement with others) and positive features (deviating set of values, aims and ambitions, imaginative not real-world-oriented activity) (Stanghellini and Ballerini 2007b).

Previously (Stanghellini and Ballerini 2004), four analytical categories were selected to account for the structure of autism in schizophrenia. They were the *cognitive categorization processes*, the *system of values*, the *social attunement*, and the *self setting-up process*. Each category represents a facet of *common sense*, the basic link that bonds each individual to the shared social system. The common sense is the grounding element and the condition of possibility of the social life (Gadamer 1960). Normally transparent is the root of our sense of reality; it possesses a moral and emotional power and each deviation induces perplexity and blame (Schutz 1962; Garfinkel 1967). Schizophrenia involves a deep disturbance in common sense experience.

15.2.2 The Semantic Drift

The secret life of patient E is a resounding deflagration of all commonsensical meanings, symbols, and causalities. The patient's ultimate declaration defeats the basic properties of *personal narratives*: here are disrupted both the *internal coherence* (Lysaker et al. 2002) as it lacks consistency, logical connections, and plausibility and the *external coherence* (van Dijk 1980) since it overwhelms any pattern of social shared knowledge, symbolism, standards, values, and frames of action. It conveys all the imaginable oddity and strangeness, with a sort of fantastic and terrific journey through space and time. It is populated by distorted representations of childhood comic heroes, slipstreamed, and absorbed in the gloomy atmosphere of a rambling *dark metal* saga. All the everyday logics and all the shared symbolism, including the universal representation of the patient's saga characters, are distorted in a paradoxical taint. The final outcome is a grotesque and bewildering *semantic drift*. How is it possible to have built up such as an alienated world?

Patient E seems to apprehend events and situations through *revelation-like experiences* (Kraus 1983). He receives from an unknown entity messages concerning the transformation of the world. He seems to experience the *revelation* with a sense of passivity; the whole existence acquires abruptly new idiosyncratic values and connotations. *Revelation* is the *existential* structure of schizophrenic delusion (Kraus 1983). In the patient's narrative, the symbolic register and the metaphors lose their public use. Meanings become semi-independent objects; biographical fragments and memories are de-situated and decontextualized. All of these *materialize* into something hard, real, and concrete. The words do not work anymore to share a world but to create a new *solipsistic* world (Stanghellini 2004a): an alien reality, provided with a *proper ontology*.

Schizophrenic phenomena give us the immediate feeling of an alien world, in which facts, events, and situations are arranged in a morbid structure, qualitatively diverse—*ontologically* divergent—from ordinary experience (Bovet and Parnas 1993; Stanghellini 2004a; Ballerini 2004; Cermolacce et al. 2010).

This is *solipsism*, where reality, provided with its perceptive consistency, is the idiosyncratic product of the individual mind (Parnas and Sass 2001).

This is the world of bizarreness. *Semantic drift*, with the peculiar arrangement of the system of values, may account for the typical taint of bizarreness of schizophrenia. Bizarreness should not only be applied to a particular form of delusion; it invests manifolds of phenomena of experience (Cermolacce et al. 2010). The patient's tenets sound assumptions of reality as they appear to us as concrete, "distorted metaphor" (Stanghellini 2004a; Cermolacce et al. 2010); they witness the derangement of basic structure of subjectivity resulting in a strange, aloof, uncanny solipsistic private world.

15.2.3 The Epistemic Eccentricity

Ethic and epistemic eccentricity in schizophrenia are rooted in a peculiar system of values. Values are attitudes, dispositions, or tendencies that guide our actions (Weber 1922). Values are articulated in concepts, but they are not logical abstractions since they are inseparably tied to emotional experience (Scheler 1973). They transcend single events and organize themselves in a personal *structure*; finally values convey the personal standpoint toward existence (Stanghellini 2004a; Stanghellini and Ballerini 2007a; Schwartz 2012).

Patients with schizophrenia are animated by (Stanghellini and Ballerini 2007a) an *immediate feeling of radical diversity*, claiming to be completely diverse from all other people. This may be felt as destiny, a fate befallen on them, or—on the contrary—the free choice to take distance from commonsensical ways of thinking, to act and to attribute value to facts and events. The emotional climate may change from astonishment to fascination including a possible strong resistance toward this sort of predestination. During adolescence, patient E developed suspicion for the common ways people think and behave, which he considered a dangerous loss of originality. In the subsequent years, he was progressively engaged in a marked interest toward a deeper comprehension of the reality, beyond the mere appearances of everyday life; the final step has been the incredible story of which he is the protagonist. Patient E is well aware of his diversity and the exceptionality of the events he lives; he does not provide any explanation. He feels it is something like a destiny, a fate, or—in his words—*a predestination.* He is absorbed in the overall meaning of his ultimate mission: the sake of humanity. It is surprising that patient E, completely absorbed in a gloomy private world, is moved by a sort of *utopian humanitarianism.*

In a previous contribution (Stanghellini and Ballerini 2007a), the system of values of patients with schizophrenia displayed two instances (constructs): *antagonomia* and *idionomia* (Stanghellini 2001, 2004a; Ballerini 2004).

The first is the disdainful refusal or the deliberate choice to take distance from social shared knowledge and commonsensical assumptions, including the intimate relationship with others: all of these are felt as a dangerous attack on originality and diversity by which patients are animated (Stanghellini 2001, 2004a; Stanghellini and Ballerini 2007a). Patient E in the course of adolescence and the premorbid period displayed a marked *antagonomic* standpoint. Conversely, he developed a marked interest for what moves behind the appearance, searching for this in occultism and mythology. The final step has been the incredible story where he is provided with special powers and he is invested by a mission. All of these recall the second construct, *idionomia* (Ballerini 2004; Stanghellini and Ballerini 2007a): this is the absolute exaltation of the personal rules, principles, vision of the world, and life questions, all detached from the social shared world, including restricted—religious, political, and moral—groups of people. *Idionomia* encompasses two constructs (Stanghellini and Ballerini 2007a): *metaphysical concern* is a profound fascination for the perplexing or astonishing complexity of existence and what effectively happens behind the appearances. Patients may be engaged in personal studies and endless lectures. They may ruminate about philosophical, religious, or sociological assumptions, subverting the tenets and the methodology of the considered disciplines. *Charismatic attitude* is the feel to be invested by superior spiritual or intellectual, material or existential powers; in other cases patients feel to be invested by an ultimate eschatological mission. Usually the special powers or the eschatological mission are comprehended by the means of a *revelation* or an *illumination*, an intuitive holistic vision that operates a transformation of the lived world. Interestingly, patient E displays all of these attitudes. *Antagonomia* may be represented in schizotypy or in the premorbid phase of disease, being *idionomia* typical of the active phase of psychosis. *Idionomia* is a key to illuminate the phenomenon of bizarreness. Bizarreness in schizophrenia is rooted in the crisis of commonsensical understanding of the world and in a consistent set of values and emotions. Taken together, they give rise to *an alien private world* marked by new meanings and causalities, all arranged in a new but peculiar and idiosyncratic order (Stanghellini 2004a; Stanghellini and Ballerini 2004, 2007a). Finally, despite the autistic standpoint, patients may display a marked interest in the human race with a strongly *utopian or humanitarian value*, where the effective engagements with others is replaced by a utopian ideology detached by the effective relationship with others (Stanghellini and Ballerini 2011a).

15.2.4 The Vanishing of Others

Attunement with Others, in an everyday transaction, is a fluid and immediate form of intersubjectivity: immediate and intuitive, enacted (dependent to the context and to the pragmatic value of interaction), and tied to social affordances; in particular circumstances, we adopt a more cognitive engagement with others, a higher-order strategy based on *inferential perspective taking* (Hutto 2013; Gallagher 2013b). On the contrary, cognitive science's notion of intersubjectivity is based on the theory of mind (ToM) mechanism, the ability to infer the mental states subtending human behavior by adopting a general *folk theory* of human interactions or by running in ourselves' simulations of the behavior of others (Gopnik and Wellman 1992; Gordon 1986). Phenomenology maintains ToM as *particular—non-prevalent—* form of intersubjectivity (Hutto 2013; Gallagher 2013b). When he was younger, patient E became more and more detached from sociality displaying—apparently—a poor form of autism. Nowadays the therapeutic sessions are marked by a sense of barrier and distance, with sporadic declarations. Beyond the negative symptomatology, patient E appears to be *dis-attuned* from other people and from the social world. Yet in a family context, he seems distant. Social contacts have been a problem for him since adolescence. He claims that the social world appears to him as unnatural and someway enigmatic. He complains of being ineffective when he tries to grasp the intentions of other people. The ordinary meaning of everyday transactions is elusive for him. Patient E displays a disorder of immediate *social attunement*. But patient E maintains a fascination for the sociality; he looks as an *ethologist*, going lonely to observe with interest ordinary people in everyday transactions searching for—perhaps—the *secret* of human *intersubjectivity*. People with schizophrenia display impairment of ToM in several diverse laboratory paradigms (Bora et al. 2009): previously (Stanghellini and Ballerini 2011b) we noted that ToM tasks rely on different aspects of empathy (i.e., inferential perspective taking and immediate emotional sharing). They are charged—at least partially—by neurocognitive abilities and they display inconsistent ecological validity: in a real-life clinical setting, patients displayed intact ToM skills (McCabe et al. 2004). Phenomenological literature erected the crisis of *intersubjectivity* as a milestone of schizophrenia. (Minkowski 1927; Binswanger 1956; Blankenburg

1971; Parnas et al. 2002; Stanghellini and Ballerini 2002; 2004; 2007b; 2011a; 2011b; Stanghellini 2004a). We, Stanghellini and Ballerini (2011a), conducted an empirical research into people with schizophrenia to depict the overall features of social relationship experience. Patients displayed an impaired ability to directly contact and intuitively decipher others' behaviors and social situations. This phenomenon was termed *hypo-attunement*). Some patients, as such patient E, adopted a peculiar strategy named ***al****gorithmic conception of sociality* to discover and elaborate a method for understanding other people by observing them when engaged in everyday activities or by elaborating a general theory from books and reports. *Algorithmic conception of sociality* may be an attempt to cope with the impairment sustained by *hypo-attunement*. Less impaired patients, without or with a lesser neuropsychological impairment, may be efficacious in adopting this inferential standpoint. Patient E has probably been able to manage social relationships for some years prior to the onset of psychosis, adopting this reparative mechanism. Besides *hypo-attunement* and *algorithmic attitude*, some patients complained, when in front of others, to be oppressed or invaded. They experienced a persistent sense of being somewhat exposed, constrained, or overrun. In other cases, they felt invaded, penetrated by glances, gestures, and/or physical contacts. Yet during interactions with others, patients felt submerged by their own emotions or by uncanny and incomprehensible bodily sensations (Stanghellini and Ballerini 2011a). Taken together, the results depicted experiences of others in people with schizophrenia as a paradoxical mixture of *painful distance* and *fearful proximity* (Stanghellini and Ballerini 2011a). Disorder of embodiment is the root for disordered *intersubjectivity*. It is the experience of the body, similar for me as for others, to consent to the development of the capability to understand others (Merleau-Ponty 1945).

15.2.5 The Time of a Lived *Cyborg*

Personal identity is grounded on a primordial, basic, immediate-nonpropositional pre-reflective instance: the *ipseity* or *basic, minimal, core self* (Henry 1990; Damasio 2000; Zahavi 2005; Gallagher 2013a).

It is a *self-affection the* immediate *presence to ourselves*, the sense of existing, pure subjectivity, the first-person perspective, automatically imprinted in every experience we have (Stanghellini 2004a; Sass and Parnas 2003; Zahavi 2005; Gallagher 2013a), the sense of *ownership* and *agency* (Damasio 2000) we live with in every experience we have. *Ipseity* is enrooted in the lived-body and in the pre-reflective temporality (Zahavi 2005; Fuchs 2007, 2010). *Ipseity* is the pre-reflective condition of the possibility of subjectivity: it organizes the field of experience, including our attunement and the spontaneous sense of immersion in the world. Schizophrenia implies a deep disturbance of *ipseity* (Parnas and Sass 2001; Sass and Parnas 2003; Stanghellini 2004a).

The panic attacks described by patient E are not *mere panic attacks*, but a persistent crisis of *ipseity*, a morbid experience of *diminished self-affection*. This morbid experience seems to fluctuate in time. This is not surprising given its nature of self-affection (Sass 2014). The Ipseity Disturbance Model (IDM) (Sass and Parnas 2003; Sass 2014; Nelson et al. 2014) recognizes two basic "complementary aspects": *diminished self-affection*, resulting in pervasive, fastidious sense of inner void, anonymity, inability to feel ourselves, diminished sense of subjectivity (Parnas and Sass 2001; Sass and Parnas 2003) and *hyper-reflectivity* where the subject is excessively involved in observing his mental activity, being at the same time engaged in the world; the subject is constrained in self-monitoring where the theme is not the content of experience but the constitutive mechanisms of experience (Sass 1992, 2014; Sass and Parnas 2003).

A manifold of morbid experience emerge from this basic disturbance.

They involve a set of prepsychotic symptoms regarding the sphere of action cognition, perception, affectivity, and body experience (Parnas and Sass 2001). *Anomalous self-experiences* represent an early phenotype of the schizophrenia spectrum (Sass and Parnas 2003). Following this model, a semi-structured interview was designed to assess the field of *anomalous self-experiences* (Parnas et al. 2005). The Examination of Anomalous Self-Experience (EASE) encompasses five domains: cognition and stream of consciousness (i.e., an inability to discriminate between forms of intentionality); self-affection and presence (i.e., diminished sense of basic-self; hyper-reflectivity); bodily experiences, demarcation, and transitivism (i.e., confusion with other); and existential reorientation (i.e., solipsism). Disturbances of self-affection are the root of full-blown psychotic symptoms in the three domains of positive, negative, and disorganized (Sass and Parnas 2003). Considering the ultimate declaration of patient E, a marked disorganization of thoughts is evident; *diminishment of self-affection* deprives him from the "lived point of orientation" (Sass and Parnas 2003) for thought coherency and pragmatic efficacy; negative symptoms displayed by patient E reside in the loss of the vitality derived from impaired ipseity, while the positive symptoms are endowed in the alteration of stream of consciousness (i.e., the inability to differentiate memory from imagery, the perceptualization of inner speech, etc.) (Sass and Parnas 2003). Impairment of the *basic-self* has been documented empirically in people with schizophrenia and schizophrenia spectrum disorders, differentiating them from psychotic bipolar disorder (Haug et al. 2012; Raballo et al. 2011; Nordgaard and Parnas 2014); it is predictive for the development of a schizophrenic spectrum disorder in *at-risk* population (Nelson et al. 2012). A recent meta-analysis confirmed these results (Hur et al. 2014).

But as recently stated, temporality is strictly connected to the constitutive process of *basic-self* and, conversely, the *basic-self* is a prerequisite for temporalization (Zahavi 2005; Fuchs 2007). Fuchs (2007) suggested that schizophrenia is characterized by a disruption of the pre-reflective structure of temporality. Following the Husserlian lesson (Husserl 1991), the temporalization of experience is operated by a continuous (moment by moment) automatic, fluid integration (passive synthesis) of *retention* (the immediate past), *protention* (the immediate future), and *primal impression* (the now). As when we listen a melody, each moment contains a *retention* of the preceding notes tied to the anticipation of the following.

The disruption of such a process is the milestone for a loss of coherence of experience in time: the grounding functions of *ipseity* are now altered, leading to psychotic symptoms, especially disturbances of *agency* (Fuchs 2007). As argued by Sass and Pienkos (2013), the disruption of *basic temporalization*, besides disturbances in everyday fluidity of action and perception, may induce disturbances in more cognitively charged processes as the biographical arrangements of events. The incredible story of patient E prefigures a temporal connotation.

Firstly, it seems a chaotic conglomerate of symbols coming from childhood, absorbed and remixed or *shaken* in adolescent *rebellious* taint. Minkowsky, in his seminal contribution (Minkowsky 1933), described in schizophrenia the blockade of *temporal becoming*, as a consequence of the *loss of the vital contact with reality*. The patient's narrative emerged as a conglomerate of de-situated, de-temporalized, and decontextualized fragments of memory. Secondly, the ultimate mission the patient is invested in displays a temporal articulation we may label *premonition* (Stanghellini et al. 2016) or *anticipation* (Kimura 1985). Patient E has lived the revelation of the mission as a *prophecy*; the mission is *something is going to*, since it is thrown into a future; now impends the wait, the wait for its fulfillment. Kimura established *anticipation* is the typical *temporalization* of patients with schizophrenia (Kimura 1985); taking the concept of *temporalization ante-festum*, used in other contexts by Gabel (Gabel 1962), he described the patients as fixed in a sort of cramp-like time, waiting for the fulfillment of a destiny. Kimura maintains the experience of time strictly linked to the establishment of the self. The defective constitution of the self is directly experienced by the patient, reverberating in the wait for its final outcome. The patient is dominated by the anxiety of not being able to become a self. The completion of this process is thrown into the uncertain future: the disaster of annihilation or the miracle of its constitution (Kimura 1985). Recently we have studied the experience of lived time in a large cohort of patients with acute and chronic schizophrenia (Stanghellini et al. 2016); especially the first sample exhibited significant alteration of *time coherence*. Within this category, we have patients with *perifrastichal* temporal arrangement of delusional experience (I'm going to . . .); we termed it *premonition*. In our view it reflects an eruption of *protention* in *primal impression*. This is the case of patient E, whose ultimate declaration is dominated by the impending mission to accomplish.

Interestingly, patient E has reported concomitant abnormal bodily sensations. He was conducted to a laboratory to become a cyborg. The cyborg is a fantastic creature, half man and half machine: human in his origin, he/it is provided with bionic grafts. Patient E *materializes* literally this character *within himself*, decontextualizing cyborg from his *natural* environment (the world of cinema, comics, heavy metal epics) and providing it with *effective* reality. This is not the only morbid experience in the domain of the body: patient E complained to be submitted to brain surgery, since he felt external forces operating in his head. Abnormal bodily sensations were considered by classical psychopathology as disorders of coenesthesis: "the general sense of bodily existence (and especially the general feeling of well-being or malaise) presumably dependent on multiple stimuli coming from various parts of the body, including sensations of internal organ activity even though these are not necessarily on a conscious level" (Campbell 1989). A list of abnormal bodily phenomena is comprised in well-established checklist for schizophrenia vulnerability (Gross et al. 1987; Parnas et al. 2005), but they displayed little predictive value (Klosterkötter et al. 2001), probably since they encompass a large manifold of phenomena including several nonspecific bodily disturbances (Stanghellini et al. 2012). Patient E's morbid bodily experiences may be assumed as a disorder of the *lived-body* (Fuchs 2007; Stanghellini 2009b), *which is* the origin of our primordial sense of being (see above).

My colleagues and I investigated disorders of the *lived-body* in first-episode patients (Stanghellini et al. 2012) and in a cohort of acute and chronic patients (Stanghellini et al. 2014a). Morbid experiences were reported by patients in terms of their features, in terms of their causes, and in terms of neologisms; they were *psychotic*—when they overstepped the "as if" condition; qualitatively, their core properties resided in the paradoxical dyad *dynamization/mechanization—morbid objectivation*.

Dynamization implies *anomalous experience of movement,* involving the body limits or the body constructs: patients reported to be invaded by strange uncanny forces, energies, or entities; in other cases, patients claimed uncanny perplexing movements inside the body, organ transformations, or the externalization of body components or vital functions; in the second case, the body or subcomponents became mechanical or substituted by inert materials; finally, organs or sub-components usually silently at work assumed a clear spatial objectivation (*morbid objectivation*). Patient E, in both the cases, provides a cognitive (delusional) elaboration of a primary lived-body morbid experience. He referred experiences of *mechanization* and *violation* (the body limits). These abnormal phenomena seem to run in parallel with ipseity disturbances: on the one hand, the crisis of minimal self and, on the other hand, the sensation to be *materially* (not *metaphorically*) nonhuman (the cyborg).

15.2.6 The *Dark Side* of the Space

The lived space may be accounted as a further feature of common sense. Usually we feel immersed in and attuned to our environment. Each person is situated and immersed in a world-ambient, shared with others. The body-subject is the source of the natural sense of immersion in the world (Merleau-Ponty 1945). Secondly, as noted (Uhlhaas and Mishara 2007) the coherent texture of the lived space is dependent too on the background of a social shared competence. The sinister sarabande, of which the patient is the protagonist, is enacted in a peculiar form of space; following Minkowsky, this kind of solipsistic space is the *dark space* (Minkowsky 1933).

The incredible story of patient E is consumed in a space entirely devoid of a geographical configuration, without definite extension or spatial relations (distance, closeness, etc.); the rules of physics and the transcendent objectivity of space, events, and objects are clamorously ignored. It is a space indistinct, without the possibility of perspective: to be here or to be there seems to change, minimally, the perception of the places—a dramatically private solipsistic space. The characters that populate it are ominous strains of heroes, completely detached from their shared symbolism; but it also displays an own intrinsic depth that seems to embrace or contain all the things you can imagine, without order and succession. It is a space provided with a dense, heavy atmosphere and an emotional climate: however, from the dark to the terrifying, from the enigmatic to the disconcerting, and finally to the magnetically fascinating, it is a space that pervades and permeates the ordinary space. (The events of the story materialize themselves in the few places actually experienced by the patient.) It seems to menace, siege, and assault the ordinary space (Binswanger 1957). This space is dark since it resembles the night, without profiles, but provided with an apparent density. It is the sieging space where psychotic experience came from. These features give us the immediate sense of the strangeness, bizarreness, oddity, and the grotesque. On the contrary, the clear space (Minkowsky 1933) is a geographical space with extension and spatial relations; it is intersubjective and everyone is an entity between entities; this is visible, provided with a clear light and thin climate; it possesses an effective prospectivity (Sass and Pienkos 2013). But *everyone* possesses a proper *dark space*—imagine to be traveling in another continent, to be sailing along a river in a region completely covered by monsoon forest: you can appreciate the dense, enigmatic space standing right beside you. The dark space is normally beside the clear space: in psychosis the *dark space* bypasses the *clear space* (Minkowsky 1933). People with psychosis are unable *to cross the horizon of private space* failing to return to intersubjective lived space, the *geographical space* (Straus 1935); patients appear to be trapped in the *dark space*. This is the case of patient E; a one-way journey to the hell, the hell he tried to escape from. Anomalies of the body-subject disrupt our natural experience of the world, or what we might describe as our "grip" on the world (Merleau-Ponty 1945). In schizophrenia the spontaneous immersion in the world is disrupted. As noted by Merleau-Ponty (Merleau-Ponty 1945), patients live in a private space, without the possibility to cross the horizon of their solipsistic space.

15.3 Conclusion

In his ultimate declaration, patient E tells the story of his life; the onset of psychosis *has frozen* the *becoming* of his life confining it *beside* the social world: only few connections remain active. The corrosion of pre-reflective basic structures of subjectivity—directly experienced by the patient—detaches himself from the social life.

His *incredible adventure* is a spatiotemporal distorted resume of his previous seasons of life, mixed with a taint of *premonition*, that is, the waiting for the future, where the fulfillment of his mission is *located*; naturally the waiting is dilated in a sort of *time-less* dimension. We see the symbolic value of the story, including the yearning for a miraculous recovery of meaning (the fulfillment of the mission), while he lives his *solipsistic creation* as a *concrete reality*.

15.3.1 Autism and Detachment from the *Common Sense*

The man is a set of solitude and sociality (Zaner 1973): each of us is permeated by an immediate feeling of individuality, rooted in the personal biography and in the unique arrangement of habits, interests, values, cognitive, and affective styles—nonetheless, each *personal world* is endowed, situated within the *extensional constraints* established by common sense. Common sense may be conceptualized as an incredible amount of taken-for-granted, social shared meanings, explanations, and principles of causality, necessary for pragmatic orientation in everyday life; a set of standards, aims, ambitions, and values, basically shared by all; the low-/high-level mechanisms of intersubjectivity, the milestone of everyday transactions with others; finally the ontological constitution of the self, necessary for the stability of subjectivity and the self/other demarcation (Stanghellini and Ballerini 2004). A further facet of common sense is the *lived space*, the spatial (geographical) configuration of our proper being-in-the-world, as we live in a common space shared with all the others (Fig. 15.2). Schizophrenic disturbance of common sense experience results in the *autistic configuration* of existence: a *semantic drift*, an *epistemic eccentricity*, a *crisis of attunement*, a spatial *derailment*, and finally an *ontological instability*—there is a circular relationship between all these categories (Stanghellini and Ballerini 2004). In every case disorder of *embodiment* (*dis-embodiment*) is the common, generative root (Stanghellini 2004a, 2009b; Stanghellini and Ballerini 2004; Fuchs and Schlimme 2009).

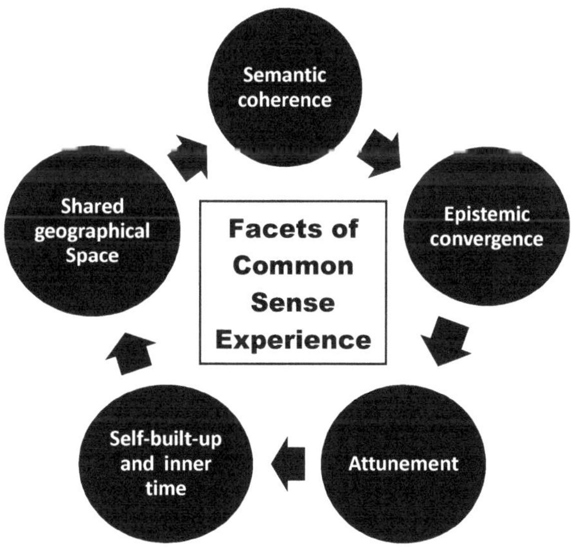

Fig. 15.2 Circular relationship between facets of normal common sense experience

15.3.2 Schizophrenia as Disorder of *Embodiment*

Dis-embodiment implies the dramatic corrosion of the pre-reflective basic structures of subjectivity. *Dis-embodiment* posses *inductive power:* as in a cascade, the impairment is reflected in the *morbid arrangement* of the higher-order *existentialia*, i.e., the symbolization processes and the system of values. *Dis-embodiment* informs and imbues the clinical picture providing its distinctive feature. On the other hand, patients' morbid experiences reveal in their structure the disturbance of embodiment (i.e., self and temporalization, the pre-reflective attunement, the indwelling in the world). The result is dramatic: an impressive private world far from the intersubjective horizon of life (Fig. 15.3).

15.3.3 The *ETHOS* of People with Schizophrenia

Real-world clinical phenotype of schizophrenia, as depicted by accurate recollection of the patients' lived experiences, seems to possess a larger breadth and depth than the one crystallized in diagnostic criteria (Stanghellini and Rossi 2014). Autism, as depicted by classical and recent-years psychopathology, seems to capture the wholeness of the life-world of patients with schizophrenia. It seems to grasp the ETHOS of patients. ETHOS may serve as a *candidate acronym* to encompass Embodiment and the Self, Time and Space experience, Hierarchy of Values, Others experience, Symbolization: ETHOS recalls the existential categories employed in the above discussion. My colleagues and I undertook the qualitative study of the lived-world of patients with schizophrenia, investigating the morbid arrangement of *existentialia*; we have studied empirically the *system of values* (Stanghellini and Ballerini 2007a), the *experience of others* (Stanghellini and Ballerini 2011a), the experience of the *lived-body* (Stanghellini et al. 2012,

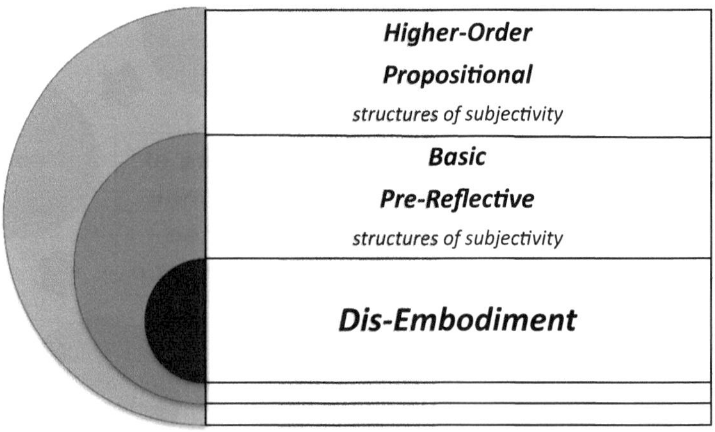

Fig. 15.3 Schizophrenia, dis-embodiment, and the impairment of the structures of subjectivity

2014a), and the experience of *time* (Stanghellini et al. 2016); we have also provided two rating scales, concerning the *experience of others* and the *system of values* (Stanghellini et al. 2014c)—the *lived-body* (Stanghellini et al. 2014b).

15.3.4 Future Research

Disturbances of *existentialia* may *be* regarded as *trait markers*, probably *state-dependent trait markers*, since they may be exacerbated during active, acute, phases of illness. Disturbances of *minimal self* have been demonstrated in schizophrenic spectrum disorders (Haug et al. 2012) and in a cohort of people at risk of developing schizophrenia (Nelson et al. 2012) displaying predictive value. Longitudinal researches are needed: what we need is the extensive study of all the *existentialia* throughout the course of schizophrenia since the prodromic phase, using other psychiatric disorders, namely, bipolar disorder, as control. Longitudinal studies are needed to draw definitive conclusions. Finally a constant dialogue with neuroscience is needed. All the theoretical models we propose need to obtain validation through the supervening data from functional neuroimaging and electrophysiologic techniques. Some empirical data are emerging from the field of neuroscience, as the Cortical Midline System (CMS) (Northoff et al. 2006) and the Default-mode system (Broyd et al. 2009) that seems to substantiate the self-experience: in the more recent years, there is a growing amount of studies documenting their impairment in schizophrenia [see, i.e., Bastos-Leite et al. (2015)].

Acknowledgments The author would like to thank Nicholas Barrett and Barbara Ciomei, European University Institute, Florence, Italy, for the linguistic revision of the chapter.

I made every efforts in order to make the case presentation not recognizable.

References

American Psychiatric Association. (2013). *Diagnostic and statistical manual of mental disorders* (5th ed.). Washington, DC.

Ballerini, A. (2002). *Patologia di un eremitaggio. Uno studio sull'autismo schizofrenico*. Torrino: Bollati Boringhieri.

Ballerini, M. (2004). Schizofrenia, Autismo, Dis-socialitá/dionomia. *Minerva Psichiatrica, 45*, 19–30.

Bastos-Leite, A. J., Ridgway, G. R., Silveira, C., Norton, A., Reis, S., & Friston, K. J. (2015). Dysconnectivity within the default mode in first-episode schizophrenia: A stochastic dynamic causal modeling study with functional magnetic resonance imaging. *Schizophrenia Bulletin, 41*(1), 144–53.

Binswanger, L. (1956). *Drei Formen Missglueckten Daseins*. Tubingen: Niemeyer.

Binswanger, L. (1957). *Schizophrenie*. Pfullingen Neske.

Blankenburg, W. (1971). *Der Verlust der natuerlichen Selbstverstaendlichkeit*. Stuttgart: Enke.

Bleuler, E. (1911). *Dementia Praecox oder Gruppe der Schizophrenien*. Leipzig: Deuticke.

Bora, E., Yucel, M., & Pantelis, C. (2009). Theory of mind impairment in schizophrenia: Meta-analysis. *Schizophrenia Research, 109*, 1–9.

Bovet, P., & Parnas, J. (1993). Schizophrenic delusions: A phenomenological approach. *Schizophrenia Bulletin, 19*(3), 579–597.
Broyd, S. J., et al. (2009). Default-mode brain dysfunction in mental disorders: A systematic review. *Neuroscience and Biobehavioral Reviews, 33*(3), 279–96.
Campbell, R. J. (1989). *Psychiatric dictionary* (6th ed.). Oxford: Oxford University Press.
Cermolacce, E., Sass, L., & Parnas, J. (2010). What is bizarre in bizarre delusions? A critical review. *Schizophrenia Bulletin, 36*(4), 667–679.
Damasio, A. (2000). *What happens: Body, emotion and the making of consciousness*. London: Vintage.
Fuchs, T. (2007). The temporal structure of intentionality and its disturbance in schizophrenia. *Psychopathology, 40*, 229–235.
Fuchs, T. (2010). Phenomenology and psychopathology. In D. Schmicking & S. Gallagher (Eds.), *Handbook of phenomenology and cognitive science* (pp. 547–573). Berlin: Springer.
Fuchs, T., & Schlimme, J. E. (2009). Embodiment and psychopathology: A phenomenological perspective. *Current Opinion in Psychiatry, 22*, 570–575.
Gabel, J. (1962). *La Fausse Conscience : essai sur la réification*. Paris: Éditions de Minuit, « Arguments ».
Gadamer, H. G. (1960). *Warheit und Methode*. Tuebingen: Mohr.
Gallagher, S. (2013a). A pattern theory of self. *Frontiers in Human Neuroscience, 7*, 1–7.
Gallagher, S. (2013b). Intersubjectivity and psychopathology. In K. W. M. Fulford, M. Davies, R. G. T. Gipps, G. Graham, J. Z. Sadler, G. Stanghellini, et al. (Eds.), *Handbook of philosophy and psychiatry* (pp. 258–274). Oxford: Oxford University Press.
Gallese, V., & Sinigaglia, C. (2011). What is so special about embodied simulation? *Trends in Cognitive Sciences, 15*(11), 512-519.
Garfinkel, H. (1967). *Studies in ethnomethodology*. New York: Englewood Cliffs.
Gopnik, A., & Wellman, H. (1992). Why the child's theory of mind really is a theory. *Mind and Language, 7*, 145–171.
Gordon, R. (1986). Folk psychology as simulation. *Mind and Language, 1*, 158–171.
Gross, G., Huber, G., Klosterkötter, J., & Linz, M. (1987). *BSABS Bonner Skala fur die Beurteilung von Basissymptomen*. Berlin: Springer.
Gundell, H., & Rudolf, G. A. E. (1993). Schizophrenic Autism, 1. Historical evaluation and perspectives. *Psychopathology, 26*, 294–303.
Haug, E., Lien, L., Raballo, A., et al. (2012). Selective aggregation of selfdisorders in first-treatment DSM-IV schizophrenia spectrum disorders. *The Journal of Nervous and Mental Disease, 200*, 632–636.
Heidegger, M. (1963). *Sein und Zeit*. Tubingen: Niemeyer.
Henry, M. (1990). *Phénoménologie materielle*. Paris: P.U.F.
Hjelmslev, L. (1971). *Linguistic essays*. Paris: Minuit.
Hur, J-W., Kwon, J. S., Lee, T. Y., & Park, S. (2014). The crisis of minimal self-awareness in schizophrenia: A meta-analytic review. *Schizophrenia Research, 152*, 58–64.
Husserl, E. (1991). On the phenomenology of the consciousness of internal time. In Brough JB, trans-ed. Dordrecht, Kluwer Academic Publishers, Boston, 1991.
Hutto, D. D. (2013). Interpersonal relating. In K. W. M. Fulford, M. Davies, R. G. T. Gipps, G. Graham, J. Z. Sadler, G. Stanghellini, et al. (Eds.), *Handbook of philosophy and psychiatry* (pp. 249–257). Oxford: Oxford University Press.
Jaspers, K. (1913). *Allgemeine Psychopathologie*. Berlin: Springer.
Kimura, B. (1985). Time and Anxiety. *Zeitschrift fur klinische Psychologie, Psychopathologie und Psychotherapie, 33*(1), 41–50.
Klosterkötter, J., Hellmich, M., Steinmeyer, E. M., & Schultze-Lutter, F. (2001). Diagnosing schizophrenia in the initial prodromal phase. *Archives of General Psychiatry, 58*, 158–164.
Kraus, A. (1983). Schizo-affective psychoses from a phenomenologicaò-anthropological point of view. *Psychiatria Clinica (Basel), 16*(2–4), 265–274.
Kretschmer, E. (1921–1961). *Korperbau und Charakter*. Berlin: Springer.

Lysaker, P. H., Clements, C. A., Plascak-hallberg, C. D., Kinpscheer, S. J., & Wright, D. E. (2002). Insight and personal narratives of illness in schizophrenia. *Psychiatry, 65*(3), 197–206.
McCabe, R., Leudar, I., & Antaki, C. (2004). Do people with schizophrenia display theory of mind deficits in clinical interactions? *Psychological Medicine, 34*, 401–412.
Merleau-Ponty, M. (1945). *Phénoménologie de la perception*. Paris: Gallimard.
Minkowski, E. (1927). *La schizophrénie. Psychopathologie des schizoïdes et des schizophrènes*. Paris: Payot.
Minkowsky, E. (1933). *Le Temps vécu. Étude phénoménologique et psychopathologiques*. Paris: D'Artrey.
Nelson, B., Parnas, J., & Sass, L. A. (2014). Disturbance of minimal self (Ipseity) in schizophrenia: Clarification and current status. *Schizophrenia Bulletin, 40*(3), 479–82.
Nelson, B., Thompson, A., & Yung, A. R. (2012). Basic self-disturbance predicts psychosis onset in the ultra high risk for psychosis "prodromal" population. *Schizophrenia Bulletin, 38*, 1277–1287.
Nordgaard, J., & Parnas, J. (2014). Self-disorders and the schizophrenia spectrum: A study of 100 first hospital admissions. *Schizophrenia Bulletin, 40*(6), 1300–1307.
Nordgaard, J., Sass, L. A., & Parnas, J. (2013). The psychiatric interview: Validity, structure, and subjectivity. *European Archives of Psychiatry and Clinical Neuroscience, 263*(4), 353–364.
Northoff, G., Alexander Heinzel, A., de Greck, M., Bermpohl, F., Dobrowolny, H., & Jaak Panksepp, J. (2006). Self-referential processing in our brain—A meta-analysis of imaging studies on the self. *NeuroImage, 31*, 440–457.
Parnas, J. (2011). A disappearing heritage: The clinical core of schizophrenia. *Schizophrenia Bulletin, 37*(6), 1121–1130.
Parnas, J., & Sass, L. A. (2001). Self, solipsism, and schizophrenic delusions. *Philosophy, Psychiatry, and Psychology, 8*(2/3), 101–120.
Parnas, J., Bovet, P., & Zahavi, D. (2002). Schizophrenic autism: Clinical phenomenology and pathogenetic implication. *World Psychiatry, 1*(3), 131–136.
Parnas, J., Møller, P., Kircher, T., et al. (2005). EASE: Examination of anomalous self-experience. *Psychopathology, 38*, 236–258.
Raballo, A., Sæbye, D., & Parnas, J. (2011). Looking at the schizophrenia spectrum through the prism of self-disorders: An empirical study. *Schizophrenia Bulletin, 37*, 344–351.
Sass, L. A. (1992). *Madness and modernism: Insanity in the light of modern art, literature, and thought*. Cambridge, MA: Harvard University Press.
Sass, L. A. (2014). Self-disturbance and schizophrenia: Structure, specificity, pathogenesis (Current issues, New directions). *Schizophrenia Research, 152*(1), 5–11.
Sass, L. A., & Parnas, J. (2003). Schizophrenia, consciousness, and the self. *Schizophrenia Bulletin, 29*(3), 427–444.
Sass, L. A., & Pienkos, E. (2013). Space, time, and atmosphere. A comparative phenomenology of melancholia, mania, and schizophrenia, Part II. *Journal of Consciousness Studies, 20*(7–8), 131–152.
Scheler, M. (1973). *Wesen und Formen der Sympathie*. Bern-Munchen: Francke.
Schneider, K. (1950). *Klinische Psychopathologie*. Stuttgart: Thieme Verlag.
Schutz, A. (1962). Common sense and scientific interpretation of human action. In A. Schutz, Collected Papers vol. I, M. Nijhoff, Den Haag.
Schwartz, S. H. (2012). An overview of the schwartz theory of basic values. Online Readings in *Psychology and Culture, 2*(1). doi:10.9707/2307-0919.1116.
Stanghellini, G. (2001). Psychopathology of common sense. *Philosophy, Psychiatry and Psychology, 8*(2/3), 201–218.
Stanghellini, G. (2004a). *Disembodied spirits and deanimatied bodies: The psychopathology of common sense*. Oxford: Oxford University Press.
Stanghellini, G. (2004b). The puzzle of the psychiatric interview. *Journal of Phenomenological Psychology, 35*(2), 173–195.

Stanghellini, G. (2009a). The meanings of psychopathology. *Current Opinion in Psychiatry, 22*(6), 559–564.
Stanghellini, G. (2009b). Embodiment and schizophrenia. *World Psychiatry, 8*, 56–59.
Stanghellini, G., & Ballerini, M. (2002). Dis-sociality: The phenomenological approach to social dysfunction in schizophrenia. *World Psychiatry, 1*, 102–6.
Stanghellini, G., & Ballerini, M. (2004). Autism: Disembodied existence. *Philosophy, Psychiatry, and Psychology, 11*(3), 259–268.
Stanghellini, G., & Ballerini, M. (2007a). Values in persons with schizophrenia. *Schizophrenia Bulletin, 33*(1), 131–141.
Stanghellini, G., & Ballerini, M. (2007b). Criterion B (social dysfunction) in persons with schizophrenia: The puzzle. *Current Opinion in Psychiatry, 20*, 582–587.
Stanghellini, G., & Ballerini, M. (2008). Qualitative analysis. Its use in psychopathological research. *Acta Psychiatrica Scandinavica, 117*(3), 161–3.
Stanghellini, G., & Ballerini, M. (2011a). What is it like to be a person with Schizophrenia in the social world? A first-person perspective study on Schizophrenic Dissociality--part2: Methodological issues and empirical findings. *Psychopathology, 44*(3), 183–192.
Stanghellini, G., & Ballerini, M. (2011b). What is it like to be a person with schizophrenia in the social world? A first-person perspective study on Schizophrenic dissociality-part 1: State of the art. *Psychopathology, 44*(3), 172–182.
Stanghellini, G., Ballerini, M., Fusar-Poli, P., & Cutting, J. (2012). Abnormal bodily experiences may be a marker of early schizophrenia? *Current Pharmaceutical Design, 18*(4), 392–398.
Stanghellini, G., Ballerini, M., Blasi, S., Blasi, S., Mancini, M., Presenza, S., et al. (2014a). The bodily self: A qualitative study of abnormal bodily phenomena in persons with schizophrenia. Comprehensive. *Psychiatry, 55*(7), 1703–1711.
Stanghellini, G., Ballerini, M., & Cutting, J. (2014b). Abnormal bodily phenomena questionnaire. *Journal of Psychopathology, 20*, 138–143.
Stanghellini, G., Ballerini, M., & Lysaker, P. H. (2014c). Autism rating scale. *Journal of Psychopathology, 20*, 273–285.
Stanghellini, G., & Rossi, R. (2014). Pheno-phenotypes: A holistic approach to the psychopathology of schizophrenia. *Current Opinion in Psychiatry, 27*(3), 236–241.
Stanghellini, G., Ballerini, M., Presenza, S., Mancini, M., Raballo, A., Blasi, S., et al. (2016). Psychopathology of lived time: Abnormal time experience in persons with schizophrenia. *Schizophrenia Bulletin, 42*(1), 45–55.
Straus, E. (1935). *Von Sinn der Sinne*. Berlin: Springer.
Uhlhaas, P. J., & Mishara, A. L. (2007). Perceptual anomalies in schizophrenia: Integrating phenomenology and cognitive neuroscience. *Schizophrenia Bulletin, 33*(1), 142–156.
van Dijk, T. A. (1980). *Macrostructures: An interdisciplinary study of global structures in discourse, interaction, and cognition*. Hillsdale: Erlbaum.
Varela, F. J., Thompson, E., & Rosch, E. (1991). *The embodied mind: Cognitive science and human experience*. Cambridge: MIT Press.
Weber, M. (1922). *Wirtschaft und Gesellschaft*. Tuebingen: Mohr.
Zahavi, D. (2005). *Subjectivity and selfhood: Investigating the first-person perspective*. Cambridge, MA: MIT.
Zaner, R. M. (1973). Solitude and sociality: The critical foundations of social sciences. In G. Psathas (Ed.), *Phenomenological sociology: Issues and applications* (pp. 25–43). New York: Wiley.

Hallucination

16

J. Cutting

16.1 Introduction

Hallucinations are protean: in form, content and modality. They occur in normal people in normal situations; they occur in normal people in anomalous physiological and psychological situations, e.g. sleep deprivation, widowhood; they occur in all psychotic states—schizophrenia, depressive psychosis, mania, delirium, drug-induced states and dementia; and they occur in the context of focal brain damage, particularly occipital and temporal lesions.

After more than a century of phenomenological study, however, there is still an influential body of opinion denying any specific pattern to any group. The thesis promoted in this chapter is that specific patterns in at least some of the above-mentioned states *are* identifiable and that attention to the phenomenological features of hallucinations can open a window on the very nature of the psychoses themselves.

I have had people referred to me worried that they were schizophrenic because they were hearing a voice of a known person uttering a few words just as they were falling asleep: these were hypnagogic hallucinations—normal in a normal situation. Knowing something about the phenomenology of hallucinations had a reassuring effect here. Yet there is a contemporary trend, promoted by Romme and Escher (1993) and Leudar and Thomas (2000), for example, to accommodate all morbid varieties of hallucination within the normal range of experience. This thesis both denies the normal person the satisfaction of knowing that they are normal *and* the psychotic the access to specialist services for his or her anomalous experiences. It is furthermore false, as we shall see.

I shall present brief vignettes of hallucinatory experiences in different situations and different nosological conditions. Before doing so, however, the reader needs to

J. Cutting (✉)
Institute of Psychiatry, London, UK
e-mail: jccutting@outlook.com; zoejeffcoat@aol.com

G. Stanghellini, M. Aragona (eds.), *An Experiential Approach to Psychopathology*,
DOI 10.1007/978-3-319-29945-7_16

be convinced that such vignettes are typical of the situations or nosological conditions exemplified, and, to this purpose, I shall present data from my series of functional psychotics (Cutting 1997)—25 acute schizophrenics, 100 psychotic depressives and 100 manics, along with those from 74 delirious subjects (Cutting 1987). For dementia, Burns et al.'s (1990) study of 177 patients with Alzheimer's disease is the best to my knowledge. Drug-induced psychosis is variously regarded as schizophrenia-like, as a specific nosological entity in its own right and as a heterogeneous collection of several psychotic forms depending on which drug is involved; it is helpful in this context, therefore, to include a phenomenological study of cocaine psychosis (Unnithan and Cutting 1992) which might help refute one of these hypotheses. The hallucinations of the normal in a wide range of anomalous circumstances—sensory deprivation (Schulman et al. 1967), solitary confinement (Grassian 1983), sensory overload (Ludwig 1972), sleep deprivation (Bliss et al. 1959) and visual failure (Holroyd et al. 1992)—are very similar inter alia, and I shall rely on Schulman and colleagues' account of the sensory-deprived state as typical of this genre. The pattern of hallucination accompanying different locations of brain damage is beyond the scope of this article, but see Cutting (2012) for details. Finally, the pattern in a normal person in normal circumstances, promoted by certain authors as the model for all sorts of hallucinations, will be examined by recourse to the study of Tien (1991), which advocates of this 'hallucination-as-normal' thesis themselves rely upon.

16.2 Descriptive Psychopathology of Hallucination

The most basic analysis of hallucination is the descriptive level. This charts (Table 16.1) the modality in which hallucination occurs and, in the case of auditory hallucination, whether it is a voice or some nonverbal experience.

It is clear from the table that to be diagnosed as schizophrenic is a situation in which a subject is most likely, relative to all other situations, to experience hallucinations, particularly auditory hallucinations of voices and tactile hallucinations. The other two groups of functional psychotics—manics and depressives—have a substantial rate of auditory hallucinations as well, but a much lower rate of tactile hallucinations. In delirium and dementia, there is the well-known preponderance of visual hallucinations relative to auditory hallucinations, a reversal of the pattern in functional psychosis. Cocaine psychosis, sensory deprivation (as our chosen example of the normal in an anomalous situation) and the oft-quoted survey of normals revealed a tiny proportion of hallucinators.

Table 16.1 Descriptive psychopathology of hallucinations

% Hallucinations	Schizophrenia $n = 250$	Mania $n = 10C$	Depressive psychosis $n = 100$	Delirium $n = 74$	Dementia $n = 177$	Cocaine psychosis $n = 18$	Sensory deprivation $n = 71$	'Normal' $n = 15{,}258$
Auditory	75	43	37	18	10	0	6	2
Voices	74	43	36	16	10	0	3	?
Non-verbal	7	1	1	2	0	0	3	?
Visual	28	28	12	34	13	0	3	2
Tactile	29	16	0	4	0	6	1	2
Gustatory	1	0	1	0	0	0	0	?
Olfactory	6	3	3	0	0	0	10	1

? unknown

16.3 Phenomenological Psychopathology of Hallucination

Everything depends on what aspect of hallucination is addressed. In the past too much emphasis was placed on whether a subject took the hallucination for 'real' or not, resulting in a sterile discussion about true hallucinations versus pseudo-hallucinations. This led nowhere and is anyway un-phenomenological. The phenomenologist's motto is: *An die Sachen selbst* [loosely translated as 'look at what is being experienced, not whether it is taken as actually there or possibly there'].

Phenomenological psychopathology, as opposed to descriptive psychopathology, is, at the very least, a more nuanced analysis of what someone experiences and, at most, an attempt to categorise such experiences in *philosophical* terms. My reading of what the so-called phenomenological psychopathologists of the last century—e.g. Minkowski, Binswanger, Straus and von Gebsattel—were aiming at was a philosophical or even metaphysical analysis of psychopathology. What we are hoping for in a phenomenological account of hallucination, therefore, is a more profound view of the subject matter than can be provided by the descriptive version presented above.

Recent in-depth studies of auditory hallucinations (Nayani and David 1996; Leudar et al. 1997; Garrett and Silva 2003), although valuable for our purposes, lack any theoretical motive, whereas here, however, I intend to justify each sort of analysis by setting it in a philosophical context. In particular, I shall rely on the writings of a philosopher central to the philosophical phenomenology movement—Max Scheler (1874–1928)—one of the trio, alongside Husserl and Heidegger, whose work his crucial to any understanding of what phenomenology is. Phenomenological psychopathology itself, debased by equating it with descriptive psychopathology, is nothing if not linked with phenomenological philosophy in some way.

I shall restrict my analysis of the data to only two aspects of phenomenological philosophy, both unique to Max Scheler:

1. The separation of human experience into *zufälliges Sosein* [the coincidental nature of something—its where-, when-, whose- and thisness] and its *Wassein* or *Wesensein* [its whatness or essence]
2. The value that some experience obtains for a subject

So, in the case of a voice-hearer, one can ask: Where is the voice? When is the voice referring to—past, present or future? And whose voice is it? Further, one can enquire into the value which the message conveys for the voice-hearer: pleasant or unpleasant, life-threatening or life-enhancing, imputing morality or immorality and concerning a spiritual or materialistic realm? [Scheler set out a hierarchical scheme of values—positive and negative at each level—and concomitant emotions, also positive and negative at each level, which constituted the entirety of the human being. This was the main thrust of his *Formalism* (Scheler 1913–1916/1973). The classes of values unique to the human being were spiritual and mental, and those shared by the human being and the animal were those of vitality and agreeableness. Respective examples of positive and negative emotions were bliss and despair (spiritual), joy and sorrow (mental), liveliness and languor (vital) and pleasure and pain (agreeableness)].

In the case of visual hallucinations, the phenomenological parameters in respect of the above are restricted to two issues: (1) the 'thisness' of the image (is it unique and plausible within anyone's everyday experience, or is it something that no one could ever experience in the natural world because it is abstract or surreal?) and (2) its value as a spiritual image or otherwise.

Tactile hallucinations, occurring in a third of schizophrenics and a sixth of manics but virtually absent in any other group, are crying out for some explanation, something that I shall tackle later. Gustatory and olfactory hallucinations are too rare in any group to be properly analysed.

The pattern of voices with respect to their coincidental qualities (Table 16.2) is presented for schizophrenics, manics, depressives and delirious subjects only, as the incidence in cocaine psychosis was nil (which undermines its status as a model for schizophrenia), and no details are given in the studies on dements, sensory-deprived subjects or normals.

What emerges in terms of the coincidental qualities of the experience is that schizophrenics tend, relative to the other groups, to hear a specific, non-religious person's voice and to hear it in a specific place outside their head. Most strikingly, the temporal framework of the voice is the *present*, sometimes the future, but rarely the past. The manics are characterised by hearing a religious voice without much specificity as to its 'where' and 'when'. The depressives differentiate from the other psychotic groups by hearing voices referring to the past or future, i.e., within a temporal context. The delirious subjects had too few voices to bear analysis.

The value of the voice as a communication (Table 16.3) splits the groups in the following way. Schizophrenics have no overwhelmingly characteristic message. Most of their voices convey banal (e.g. 'tatty-bye, nighty-night') communications

Table 16.2 Phenomenological psychopathology of voices: coincidental qualities

% of entire group with voices of the specified variety	Schizophrenia $n = 250$	Mania $n = 100$	Depressive psychosis $n = 100$	Delirium $n = 74$
Where is the voice?				
In head	3	3	2	0
Elsewhere	9	5	2	1
Whose voice is it?				
Religious figure	4	11	2	1
Specific non-religious figure	12	9	3	3
When is the voice referring to?				
Past	1	0	6	0
Present	26	2	5	1
Future	8	3	12	1

Table 16.3 Phenomenological psychopathology of voices: value of message

% of the entire group with voices of the specified variety		Schizophrenia $n = 250$	Mania $n = 100$	Depressive psychosis $n = 100$	Delirium $n = 74$
What value is conveyed?					
Spiritual?	Religious	4	11	2	1
	Specifically non-religious	12	9	3	3
Mental?	Moral person	0	1	0	0
	Immoral person	4	0	16	3
Vital?	Life-enhancing	0	0	0	0
	Life-threatening	3	0	12	1
Agreeableness?	Pleasant	1	5	0	0
	Unpleasant	5	2	26	3

Table 16.4 Phenomenological psychopathology of visual hallucinations

% of entire group with visual hallucinations of the specified variety	Schizophrenia $n = 250$	Mania $n = 100$	Depressive psychosis $n = 100$	Delirium $n = 74$
People	16	14	6	21
Animals	8	2	4	15
Things	5	1	3	4
Abstract patterns	5	0	0	0
Surreal/part objects	9	0	0	0
Religious themes	2	10	0	0

or call their name (e.g. 'Colin') or talk about what they are doing (e.g. 'she is taking a bath'). Manics hear a positive tone in the voice, with a religious flavour. Depressives hear a voice accusing them of immoral acts, threatening their very life and always having a disagreeable tone. The few voices that delirious subjects hear are not typecast in this respect.

Visual hallucinations (Table 16.4) were quite aberrant in schizophrenics relative to the other groups, with part objects (e.g. 'leg on bedroom wall', 'heads and fists suspended in air'), unreal or surreal items (e.g. 'legless spiders shimmering on floor', 'gifted people in the world talking to each other') or abstract images (e.g. 'abstract patterns like on a church window', 'blue circles and yellow, red and mauve circles on ceiling') dominating their experience. The only other notable point in the table is the religious theme of the manics.

16.4 Vignettes

As one who likes puzzles and as one who is constantly confronted with the difficulties in diagnosis as part of medicolegal practice, I shall now present eight vignettes of hallucinators. These are semi-authentic in that the vignette contains actual experiences from subjects with the same nosological or circumstantial condition, but not all from one subject. The eight vignettes are of people diagnosed with schizophrenia, mania, depressive psychosis, delirium, dementia or cocaine psychosis or in a state of sensory deprivation or 'normality'. They are presented in a different order from the above to create a puzzle, and the solution is given at the end of the chapter.

Vignette 1. A man of 23 reported that he had felt 'a crawling in the skin'.

Vignette 2. A woman of 45 heard voices saying that she was a coward, and that she had not helped her husband, that she'd stolen from a supermarket and that she had killed a cat. The voices said that she was going to be thrown into the water and killed. She saw a vision of two men being electrocuted from a light under her bed and saw a film star with blood coming out of her mouth.

Vignette 3. A man of 37 heard his mother's voice telling him to be good. The voice occurred at night as he was falling asleep.

Vignette 4. A man of 34 heard voices calling his name, saying words like 'epilepsy', or 'smack it on the head', and asking what he was doing during the day. The voices fell into two groups—those that 'kept him down' and those that were fighting to 'hold him up'. The voices came from his sternum or above his right ear. They were male and female, spoke in English and Russian, sometimes seemed to be Aborigines and sometimes seemed to be like the voice that read the Nine-o-clock News. There were visual hallucinations—'rows of indistinguishable people', 'thousands of wasps', a 'pair of eyes above a normal pair' and bright lights. He had 'thumps' on his back, a 'pneumonia' smell and a taste of 'staphylococci' on his toothbrush.

Vignette 5. A woman of 39 heard God's voice saying that 'she will never understand'. She heard God's voice telling her to pray and heard good and evil forces fighting over her. She saw Christ's face, a guardian angel and a face in a curtain like a devil's face.

Vignette 6. A woman of 67 heard the sounds of, and saw actual belongings of, someone in her house.

Vignette 7. A woman of 37 heard falling rain, the hum of heavy machinery and high-pitched whining sounds. She felt the mattress underneath her move and felt pressure on her face. She smelled oranges and burnt coffee. She felt her friend in front of her and saw people's faces in the window.

Vignette 8. A man of 68 heard bagpipes, babies crying and lovers' tiffs. He saw animals, felt something crawling on him and felt the bed was wet and moving.

16.5 Discussion

16.5.1 Are Hallucinations Heterogeneous in Nature?

What emerges from the analyses in this chapter, particularly Tables 16.1, 16.2 and 16.3, is that to be diagnosed with schizophrenia or psychotic depression guarantees that if there are hallucinations, then these will generally have a unique pattern with respect to the other situations in which hallucinations occur. Three groups of hallucinators can be identified from all this—schizophrenic, psychotic depressive and 'the remainder'. This last group has some claim to be heterogeneous in itself—manics and the pervasive religious theme in their hallucinations, delirious subjects and their preponderance of visual hallucinations of animals—but these are far from specific. What is clear is that the 'normal' hallucinators are not an appropriate standard against which to measure all other sorts of hallucinators. Hallucinations in 'normal' people are very rare—around 2 %—and nothing in the literature links these with the bizarre content of the visual hallucinations in schizophrenia or the consistent demoralising tone of the hallucinations in the psychotic depressions, among other features.

16.5.2 What Is the Contribution of Descriptive Psychopathology?

The best studies have taken specific diagnostic groups and looked at the pattern of hallucinations. Leudar et al. (1997), for example, compared schizophrenics with 'normal' university students, and Garrett and Silva (2003) compared schizophrenics with drug-induced psychotics. Leudar and colleagues found that schizophrenics were less likely to hear the voice of a family member and more likely to hear the voice of a public figure than normals, which schizophrenics more often than normals experienced expressed violence in the voice and that schizophrenics were less likely than were normals to be bothered about the value contained in the voice. Garrett and Silva discovered that schizophrenics held more strongly to an objectivity about the voice than did those with drug-induced psychoses. Nayani and David's (1996) study deserves equal place alongside these descriptive psychopathological studies of voices because it tackles the nature of the voice producing the hallucination, though it falls short of the others because it brings together hallucinators from various diagnostic categories.

Altogether, these three studies exemplify the best of descriptive psychopathology, as they tackle critical aspects of the experience of hallucinators. They even illuminate some areas of phenomenological psychopathology, as we shall see below.

There is no comparable descriptive psychopathology of visual or tactile hallucinations, which are crying out for such treatment.

16.5.3 What Does Psychological Psychopathology Contribute?

The thrust of psychological studies on voices, and there is nothing on visual or tactile hallucinations, is the promotion of the thesis that an abnormality in one or other conventional mental functions underlies them. All the mental functions recognised by psychologists—attention, consciousness, emotion, language, memory, perception, thinking and even movement initiation—have been incriminated.

Frith (1979), for example, formulated voices as the inappropriate incursion into consciousness of fragments of preconscious processing. Hoffman (1986) saw them as premature, inchoate precursors of what would eventually be a final utterance, but somehow projected into external space in this half-baked form. Jarvik (1970) conceived them as a muddled up chimaera of memory and perception. Heilbrun (1993) focused on an incompetent attentional strategy. Slade and Bentall (1988) thought that voices stemmed from some emotional conflict. Bazhin et al. (1975) claimed that voices were misperceptions of an actual world event.

None of these suggestions is true to the facts of the matter, in schizophrenics at least, which they all purport to explain. If someone hears a voice in his breastbone, in a foreign language, or with an accent different from his own, belonging to a public figure—which my subjects and those reported in the descriptive psychopathology literature often did—how can the voice be a misperception of some everyday occurrence? How can it be a mere attentional hiccough? How can it stem from an emotional conflict between different lifestyles? How can it even be the intrusion into *my* consciousness, externalised or not, of a precursor to some utterance? What is experienced as a voice is, in schizophrenics at least, something *alien* to me and nothing in the way of an everyday event which is picked up wrongly by some component of my mental apparatus. Psychological psychopathology assumes a naively realist philosophical perspective on everything and is perpetually undone by the actual facts of phenomenological and even descriptive psychopathology.

16.5.4 Why Is Phenomenological Psychopathology the Only Valid Approach?

Merleau-Ponty (1945/1962), who had studied the phenomenological literature, concluded:

> Hallucinations are played out on a stage different from that of the perceived world and are in a way superimposed.

Schröder (1926) and Minkowski (1932) had provided accounts, which Merleau-Ponty read, which allowed him to come to this view:

> It is as if I heard with my mouth.
> (Schröder 1926)

> A voice as if a German were trying to talk Yiddish.
> A young man imitating an old man's voice.
> A voice of a person pretending to be uncouth.
> (Minkowski 1932/1970)

Here we see that a handful of facts about the actual hallucinations undermine psychological theory after psychological theory about the nature of hallucination.

16.5.5 What Is the Nature of Schizophrenic Hallucinations?

To recap the salient facts of the matter, *schizophrenic voices* occur in three quarters of subjects given this diagnosis as opposed to 2 % of normals. They emanate from odd places (e.g. breastbone), may be spoken in a strange accent ('as if a German were trying to speak Yiddish') and have the physical characteristics, not of the hallucinator but of a public figure (Nayani and David 1996; Leudar et al. 1997). In Nayani and David's study, although a minority were not schizophrenic, most were, and the voices were predominantly those of a white, male, middle-aged, middle-class and middle-England person, regardless of whether the voice-hearer were black, female, young, lower class or a Londoner. Moreover, the content of the voice is largely confined to what is going on in the *present*, the voice taking on the role of a commentator here and now.

It is difficult to bring all this together in one viable concept, but one parsimonious explanation, which Stanghellini and myself (Stanghellini and Cutting 2003) proposed, and which is a phenomenological version of the psychological theories of Frith (1979) and Hoffman (1986), is that voices are a morbid objectivisation of some inner dialogue about the goings-on of their life. Why the peculiar sites and ownerships of the voices? My answer is that once the morbid objectivisation has taken place, the character of the experience—'the voice'—must be self-alien; it must take on the features that anything in the external world has a penumbra of qualities that gives it a 'thisness' alien to the self. The particular characteristics—whether it emanates from the breastbone or whether it sounds Russian or Yiddish—are the consequence of the experience's being an invention of the mind but given spurious actuality in the external world, where, like dreams, hitherto non-experienced images can take root as if they were everyday experiences.

The schizophrenics' visual hallucinations are of a similar ilk. They are generally experiences which no person in an everyday world *could* experience, because they are denatured fragments of those very experiences—'legs on bedroom wall'—but they are experienced in the same region as hitherto everyday experiences because the workings of the mind are projected out in the process of morbid objectivisation to look like actual everyday experiences.

The same goes for tactile hallucinations, which were common in my series, in line with the account of a schizophrenic called Lang (1938), who, in his autobiographical account, bemoaned the fact that his 'hallucinatory pain' troubled him more than any other sort of hallucination. This again appears to be a morbid objectification of the subconscious exposure to all sorts of normally unacknowledged influences.

In summary, only the schizophrenic, among the various sorts of hallucinators, experiences such aberrant images of what populates their world, relative to the images of things which are depicted in a normal frame of mind. Moreover, these images unfold in the course of their on-going life as an objectivisation or 'presentification' of matters normally remaining subconscious.

16.5.6 What Is the Nature of Depressive Hallucinations?

Psychotic depressives experience voices and visual hallucinations to a substantial extent, and although this is half the rate in schizophrenics, it is still nearly 20 times the rate in normals. What is going on here? Our phenomenological analysis uncovered a different pattern from that obtaining in schizophrenics. The depressive 'voice' is generally nonobjectivised and non-specific—its 'whoness' and 'whereness' are not revealed. Nevertheless, it conveys powerful messages for the voice-hearer—accusatory and incitory, incriminating past actions and threatening future retribution. This is quite unlike the schizophrenic or any other pattern.

In trying to explain this, a simple morbid objectivisation thesis, as in the schizophrenic case, makes no sense, because what is being communicated is something that is *not in the present*, but is steeped in the temporality of past and future and, moreover, calls the voice-hearer to account much more so than is evident in the schizophrenic.

There is nothing in the psychopathological literature of any sort to guide us here. But, as in the framework for our phenomenological analysis, when we turned to Max Scheler, one of the original trios of phenomenological philosophers, we can again derive insight from phenomenological philosophy, but, here, it is Heidegger who has most to say about our problem. He himself would deny that his trailblazing book *Sein und Zeit* [*Being and Time*, Heidegger 1927/1962] had anything whatsoever to do with a morbid state of the human being, as he was trying to depict some original status of the human being—*Dasein*—which was not only normal but more authentic, i.e. 'supernormal', than the dilapidated, human being that he saw as modern man. Yet there are reasons to interpret what he wrote about *Dasein* as more applicable to a depressive state of mind than to a normal human state. (There are further reasons to accommodate both Heidegger's notion of *Dasein* as some sort of primitive man's normal take on everything *and* our interpretation of his description as a brilliant phenomenological account of depression, but I shall deal with this in the last section of this chapter.)

Before considering Heidegger's writings, there is another author whose views on the nature of hallucinations are uncannily in tune with what the depressive experiences, and like Heidegger, the author would deny that his thesis had anything to do with the depressive state. The author is an American psychologist Jaynes, whose wide-ranging book *The Origin of Consciousness in the Breakdown of the Bicameral Mind* (Jaynes 1976) puts forward a number of suggestions about the nature of consciousness, primitive societies, auditory hallucination and the neuropsychological basis for hallucinations. For our purposes, his thesis is that in primitive societies, the 'mind' has two chambers—hence his term bicameral; one of them issues a god's commands and the other unquestioningly obeys them; when this dissipates or 'breaks down' in more modern societies, the impetus for action becomes my responsibility and not a god's; my consciousness then evolves as a replacement for the alien command, giver; the 'voices' that the god invoked and which the primitive person experienced as spurs to action are, according to Jaynes, then re-experienced in the morbid state of schizophrenia as an atavistic throwback to a primitive state. Here is Jaynes summarising his own argument:

> I have endeavoured to examine the record of a huge time span to reveal the plausibility that man and his early civilizations had a profoundly different mentality from our own, that in fact men and women were not conscious as are we, were not responsible for their actions, and therefore cannot be given the credit or blame for anything that were done over these vast millenia of time, that instead each person had part of his nervous system which was divine, by which he was ordered about like any slave, a voice or voices which were indeed what we call volition and empowered what they commanded and were related to the hallucinated voices of others in a careful, established hierarchy.

Setting aside the fact that he thought this atavistic state of affairs pertained to schizophrenics, Jaynes' thesis that auditory hallucinations (he says schizophrenic, I say depressive) are a throwback to earlier human states of mind is a gem of a theory in a relatively barren field.

Heidegger's account of *Dasein*, however, is even more resonant with what we have uncovered about depressive voices.

> Conscience is the call of care from the uncanniness of Being-in-the-world—the call which summons Dasein to its ownmost potentiality-for-Being-guilty... Conscience summons Dasein's Self from its lostness in the 'they'. The Self to which the appeal is made remains indefinite and empty ... and yet the Self has been reached unequivocally and unmistakably... In the call Dasein 'is' ahead of itself in such a way that at the same time it directs itself back to its thrownness.

What we have here are precisely the three characteristics which differentiate the depressive's voices from all others—an uncanny message that the person is guilty, the indefiniteness of who the caller is and where the call comes from and the joint futural and pastness of what the voice alludes to. Of course, as I say, one can dismiss my analogy of depressive voices with Heidegger's account of some primitive state of human being as unfair to Heidegger, who had no intention of writing about a psychopathological state of affairs. But there are both philosophers and psychopathologists (Scheler 1928; Hartmann 1935/1948; G. Owen, personal communication, 2014) who have interpreted Heidegger's treatise on Dasein as more applicable to a morbid state than to a normal one, even though, as I shall return to in the next but one section, this by no means belittles Heidegger's efforts, if, as I believe, the depressive condition as a whole is an atavistic throwback (Andersch and Cutting 2013).

In summary, depressive voices bear some resemblance to a hypothetical atavistic state of human being, commanding and accusing their subject, eerily proclaiming this subject guilty of past misdemeanours and threatening future retribution.

16.5.7 What Is the Nature of Non-Schizophrenic, Nondepressive Hallucinations?

There are either too few case studies or too little phenomenological analysis in the extant studies to make any pronouncement here. Some of the groupings I tentatively analysed are themselves heterogeneous—there are various kinds of dementia and numerous psychosis-inducing drugs—and no specific sorts of hallucinations would be expected in these generic groups.

What is *not* supported in this chapter is a bland thesis to the effect that because 'normals' experience voices, then normality is a suitable standard with which to compare voices in other situations and well-established nosological conditions.

16.5.8 What Do Hallucinations Tell Us About the Nature of Psychosis?

Despite the best endeavours of twentieth-century psychopathologists, schizophrenia and depressive illness are still poorly understood, even at the descriptive level. Aside from the habit among psychologists to blur psychosis with normality, which we have castigated here, there is the equally misleading tendency among some psychiatrists to revive the nineteenth-century concept of a unitary psychosis. The findings presented in this chapter should help to scotch both such theses: if 'normals' experience hallucinations, then they are unlike those of schizophrenics or depressives, and schizophrenics and depressives differ between themselves in the sort of hallucinations they experience.

By and large, *schizophrenics* are plagued by an overwhelming sense of the present. Minkowski (1927/1987) saw this nearly a century ago and called it a morbid preoccupation with geometry, perhaps more accurately deemed morbid objectivisation (Cutting 1999), or, using Heidegger's (1927/1962) human realms of ready to hand and present at hand, a shift *from* the former *to* the latter (Kuhn 1952; Kraus 2007). The voices schizophrenics hear are often, and more so than any other group of hallucinators, a 'presentification' of what is going on too—thoughts simultaneously experienced as 'present at hand' spoken by someone in the external world, activities contemporaneously commented upon by someone outside of the person.

Depressives, by contrast, are generally preoccupied with past and futural dimensions of time. This can be discerned in the pattern of their delusions, where guilt for some *past* action is the commonest sort (Kuhs 1991), but a conviction that something awful is going to happen in the *future* is also common (Minkowski 1923/1958). In fact nihilistic delusions, which are the second commonest delusion in depressives, were rightly identified by Cotard (1880) and Toulouse (1893) not as a belief that one is dead but as a conviction that they are immortal and cannot die:

> They feel oppressed by their immortality and plead for someone to deliver them from it. (Cotard 1880)

Their voices, too, as we demonstrated, are concerned largely with past and future, not the present. Not only this, but there are reasons, other than the nature of their voices, for linking the depressive state to that of the 'normal' human being of past millennia (Andersch and Cutting 2013), and so Heidegger's claim that the original situation of the human being—privy to a call to care (for other human beings) by means of a *Stimme* [voice] which conveys guilt—which is what he largely means by his term *Dasein*, is both consistent with a depressive state *and* is an inspired depiction of a primitive human.

[Solution to vignette puzzle: (1) cocaine psychosis, (2) depressive psychosis, (3) normal, (4) schizophrenia, (5) mania, (6) dementia, (7) sensory deprivation and (8) delirium].

References

Andersch, N., & Cutting, J. (2013). *Schizofrenia e malinconia*. Rome: Giovanni Fioriti Editore.

Bazhin, E. F., Wasserman, L. I., & Tonkonogii, I. M. (1975). Auditory hallucinations and left temporal lobe pathology. *Neuropsychology, 13*, 481–487.

Bliss, E. L., Clark, L. D., & West, C. D. (1959). Studies of sleep deprivation: Relationship to schizophrenia. *Archives of Neurology and Psychiatry, 81*, 348–359.

Burns, A., Jacoby, R., & Levy, R. (1990). Psychiatric phenomena in Alzheimer's disease. *British Journal of Psychiatry, 157*, 72–94.

Cotard, J. (1880). Du délitre hypochondriaque dans une forme grave de la mélancholie anxieuse. *Annales Médico-Psychologiques, 38*, 168–174.

Cutting, J. (1987). The phenomenology of acute organic psychosis: Comparison with acute schizophrenia. *British Journal of Psychiatry, 151*, 324–332.

Cutting, J. (1997). *The principles of psychopathology*. Oxford: Oxford University Press.

Cutting, J. (1999). Morbid objectivization in psychopathology. *Acta Psychiatrica Scandinavica. Supplementum, 395*, 30–33.

Cutting, J. (2012). *A critique of psychopathology*. Berlin: Parodos Verlag.

Frith, C. D. (1979). Consciousness, information and schizophrenia. *British Journal of Psychiatry, 134*, 225–235.

Garrett, M., & Silva, R. (2003). Auditory hallucinations, source monitoring, and the belief that 'voices' are real. *Schizophrenia Bulletin, 29*, 445–457.

Grassian, S. (1983). Psychopathological effects of solitary confinement. *American Journal of Psychiatry, 140*, 1450–1454.

Hartmann, N. (1935/1948). *Zur Grundlegung der Ontologie* (3rd ed., p. 197). Berlin: Walter de Gruyter.

Heidegger, M. (1927/1962). *Being and time*. Oxford: Basil Blackwell.

Heilbrun, A. B. (1993). Hallucinations. In C. J. Costello (Ed.), *Symptoms of schizophrenia* (pp. 56–91). New York: Wiley.

Hoffman, R. E. (1986). Verbal hallucinations and language production processes in schizophrenia. *The Behavioral and Brain Sciences, 9*, 503–548.

Holroyd, S., Rabins, P. V., Finkelstein, D., Nicholson, M. C., Chase, G. A., & Wisniewski, S. C. (1992). Visual hallucinations in patients with macular degeneration. *American Journal of Psychiatry, 149*, 1701–1706.

Jarvik, M. (1970). Drugs, hallucinations and memory. In W. Kemp (Ed.), *Origin and mechanisms of hallucinations* (pp. 277–302). New York: Plenum Press.

Jaynes, J. (1976). *The origin of consciousness in the breakdown of the bicameral mind.* Boston, MA: Houghton Mifflin.

Kraus, A. (2007). Schizophrenic delusion and hallucination as the expression and consequence of an alteration of the existential a prioris. In M. C. Chung, K. W. M. Fulford, & G. Graham (Eds.), *Reconceiving schizophrenia.* Oxford: Oxford University Press.

Kuhn, R. (1952). Daseinsanalytische Studie über die Bedeutung von Grenzen im Wahn. *Monatsschrift fur Psychiatrie und Neurologie, 124*, 354–383.

Kuhs, H. (1991). Depressive delusion. *Psychopathology, 24*, 106–114.

Lang, J. (1938). The other side of hallucinations. *American Journal of Psychiatry, 94*, 1089–1097.

Leudar, I., & Thomas, P. (2000). *Voices of reason, voices of insanity.* London: Routledge.

Leudar, I., Thomas, P., McNally, D., & Glinski, A. (1997). What voices can do with words: Pragmatics of verbal hallucinations. *Psychological Medicine, 27*, 885–898.

Ludwig, A. M. (1972). 'Psychedelic' effects produced by sensory overload. *American Journal of Psychiatry, 128*, 1294–1297.

Merleau-Ponty, M. (1945/1962). *Phenomenology of perception.* London: Routledge and Kegan Paul.

Minkowski, E. (1923/1958). Findings in a case of schizophrenic depression. In R. May, E. Angel, & H. F. Ellenberger (Eds.), *Existence* (pp. 127–157). New York: Basic Books.

Minkowski, E. (1927/1987). The essential disorder of schizophrenia. In J. Cutting, M. Shepherd (Eds.), *The clinical roots of the schizophrenia concept* (pp. 188–212). Cambridge: Cambridge University Press.

Minkowski, E. (1932/1970). The problem of hallucinations and the problem of space. In E. Minkowski (Ed.), *Lived time* (pp. 382–398). Evanston, IL: Northwestern University Press.

Nayani, T. H., & David, A. S. (1996). The auditory hallucination: A phenomenological survey. *Psychological Medicine, 26*, 177–189.

Romme, M., & Escher, S. (1993). *Accepting voices.* London: Mind Publications.

Scheler, M. (1913–1916/1973). *Formalism in ethics and non-formal ethics of values.* Evanston, IL: Northwestern University Press.

Scheler, M. (1928/1995). *Gesammelte Werke* (Bd. 9, p. 300). Bonn: Bouvier.

Schröder, P. (1926). Das Halluzinieren. *Zeitschrift für die gesamte Neurologie und Psychiatrie, 101*, 599–614.

Schulman, C. A., Richlin, M., & Weinstein, S. (1967). Hallucinations and disturbances of affect, cognition, and physical state as a function of sensory deprivation. *Perceptual and Motor Skills, 25*, 1001–1024.

Slade, P. D., & Bentall, R. P. (1988). *Sensory deception: A scientific analysis.* London: Croom Helm.

Stanghellini, G., & Cutting, J. (2003). Auditory verbal hallucinations—breaking the silence of inner dialogue. *Psychopathology, 36*, 120–128.

Tien, A. Y. (1991). Distributions of hallucinations in the population. *Social Psychiatry and Psychiatric Epidemiology, 26*, 287–292.

Toulouse, E. (1893). Le délire des négations. *Gaz Hôpitaux, 66*, 301–309.

Unnithan, S. B., & Cutting, J. (1992). The cocaine experience: Refuting the concept of a model psychosis. *Psychopathology, 25*, 71–78.

Fear and Trembling: A Case Study of Voice Hearing in Schizophrenia as a Self-Disorder 17

Marino Pérez-Álvarez, Oscar Vallina-Fernández, José M. García-Montes, and Louis A. Sass

This chapter consists of three parts. The first part presents a case from a mental health unit for first psychotic episodes. After presenting a few biographical details, we focus on the patient's lived world, which was marked by terrifying voices, and on his attitudes toward these disturbing experiences. In the second part, the case is conceptualized from the perspective of structural phenomenology (also known as genetic-structural phenomenology) and, specifically, according to the ipseity-disturbance model (ipseity is synonymous with basic, core, or minimal self). The idea here is that psychotic symptoms indicate a more *profound* level of impairment, one that has to do with the basic structure of self-experience and one's associated way of being in the world. The third part emphasizes the implications of this phenomenological conception of schizophrenia with regard to the assessment, diagnosis, and treatment of the condition.

17.1 Case Description: Fear of Voices and Trembling

Maycon is a 17-year-old boy who was referred to the mental health service for urgent care because of a psychotic crisis, marked by auditory hallucinations and severe anxiety. His mother brought him to the service because of her concern about his behavior at home, where he was spending most of his time, hardly eating

M. Pérez-Álvarez
Department of Psychology, University of Oviedo, Oviedo, Spain

O. Vallina-Fernández
Hospital Sierrallana, Torrelavega, Spain

J.M. García-Montes
Department of Psychology, University of Almeria, Almeria, Spain

L.A. Sass (✉)
Department of Clinical Psychology, GSAPP—Rutgers University, Piscataway, NJ, USA
e-mail: lsass@rci.rutgers.edu

G. Stanghellini, M. Aragona (eds.), *An Experiential Approach to Psychopathology*,
DOI 10.1007/978-3-319-29945-7_17

(or doing so in an anarchic manner), neglecting his personal hygiene, and refusing to talk with anybody. His mother says she often heard her son talking to himself, as if he were having a conversation with someone else. If she asked him what he was doing, he shouted that she should leave him alone.

Background Maycon began to take drugs in his home country (Brazil) when he was 11; the substances he ingested included gasoline, cocaine, cannabis, and alcohol. He had his first experience with voices when he was 12. When he mentioned this to his grandmother, she told him it was because Satan was trying to possess him. At 13 he moved to Spain with his mother and became involved there with a group of substance users. The frequency of the voices increased, and he began developing referential ideas, attributing the voices to friends who were talking about him. Maycon, whose brother was born from his mother's relationship with her second partner, started to feel displaced at home and to feel distant from his mother. At 15 he began a very intense friendship with a composer of violent rap music who was involved with the occult and Satanism.

For 2 years Maycon went on the "deep Web" (this refers to the part of the World Wide Web that is not indexed or accessible to standard search engines, understood to be a dark and sometimes scary place where illegal activities are rampant), and he began mimicking the thoughts, likes, and ideas of his composer friend:

> I saw what he saw and wanted to be like him, he had an awesome vocabulary, you heard him and you said, Jesus, he knows what he's talking about! A while ago I told him I didn't want to listen to that music with him anymore. I told him I was hearing those things in my voices and I told him not to listen to that music then, and if he did it would make me go crazy and do what the voices told me to do [. . .] Like strange things started to happen to us, we saw weird things, we heard voices, we felt some very evil energies [. . .] we went on horrible Internet pages. My friend and me were like that for two years. Now I can't look at those things anymore, they do something funny to me, the picture stays with me up here [in my head] and I can't stand it.

At 16, there was an increase in Maycon's behavioral disturbance. He acted in a disorganized and suspicious manner and was aggressive toward his mother, whom he accused of favoring his brother. The intensity of his psychotic experiences increased. More and more he felt that he was being observed and controlled when outside. From the way people around him interpreted his gestures and from how they acted, he was convinced they could hear his thoughts. Maycon reacted to the distress generated by these experiences by isolating himself at home or with his friend and by using cannabis or alcohol to relax. After his mother reported the situation to the social services, he was admitted to a center for minors. There, during a 9-month stay, he stopped taking drugs, received psychiatric medication, and became religious.

At 17, after leaving the center for minors, Maycon started attending the Evangelical Church, which however he left after a few months, disillusioned with its teachings and behavioral norms: "They're too radical, nobody can live like that, they don't let you do nothin', like everything is a sin, man, of course, since they say Satan rules the earth, everything is evil." He started occasional use of alcohol and cannabis again and stopped taking his prescribed medication. His psychotic experiences intensified again, together with suspicious and aggressive behaviors. Also, his relationship with his mother worsened and he started treatment in the mental health services.

Lived World The most salient aspects of Maycon's lived world were the following: the terrifying voices he heard, experiences of "thought diffusion," feelings of being dominated by voices and Satan, and, finally, dreading that something very bad was going to happen. It was with considerable emotion that Maycon described recent experiences, as in the following statements:

> "I started to hear them calling out to me in the street, to see people watching me at home, I was afraid." "I'm at home and I hear conversations talking to me. I think it's Satan who wants to take hold of me." "I hear in my head: What? That's a dirty trick! Is that you, are you going to stay like that forever? And now what, huh?" "They speak my language, it's all very strange, I'm in the kitchen and I hear them in the living room, and when I go see, they disappear, and I hear the noise... it's like they were inside the walls." "I spend the day listening to music with the earphones on so I won't hear them. They aren't good, they want to torture my head to fuck me, and I'm really afraid of them!" "I see heads peeking out and watching me, I see them very clearly and they try to stick things in my head, give me messages. I know that voice wants to get inside my head." "At night, I know that I am not going to be able to sleep, I know something is waiting for me." "I stopped going to class because I was hearing voices that told me my classmates were saying bad things about me; they were saying that I was a fucking foreigner." "I can't be alone outside. It's fucking paranoia, the hairs stand up on the back of my neck. And I hear someone breathing around me." "The voices are like wandering souls, they call me by my name, hey, Maycon! And they whisper, they're like Hell's angels, like beings made of light, I see them shining in the night, they're like paranormal."

Maycon explained that he had a cross tattooed on his arm because a voice told him to do so: "It was an angel that told me to do it so Satan wouldn't take me." And he offered more descriptions of the voices and of the fear and trembling they caused him:

> "I told my mother because I couldn't stand it anymore, I see and hear things my mother doesn't see when I'm with her. They're like talking to each other, like planning something. It's fucking weird. I hear it so clear it frightens me." I didn't want people to think I'm crazy, because the guys'd say, I ain't goin' out with him." "My head tells me that I shouldn't come here [to the Health Center], then I feel guilty, they say, what am I coming for?"

> "I see women, I see a girl all the time, she's like a human toy, she looks at me, and she makes signs at me with her eyes. I feel people behind me. It makes me dizzy. I made some rap instrumentals, and when I get dizzy I lose reality, I'm like lost, I feel like I'm going to be possessed, I hear horror music in my house. I think there is something in my house." "I have the paranoia that I read people's minds, I know everything about them just by looking at them." "My thoughts are so fucking loud, sometimes I think my pal hears what I'm thinking."

The voices occurred during the interview itself, after the therapist had asked him whether he could elicit the voice-hearing experience in the therapeutic session. After a period of silence, he spoke: "I don't hear nothin', man, I'm cool [. . .]." Then he went on:

> Now I hear crickets, don't you hear them? [to the therapist] "What do you mean, no? Listen [. . .] They say they're gonna kill Antonio, the guy with the tattoo that I owe 70 bucks. For cryin' out loud, I forgot all about the guy [. . .] Now they're telling me they're gonna take my girl out there and fuck her . . . Shit, I can't breathe. . ." [stops to calm down] "They say you [the therapist] are cheating me, there's nothing wrong with me, what happens to me is normal and [the voices] are there because they're real." "Now they want me to sell my soul to the devil, I should go to a gypsy and have her read my palm, do a *macumba* [ritual], shit!" [He gets nervous] "What kills me the most is that when I hear them, I'm the first to laugh, but then they get mad and I'm afraid they'll do something to me."

In the second and third sessions, the nature of Maycon's voices and of his experience of them emerged in still clearer fashion. Below we describe, first, the specific characteristics of the voices and of his fearful reactions to them; second, his explanation of their meaning; and third, certain circumstances that seemed to be related to their emergence.

Characteristics of the Voices and Attitude Toward Them The voices may be those of unknown persons or may be recognizable as those of friends and his mother. Often, Maycon hears full sentences and clear dialogues, at other times just isolated words or sounds, like the word "breathing" or "crickets." The voices are loud, so much so that he can be surprised that others do not hear them. They have a "perceptual" and "objectified" quality, as if they were somehow "recorded" in his brain, leaving him "trembling":

> "I hear them out there, around me, in the walls, in the bathroom, I hear them and I say to my mother, 'Did you hear that?' They are very ugly and sound awful. I get very nervous when I hear them, they make my hair stand on end, I start to breathe fast, I can't stop moving and I have to do something." "Sometimes I feel fucking cold inside and I start to shake."

The voices threaten him and tell him to do things, sometimes terrible things, as described in the following statements:

> "They're telling me to kill that guy!" "What do you do when you hear that?", the therapist asks. "Nothing! I keep real quiet and don't move, and I just start shaking [. . .] after a while they go away, but they come back and raise the volume [. . .] other times they stay there, but talking about things that don't make sense." "If I talk to them I go crazy. Once it occurred to me to tell them, 'but what are you saying?' And they said, but I can control you kid, I'm your head, I can pull your heart right out."

One of his greatest fears, says Maycon, is that the voices "can control me and make me do things automatically." "I go into a mental collapse," he says, describing some incidents: "The other day I was dreaming about the voices, and when I woke up I was eating yogurt in the kitchen, and while I was eating it, I thought to myself, what am I doing here? How did I live?" Another day, after drinking and smoking a few joints: "I woke up the next day without remembering anything. And people said to me: look what you did, you were going down the road like crazy, and I didn't remember a thing."

Maycon adopts several strategies for dealing with the voices. On rare occasions, he talks to them out loud: "The other day I was sitting on a bench and they started up, and I said, leave me alone, I don't want to talk, why are you telling me to do those things? And they said: it's for your own good, and then you'll feel good. And I go, but what are you talking about! And then a man walked by and was staring at me." He uses other strategies as well: "What I do most often is listen to music when I hear them, I put on the earphones as high as they'll go and the music mixes with them." Sometimes he composes music to understand and express what he feels when hearing the voices. As he explained about one of these compositions, which he brought with him to the visit:

> It took me several days to do it [the musical composition], because I can't express what I feel with words and I need to express what I have in my head, but with the music it comes out better, here is everything I feel when I hear them, my paranoias, my distrust of people [...] When I finished composing it, the voices got really loud, I couldn't sleep a wink all night, I felt awful, but the next day I felt better, they had gone down a lot, and when I heard it again, it relaxed me, I felt good, it felt very peaceful. It's like the voices had stayed in the music, I flip out!

The cross tattooed on his arm, he now explained, was meant to protect against the voices.

Meaning of What Happened Maycon has his own ways of explaining or understanding what happens to him. Sometimes he connects his voices to his life and life circumstances:

> I am very angry inside because of the life I have and I have to express it [...] my mother is out of work, separated, has shared custody for my brother with my stepfather and she talks to me in a way I don't like at all, and there is where the voices come from, and it balls me because she doesn't talk to my brother like that, maybe I bother her, I don't know, it's like she's putting me down, and I understand, because she's stressed, but she takes it out on me [...] And I am very angry with God, God has let me down.

Other times he associates the voices with insanity and Satan, saying he is afraid he is going crazy because Satan wants to hurt him:

> "My grandmother said that people who were sick saw Satan or that he controlled them, and when the brain is sick, Satan takes advantage of it." "I think a lot about God. The Bible says that Satan is on earth with his demons and I think that Satan wants to hurt me so I'll go crazy. When I get dizzy it seems like I'm in Hell." "I think that when you go crazy it's something that takes hold of you, I think that sickness comes from Satan." "The other day I thought: Bah! That's not from Satan. But see, the voices are strange, voices I don't know, very strange [...] You know I make music, well now [Satan] puts effects in the voices, and

> it scares you to death. From what they tell me, it's Satan, they're very strange things that I never would have imagined. Yesterday I was with my girlfriend and I was quiet for a while, and [the voice] started to say, 'Look kid, I'm going to give you an idea you're going to love, take her out in the bushes, invite her out to eat, take a knife with you and you rape her and kill her, and then you bury her there.' Sometimes I laugh and say, come on man! But then he shouts more, Kill her! Kill her! It puts pressure on my mind and I can't stand it."

He also went so far as to wonder if his brain is "shot." "I'm sorry I smoked pot and all that [. . .] I think I started with [sniffing] gas. My mother says that everything that happens to me is because my brain is shot from all the pot in me."

At times the content of his voices seems to reflect things Maycon has heard or seen from popular culture, such as a horror film or rap lyrics. At other times, the hallucinatory experiences seem to be generated by the act of thinking alone: "When I'm alone, quiet, thinking, I begin to hear voices [. . .] Others [thoughts] are already in the way, and here they come, shit bitch, here they come, insults or strange things!"

17.2 The Case from the Perspective of the Ipseity-Disturbance Model

The case was referred to the mental health services because of the severe symptom of voice hearing; the patient entered the early attention program for psychosis. Although this program avoids using the diagnosis of schizophrenia, preferring to speak of psychotic episodes, the case does seem to merit the former diagnosis. Here we wish to offer a phenomenological/structural analysis that focuses on a fundamental disturbance of selfhood or the "I" (Akroyd 2013; Hirjak et al. 2013; Nelson et al. 2009; Sass and Parnas 2003). In the pages below, we first offer a brief characterization of structural phenomenology, differentiating it from nosographic and idiographic approaches. Then we present the ipseity-disturbance model. Finally, we formulate the case from this latter perspective.

Structural Phenomenology Although description is a primary task of phenomenology, structural phenomenology [also known as genetic-structural phenomenology (Ellenberger 1958/1967)] is not limited to a nosographic description of signs and symptoms. Nor is it satisfied with describing psychotic subjectivity as if it involved mere variations of normal experiences, albeit exaggerated. On the contrary, structural phenomenology recognizes that other people may experience themselves and the world in an entirely and qualitatively different way from the standard, and it seeks to grasp the essence of the overall abnormality of subjectivity that characterizes a given person or category of psychopathology. Recognition of these profound differences between oneself and another requires adopting what has been termed an approach of "radical empathy," namely, "a way of engaging with others' experiences that involves suspending the usual assumption that both parties share the same modal space." (Ratcliffe 2012, p. 483; see also Pienkos and Sass 2012).

Phenomenology is especially interested in "capturing" and describing the "essence" of the phenomena: their form, core, *gestalt*, or structure (Parnas 2012a; Sass and Parnas 2007). The writer Antoine de Saint-Exupéry said, in a famous line: "what is essential is invisible to the eye". Here the essence is not, however, something metaphysical, which exists *outside* of the world, nor is it merely a mental construction of the clinician or researcher. The essence of things, one might say, is to be found in the things themselves, in their being what they are: it is, for example, the pervasive quality that makes a given experience *psychotic*, or schizophrenic, and not some other form of psychosis.

Structural phenomenology is not idiographic in the sense of being interested only in the uniqueness of the individual case. Nor is it nosographic in the sense of seeking primarily to subsume the case within an abstract category, grounded in generalizations and statistical data. Its way of categorizing is, rather, *prototypical*, in the sense of attempting to identify *typical* structures, or general, basic, cross-personal forms of impairment or abnormality—even while granting the undeniable fact that each case has its particularity and that no case is quite the same as another. The prototypes in question are like Weberian ideal types, which are grounded in, and reveal, the most characteristic attributes. In this sense, for example, a cat can be said to be a more typical or exemplary mammal than is a bat or a platypus. A real case may exemplify an ideal type without necessarily capturing *all* the aspects of the type (Parnas 2012b; Schwartz and Wiggins 1987). Table 17.1 summarizes the different ways in which the project of clinical phenomenology can be conceived.

The Ipseity-Disturbance Model Phenomenological investigation, grounded in clinical experience and empirical research as well as theoretical analysis and speculation, has revealed a particular self-disorder called ipseity disturbance (Nelson et al. 2014; Sass 2014) as the possible core of schizophrenia. The essence of this model was originally proposed by Louis Sass in *Madness and Modernism* (Sass 1992) and further developed in a seminal article by Sass and Parnas called "Schizophrenia, Consciousness, and the Self" (Sass and Parnas 2003).

Ipseity refers to the most basic sense of existing as an I or a first-person perspective on the world. It refers to the most fundamental sense of selfhood, the

Table 17.1 Different versions of clinical phenomenology

Varieties of phenomenology	Focus of interest	Examples
Objectivist nosographic	Signs and symptoms	DSM; CIE
Subjectivist idiographic	Individual subjectivity (content of experiences)	Jaspers; humanist psychology (see Sass 1988)
Structural, transpersonal (gestalt prototypic)	Structures and dimensions of subjectivity (intentionality, bodily, lived time, etc.)	Minkowski; Blankenburg; Sass & Parnas; Stanghellini; Fuchs

nearly ineffable sense of existing as a *subject* of one's own experience (sense of ownership) and as an agent of one's own actions (sense of agency) (Hur et al. 2014; Nelson et al. 2014). The selfhood captured by the term ipseity is tacit, implicit, and prereflective. It serves as the foundational infrastructure of more obvious and explicit forms of selfhood that are more reflective and narrative in nature. Ipseity also grounds our tacit or implicit articulation with the world, for it serves as a sort of imperceptible background or foundational bridge that joins us seamlessly to persons, things, and the commonsense, taken-for-granted world, with its normal quality of obviousness or "natural self-evidence." Needless to say, ipseity is anchored in the body (embodied), just as the body is implicated in the world (embedded), yet it cannot be reduced to an organ or suborganic structure.

Schizophrenia as ipseity disturbance assumes a global crisis of common sense (Stanghellini 2004) or as a patient of Blankenburg put it, a "loss of natural self-evidence" (of "*natürliche Selbstverständlichkeit*"), that is, a loss of the unquestioned sense of obviousness and of the unproblematic background quality that normally enables a person to take for granted so many aspects of the social and practical world (Blankenburg 1971/2014). More specifically, the ipseity disturbance implies two aspects of anomalous self-experience: termed hyperreflexivity and diminished self-affection or diminished self-presence (Sass 2014; Sass and Parnas 2003, 2007).

Hyperreflexivity refers to intensified awareness of aspects of oneself that would normally be "inhabited" or experienced tacitly, but that now erupt into one's field of consciousness, interrupting the smooth flow of spontaneous experience and functioning. These aspects include, for example, forms of synesthesia, strange bodily sensations, and sonorization of thought, as well as de-automatization of habits such that one may have to attend consciously to each step of a routine activity (Stanghellini and Cutting 2003). Hyperreflexivity need not involve intellectual, deliberate, or volitional forms of self-consciousness, though these *reflective* forms (what can be termed hyper-*reflectivity*—as opposed to the more generic term hyper*reflexivity*) can also occur and may come to play an important role in the anomalous forms of experience and action (Sass et al. 2013a). At its most foundational level, however, hyperreflexivity seems to involve the automatic irruption into focal or conscious awareness of normally tacit aspects of experience. (One might, in fact, describe this most basic form of hyperreflexivity by using the, at first, paradoxical-sounding phrase, *prereflective* hyperreflexivity.) Diminished self-affection or self-presence refers to a concomitant weakening sense of the experience of existing as a subject of awareness or agent of action, as when the patient feels lifeless, alienated, or utterly dominated by outside forces or powers.

Whereas "hyperreflexivity" emphasizes that something normally tacit becomes focal and explicit, "diminished self-affection" or self-presence emphasizes what is probably a complementary aspect of this same process: the fact that what once was "tacit is no longer being inhabited as a medium of taken-for-granted selfhood" (Sass 2014). Despite this interdependence, there are patients, and periods of illness, in which one facet or the other emerges as more prominent. It is difficult to determine whether hyperreflexivity and diminished-self-affection are best conceived as complementary facets or tightly interacting processes; perhaps both conceptions are needed (Sass et al. 2013a).

Hyperreflexivity and diminished self-affection necessarily imply, as well, various disturbances in one's experience of or attunement to the world, referred to (following the philosopher Merleau-Ponty) as "disturbed hold" or "grip" on the world. The day-to-day world comes to appear strange, with familiar things seeming oddly decontextualized and sometimes imbued with special meaning, persons taking on an automaton-like quality, and often a sense of being watched or pursued by hostile beings. Another common aspect of disturbed grip, also grounded in abnormalities of the embodied or vital experiential self, is a sense of confusion about whether something experienced is being perceived versus imagined versus remembered (Sass 2004, 2014). Table 17.2 shows the components of the ipseity-disturbance model schematically.

Table 17.2 Components of ipseity-disturbance model

Ipseity	Ipseity disturbance	Examples
Sense of oneself as existing as a vital and self-identical *subject* of experience and action and as a first-person perspective on the world	Disturbed "mineness"; disorder of self-presence; lack of sense of self	"Consciousness gradually loses its coherence. The center cannot hold. The "me" becomes a haze, and the solid center from which one experiences reality breaks up like a bad radio signal. There is no longer a vantage point from which to look out, take things in, assess. No core holds things together, providing the lens through which we see the world" (Saks 2007). "[M]y sense of self is totally crushed when the "bubble" surrounding my self-consciousness is destroyed by this unstable permeability [...] until the entire self-experience disintegrates" (Kean 2009)
	Hyperreflexivity: intensified self-consciousness that involves self-alienation	Corporeal sensations, de-automatization, thoughts aloud, etc.
	Diminished self-affection: diminished sense of existing as the subject of one's own experience and action	Devitalization; feeling influenced; depersonalization
	"Disturbed hold" or "grip" on the world; alteration of attunement to the world	Estrangement; derealization; feeling persecuted; confusion between perception/imagination/memory; uncanny sense of "revelation"

Case Formulation Maycon exhibits anomalous experiences in all three aspects of ipseity disturbance as described in the ipseity-disturbance model. The voices breaking the silence of inner dialogue can be considered manifestations of hyper-reflexivity. For example, Maycon would hear voices in conversations addressing themselves to him. These can be interpreted as involving a bringing to explicit awareness of processes of (self-referential) inner speech that would normally be silent, even unnoticed by the person experiencing them. Some of these experiences are particularly horrifying and leave him "shaking"; they may be accompanied by equally disturbing visual images, often of faces looking back at him. Though frequently derived from recent experiences (listening and composing rap music, a movie), these voices and visions are not experienced by Maycon as returning memories or as mere images. Typically, they have an objectified and somehow perceptualized quality, and often they engender an undefined sense of unease or even terror. In this way, mental activities that would normally form part of the "stream of consciousness" come to be objectified and to take on a sort of life of their own, offering themselves as strange and fearsome quasi-realities.

The voices also suggest diminished self-affection or self-presence, a weakened sense of self as the subject of action. In fact, Maycon fears the voices because, he says, they might cause him to have a "mental collapse" or "lose his mind," that is, lose control of himself or awareness of himself—which is what already happened when he found himself doing something (e.g., walking down the street) without knowing how he came to be engaged in that action or how he got to that place. Both Maycon's experience of "thought diffusion" and his sense of "feeling controlled" when out in the public street illustrate his weakened sense of self-presence and agency.

Thus, we see, in Maycon, both hyperreflexive objectification of aspects of the normally tacit self, such as inner thoughts, and, at the same time, diminished self-affection in the form of a weakened sense of the self as active subject. The voices, along with the visions and uncanny sense of dread, certainly have the effect of undermining any normal sense of harmony either with himself or the world.

Auditory hallucinations (to use the classic psychopathological term, instead of "voices") are not mere perceptions without an object, which is how they are standardly defined. They need to be understood as involving alterations of the structure of experience itself—of consciousness and the lived world, typically involving a loss of positioning within one's social milieu. According to the phenomenological psychiatrist Alfred Kraus, both hallucinations and delusions should be understood as *secondary* phenomena. The more primary disorder, according to Kraus, involves an impairment of being in the world itself and, in particular, forms of depersonalization (Kraus 2007). In this sense, hallucinations imply a double alienation: from aspects of self-experience that are now estranged and thus felt as strange and also from the social world due to a felt loss of position and the loneliness this entails (Schwartz 2013). Auditory hallucinations can, in fact, sometimes become a sort of world in themselves that replaces the social world of real others (Rojcewick and Rojcewick 1997).

A phenomenological case analysis requires going beyond overt symptoms to this sort of more "profound" and pervasive level. The latter is not, however, the depth of the psychodynamic unconscious, of information processing, or of "deep" brain structures. It refers to a "profound and characteristic modification of schizophrenic existence or being in the world" consisting of "a typical kind of depersonalization and derealization" (Stanghellini 2011, p. 164). An *in-depth* study of persons with schizophrenia or in prodromal phases suggests, for instance, that "first-rank symptoms" (including voices) actually develop out of, and express, a prior and more fundamental transformation of subjectivity with respect to ipseity and sense of agency (Hirjak et al. 2013).

In accord with the ipseity-disturbance model, then, it can be argued that Maycon's psychotic experiences, or his symptom of voice hearing, reveal "an instability of the normally tacit, pre-reflective, and pre-predicative founding stratum of our experiential life that is property-less and that resists further qualification" (Parnas and Henriksen 2014, p. 255). This refers to an overall disturbance of what might be termed the center of *experiential* gravity, which is one way of describing the notion of ipseity or core self-experience (Nelson et al. 2008, p. 386).

There is growing evidence of a link between life adversities and psychotic symptoms (Bentall et al. 2014). Maycon's adversities, obvious in his biography, extend back to a "marginal" childhood which led him to substance abuse, including of gasoline, starting at age 11. His emigration from Brazil to Spain was yet another source of adversity, bringing him into contact with marginal environments even while he felt marginalized in his own home, with the birth of his brother. Maycon's admission to a center for minors reveals this marginalization and contributes to it at the same time. The search for meaning and social context in religious communities (Jehovah's Witnesses, Evangelical Church) turned out to be, for him, just another source of new disappointing experiences and failure. This kind of "defeat," loss of social/existential position, and associated "ontological insecurity" was captured by a similar patient, more verbally sophisticated, who wrote about her own weakened ipseity and existential permeability by referring to what she called "the dissolved, the disorientated, and the disembodied self." (Kean 2009).

The *dissolved* self involves excessive permeability between the individual and others, as shown by the voices attributed by Maycon to his friends as well as his "fusion" with his "exoteric" friend. In *disoriented* self-experience, the self has a somewhat stronger sense of existing yet is unstable and unsure of how to relate to a threatening world—as when Maycon experiences others as hostile toward him but feels helpless to respond, often associated with thought-broadcasting experiences in which he experiences his own self-critical inner thoughts as coming from other people. The *disembodied* self emerges in the experience of "made" happenings or passivity phenomena (as, e.g., when Maycon found himself in a place without knowing how he got there or feared of "losing his mind") and in "hearing voices," in which normally unconscious forms of inner speech emerge in a reified, isolated, and alienated fashion (Kean 2009, p. 1035). Figure 17.1 shows key aspects of this case formulation in schematic fashion, suggesting some possible relationships among the variables at issue.

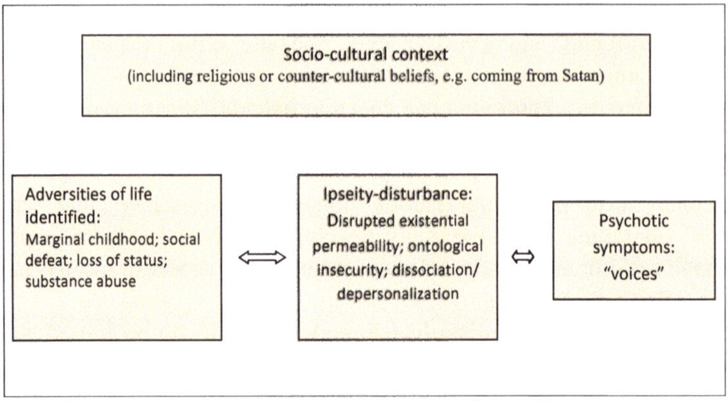

Fig. 17.1 Case formulation showing a set of interdependent factors, in constant interaction

We see here how fundamental ipseity disturbance, manifest, e.g., in a tendency toward depersonalization, stands as mediator between adversities of life, to the left, and psychotic symptoms including voices, to the right (Perona-Garcelán et al. 2014; Sass et al. 2013b).

The two-way arrow on the left indicates (1) that certain "life adversities"—together with existential or anthropological vulnerability (probably including a neurobiological component)—might play an important pathogenetic role in instigating the "ipseity disturbance" underlying the "psychotic symptoms" (a point consistent with recent findings regarding the probable pathogenetic role of trauma in schizophrenia) (Read et al. 2005; Velikonja et al. 2015); but also (2) in addition to being a partial consequence of difficult or traumatic life experiences, the impairment of core self or basic-I experience can also play a role in turning experiences that might otherwise have been merely challenging into something more truly disruptive or traumatic. The two-way arrow on the right indicates (1) that overt psychotic symptoms may be the consequence or expression of ipseity disturbance, but also that (2) once such symptoms develop, they can also exacerbate the more originary basic-I impairment—as, e.g., when attention to auditory hallucinations brings on a still more extreme sense of alienation from one's own thinking.

All this occurs, of course, in a given sociocultural environment (indicated by the overarching box at the top of the figure). The latter plays a crucial role in determining the particular nature of the life adversities (e.g., the lived meaning of loss of status, the particular feel of stigma) and also molds the way in which symptoms are expressed (e.g., in accord with religious or countercultural beliefs, as when voices are interpreted as coming from Satan, an extraterrestrial, a rock star).

Regarding the goals of therapeutic intervention, consistent with earlier publications, we would pose three main objectives: (a) the promotion of insight and understanding of voices in the context of lived experiences (Vallina-Fernández et al. 2014), (b) helping the patient find a way to "reinhabit" or reengage with his self (i.e., reinstate a sense of core self or ipseity) through the therapeutic relationship

(Stanghellini and Lysaker 2007), and (c) attempting to diminish the patient's hyper-reflexive processes by encouraging immersion in meaningful activities (work, leisure, social relations) (Nelson and Sass 2009). The practical implications are addressed below in general terms.

17.3 Implications for Assessment, Diagnosis, and Treatment

The phenomenological conception of schizophrenia has numerous implications for clinical practice, regarding assessment, diagnosis, and treatment. One might distinguish four themes, which we describe here in general terms, those pertaining to: (1) an open attitude (similar to the *epoché* characteristic of phenomenological investigation), (2) adoption of a hermeneutic orientation, (3) use of qualitative analysis, and (4) a new approach to psychotherapy for schizophrenic spectrum disorders. These issues have been discussed in a previous case study concerning a treatment involving 53 sessions over a 2-year period (Vallina-Fernández et al. 2014).

Open Attitude Conceiving schizophrenia in terms of *ipseity* provides a useful context for open exploration of lived experience and its experiential meaning. While conceptualizing schizophrenia as essentially a brain disease means viewing it as, in essence, just another chronic illness, like diabetes, the phenomenological attitude orients us toward the "things themselves"—which in this context means toward persons with their actual, lived experiences and subjective ways of being. Adopting the phenomenological attitude means accepting the experience of the other person and tolerating considerable ambiguity, without being obliged to understand everything or always provide a "diagnosis," explanation, or solution. The clinician adopts a sort of *epoché* or suspension of his own conceptions and opinions, with an attitude of openness and acceptance.

Hermeneutic Framework A hermeneutic framework, based on phenomenology, requires the clinician or interviewer to entertain, from the beginning, a series of questions that help to orient one's attempts at empathic comprehension, description, and analysis of the subjective experiences of the patient. Typical orienting questions could include, among others (Fuchs 2010, p. 271):

- What is it like to be in a certain mental state (e.g., to feel depressed or to hear voices)? What is the personal meaning of that certain state?
- How does the patient experience his or her world? How does he or she express, move, and define space as an embodied subject?
- Does the patient experience him or herself as an effective agent in the world or, rather, as only passively exposed to the world?
- Is there a sense of continuity over time, or are there breaks or fadings of self-awareness? What in fact is the subject's experience of existential time?

As already mentioned, structural phenomenology seeks to identify the "psychopathological organizers" or fundamental patterns that connect the single features; an example is, of course, the fundamental ipseity-disturbance characteristic of schizophrenia. The personal narratives by which patients themselves strive to organize and make sense of their experiences are also of great interest.

The hermeneutic/phenomenological framework aims not merely to *understand* subjective experiences but also to *explain* them by considering "meaningful connections" between phenomena—both synchronic and diachronic (Sass 2013; Sass and Parnas 2007). Of special interest are possible connections between particular *types* of psychotic experiences and the personal circumstances in the patient's present or past (Vallina-Fernández et al. 2014). The hermeneutic method involves co-construction of interpretations and narratives by both patient and therapist in the course of the clinical relationship, with the aim of reappropriating discordant or "alienated" experiences (Ricoeur 1992).

The hermeneutic framework is fundamental for diagnosis for reasons that Thomas Fuchs has aptly described as follows: "(1) the patient as a person in his or her life world can only be adequately understood through the medium of the interpersonal relationship which already unfolds during the first encounter of patient and psychiatrist, and (2) a major part of psychopathology, but also personality features relevant for diagnosis may only be grasped during and through the interaction" (Fuchs 2010, p. 272). Such a framework is particularly suited to conceptualizing psychotherapy, for it assumes the fundamental importance of a lived space or interactive field opened by the meeting of patient and therapist, a field that has the potential to create the interpersonal conditions for recovering the lost sense of being an I or a subject of action and experience (Fuchs 2007). In this sense, it offers an important alternative to the rather technological perspective of contemporary biological psychiatry (Bracken 2014; Maj 2014; Bracken et al. 2012).

Qualitative Analysis A phenomenological focus, open to experiences that are often too subtle to emerge in standard interviews or to be captured in questionnaires, requires qualitative forms of analysis. Such an analysis can be systematic, but it must also be flexible, beginning with unstructured interactive exploration of the phenomena under study. Stanghellini describes the procedure as follows:

> The phenomena under investigation may be gathered from interview transcripts, diaries or personal notes provided from patients or their relatives. Sentences reported by patients as they were made explicit during therapeutic interviews are good exemplifications of their experience about themes under investigation. [. . .] In the course of interviews, patients are encouraged to narrate, conceptualize and elaborate on these themes. In subsequent interviews, each patient is asked to reflect upon the narratives he had previously articulated and about narratives of other patients. This cycle of interpretations is set in a context of dialogical reciprocity that widens rather than restricting the range of meanings; [. . .] Elaborations of these materials and cocreation of meaningful narratives and constructs are seen as part of the treatment as well as of the inquiry. (Stanghellini 2008, 162)

A semi-structured interview covers preset themes or domains of experience (these derived from research and clinical experience) yet is open to exploration of unpredictable and unique features of the individual patient. A good example is the EASE—Examination of Anomalous Self-Experience (Parnas et al. 2005)—a qualitatively rich, 57-item semi-structured interview that operationalizes and quantifies the ipseity-disturbance model and is designed to detect sub-psychotic experiences. Each item is briefly defined and illustrated by prototypical examples of complaints. The items are aggregated into five rationally cohesive sections: (1) cognition and stream of consciousness, (2) self-awareness and presence, (3) bodily experiences, (4) demarcation/transitivism, and (5) existential reorientation. The EASE exhibits high internal consistency, a single-factor structure, and good to excellent inter-rater reliability among trained and experienced psychiatrists or clinical psychologists (Parnas and Henriksen 2014; Sass 2014). A companion to the EASE, called the EAWE (Examination of Anomalous *World* Experiences) and focusing on experiences of time, space, other persons, language, and general atmosphere is under preparation by Louis Sass, Elizabeth Pienkos, and others and should be published in the relatively near future.

New Approach to the Psychotherapy of Schizophrenia Psychological therapies are often integrated in the treatment of schizophrenia, along with medication. One might argue that an informed phenomenological psychotherapy, focusing on the person, should sometimes be the first line of approach, together with medication as deemed advisable (Pérez-Álvarez and García-Montes 2012; Pérez-Álvarez et al. 2011).

If schizophrenia is understood as a disorder of the I or core self, it is not unreasonable to think that important therapeutic work could take place in the lived space of a first- and second-person therapeutic relationship (Fuchs 2007; Stanghellini and Lysaker 2007). Though akin in important respects with other therapies, phenomenologically informed psychotherapy has (at least) two distinctive characteristics, pertaining to (1) the lived, intersubjective space of the therapeutic relationship and (2) the understanding of experiences in a biographical context.

With regard to intersubjectivity space, we would recall the four principles pointed out in an article on psychotherapy of schizophrenia by Stanghellini and Lysaker (2007):

1. Highlighting disturbances of intersubjectivity as a *core feature* of schizophrenia, *not* an epiphenomenon
2. Aiming at achievement of a shared partnership as a way to reestablish a first perspective of one's self—to reappropriate one's own experiences
3. Focusing on the here-and-now, I-and-thou relationship and using this as a "dialogical prosthesis" to help reestablish lost connections between feelings and interpersonal situations
4. Aiming to achieve a shared sense of meaningfulness refers to co-constructing narratives that are not only internally coherent but also reasonably commensurate with standard narrative structures and able to be grasped and accepted by other, sympathetic individuals

Achieving an understanding of anomalous experiences requires, among other things, a retracing of "the psychological/existential contexts in which [the patient's] abnormal experiences were generated (remote life history) and/or are aggravated (recent pathogenic situations)" (Doerr-Zegers and Stanghellini 2013, p. 232). This biographical contextualization—connecting symptoms and life experiences—not only provides *insight* but serves to *reappropriate* the experiences themselves, by making them seem less "strange," alienated, and existentially disconcerting. This sort of reframing or reconstruction of psychotic experiences may be a better therapeutic goal than focusing mainly on reducing "positive" symptoms (Irarrázaval and Sharim 2014; Vallina-Fernández et al. 2014).

A phenomenologically oriented psychotherapy would seem to have more affinity with recently developed contextual therapies referred to as "third wave" than with *traditional* cognitive behavioral therapy (the "second wave" of the behavioral tradition). Traditional cognitive behavioral therapy concentrates on reducing symptoms, as in medicine; but, paradoxically, it may actually contribute to an exacerbation of hyperreflexivity through its focusing on the abnormal *contents* of abnormal experiences such as delusions (Skodlar et al. 2013). By contrast, contextual therapies try to diminish hyperreflexivity and associated alienation from action and experience by promoting immersion in activities significant to the person, thereby fostering a sense of self-presence (Pérez-Álvarez et al. 2008). One patient described these activities as helping him to "forget" about himself. We understand this to refer to a forgetting of the self as an *objective focus* of awareness, thereby allowing the more foundational sense of oneself as a *subjective perspective* on the world to feel more grounded (Nelson and Sass 2009, p. 499).

We argue, then, that a phenomenological, person-centered orientation provides the most appropriate psychotherapeutic approach for the disorder of self-experience that seems to be at the core of schizophrenia. This is of particular importance in the context of recent studies of therapeutic outcome, which suggest that psychological approaches, appropriately conducted, may be both more effective and less costly than relying on mediation alone (Calton and Spandler 2009; Gumley and Clark 2012; Harrow et al. 2014; Morrison et al. 2012; Pérez-Álvarez and García-Montes 2012).

References

Akroyd, M. J. (2013). You can't spell schizophrenia without an 'I': How does the Early Intervention in Psychosis approach relate to the concept of schizophrenia as an ipseity disturbance? *Early Intervention in Psychiatry, 7*, 238–246.

Bentall, R. P., de Sousa, P., Varese, F., Wickham, S., Sitko, K., Haarmans, M., et al. (2014). From adversity to psychosis: Pathways and mechanisms from specific adversities to specific symptoms. *Social Psychiatry and Psychiatric Epidemiology, 49*, 1011–1022.

Blankenburg, W. (1971/2014). *La pérdida de la evidencia natural. Una contribución a la psicopatología de la esquizofrenia.* Santiago de Chile: Edicionnes de la Universidad Diego Portales.

Bracken, P. (2014). Towards a hermeneutic shift in psychiatry. *World Psychiatry, 13*, 241–243.

Bracken, P., Thomas, P., Timimi, S., Asen, E., Behr, G., Beuster, C., et al. (2012). Psychiatry beyond the current paradigm. *British Journal of Psychiatry, 201*, 430–434.

Calton, T., & Spandler, H. (2009). Minimal-medication approaches to treating schizophrenia. *Advances in Psychiatric Treatment, 15*, 209–217.

Doerr-Zegers, O., & Stanghellini, G. (2013). Clinical phenomenology and its psychotherapeutic consequences. *Journal of Psychopathology, 19*, 228–233.

Ellenberger, H. F. (1957/1967). Introducción clínica a la fenomenología psiquiátrica y al análisis existencial [Clinical introduction to psychiatric phenomenology and existential analysis]. In R. May & H. H. Ellenberger (Eds.), *Existencia* [*Existence*] (pp. 123–160). Madrid: Gredos.

Fuchs, T. (2007). Psychotherapy of the lived space. A phenomenological and ecological concept. *American Journal of Psychotherapy, 61*, 432–439.

Fuchs, T. (2010). Subjectivity and intersubjectivity in psychiatric diagnosis. *Psychopathology, 43*, 268–274.

Gumley, A., & Clark, S. (2012). Risk of arrested recovery following first episode psychosis: An integrative approach to psychotherapy. *Journal of Psychotherapy Integration, 22*, 298–313.

Harrow, M., Jobe, T. H., & Faull, R. N. (2014). Does treatment of schizophrenia with antipsychotic medications eliminate or reduce psychosis? A 20-year multi-follow-up study. *Psychological Medicine, 44*, 3007–3116.

Hirjak, D., Breyer, T., Thomann, P. A., & Fuchs, T. (2013). Disturbance of intentionality: A phenomenological study of body-affecting first-rank symptoms in schizophrenia. *PLoS One, 8*(9), e73662.

Hur, J.-W., Kwon, J. S., Lee, T. Y., & Park, S. (2014). The crisis of minimal self-awareness in schizophrenia: A meta-analytic review. *Schizophrenia Research, 152*, 58–64.

Irarrázaval, L., & Sharim, D. (2014). Intersubjectivity in schizophrenia: Life story analysis of three cases. *Frontiers in Psychology, 5*. doi:10.3389/fpsyg.2014.00100.

Kean, C. (2009). Silencing the self: Schizophrenia as a self-disturbance. *Schizophrenia Bulletin, 35*, 1034–1036.

Kraus, A. (2007). Schizophrenic delusions and hallucinations as the expression and consequence of an alteration of the existential a prioris. In M. C. Chung, K. W. M. Fulford, & G. Graham (Eds.), *Reconceiving schizophrenia* (pp. 97–111). Oxford: Oxford University Press.

Maj, M. (2014). Technical and non-technical aspects of psychiatric care: The need for a balanced view. *World Psychiatry, 13*, 209–210.

Morrison, A. P., Hutton, P., Shiers, D., & Turkington, D. (2012). Antipsychotics: Is it time to introduce patient choice? *British Journal of Psychiatry, 201*, 83–84.

Nelson, B., Parnas, J., & Sass, L. A. (2014). Disturbance of minimal self (ipseity) in schizophrenia: Clarification and current status [Editorial]. *Schizophrenia Bulletin, 40*, 479–482.

Nelson, B., & Sass, L. A. (2009). Medusa's stare: A case study of working with self-disturbance in the early phase of schizophrenia. *Clinical Case Studies, 8*, 489–504.

Nelson, B., Sass, L. A., Thompson, A., Yung, A. R., Francey, S. M., Amminger, G. P., et al. (2009). Does disturbance of self underlie social cognition deficits in schizophrenia and other psychotic disorders? *Early Intervention of Psychiatry, 3*, 83–93.

Nelson, B., Yung, A., Bechdolf, A., & McGorry, P. D. (2008). The phenomenological critique and self-disturbance: Implications for ultra-high-risk ("prodromal") research. *Schizophrenia Bulletin, 34*, 381–392.

Parnas, J. (2012a). The core gestalt of schizophrenia. *World Psychiatry, 11*, 67–69.

Parnas, J. (2012b). DSM-IV and the founding prototype of schizophrenia: Are we regressing to a pre-Kraepelinian nosology? In K. S. Kendler & J. Parnas (Eds.), *Philosophical issues in psychology II: Nosology* (pp. 237–259). Oxford: Oxford University Press.

Parnas, J., & Henriksen, M. G. (2014). Disordered self in the schizophrenia spectrum: A clinical and research perspective. *Harvard Review of Psychiatry, 22*, 251–265.

Parnas, J., Moller, P., Kircher, T., Thalbitzer, J., Jansson, L., Handest, P., et al. (2005). EASE: Examination of anomalous self-experience. *Psychopathology, 38*, 236–258.

Pérez-Álvarez, M., & García-Montes, J. M. (2012). From neurochemistry to interpersonal chemistry: Towards a psychotherapy of schizophrenia. In A. J. Lancaster & O. Sharpe (Eds.), *Psychotherapy: New research* (pp. 1–21). New York: Nova.

Pérez-Álvarez, M., García-Montes, J. M., Perona-Garcelán, S., & Vallina-Fernández, O. (2008). Changing relationship with voices: New therapeutic perspectives for treating hallucinations. *Clinical Psychology and Psychotherapy, 15*, 75–85.

Pérez-Álvarez, M., García-Montes, J. M., Vallina-Fernández, O., Perona-Garcelán, S., & Cuevas-Yust, C. (2011). New life for psychotherapy in the light of phenomenology. *Clinical Psychology and Psychotherapy, 18*, 187–201.

Perona-Garcelán, S., García-Montes, J. M., Rodríguez-Testal, J. F., López-Jiménez, A. M., Ruiz-Veguilla, M., Ductor-Recuerda, M. J., et al. (2014). Relationship between childhood trauma, mindfulness and dissociation in subjects with and without hallucination proneness. *Journal of Trauma and Dissociation, 15*, 35–51.

Pienkos, E., & Sass, L. (2012). Empathy and otherness: Humanistic and phenomenological approaches to psychotherapy of severe mental illness. *Pragmatic Case Studies in Psychotherapy, 8*, 25–35.

Ratcliffe, M. (2012). Phenomenology as a form of empathy. *Inquire, 55*, 473–495.

Read, J., van Os, J., Morrison, A. P., & Ross, C. A. (2005). Childhood trauma, psychosis and schizophrenia: A literature review with theoretical and clinical implications. *Acta Psychiatrica Scandinavica, 112*, 330–350.

Ricoeur, P. (1992). *Oneself as another*. Chicago: The University of Chicago Press.

Rojcewick, S. J., & Rojcewick, R. (1997). The 'human' voices in hallucinations. *Journal of Phenomenological Psychology, 28*, 1–41.

Saks, E. (2007). *The center cannot hold*. New York: Hyperion.

Sass, L. A. (1988). Humanism, hermeneutics, and the concept of human subject. In S. B. Messer, L. A. Sass, & R. L. Woolfolk (Eds.), *Hermeneutics and psychological theory* (pp. 222–271). New Brunswick, NJ: Rutgers University Press.

Sass, L. (1992). *Madness and modernism: Insanity in the light of modern art, literature, and thought*. New York: Basic Books. [Spanish translation: Sass, L. (1992/2014). *Locura y modernismo. La esquizofrenia a la luz del arte, la literatura y el pensamiento modernos*. Madrid: Dykinson.]

Sass, L. A. (2004). Schizophrenia: A disturbance of the thematic field. In L. Embree (Ed.), *Gurwitch's relevancy for the cognitive sciences* (pp. 59–78). Dordrecht: Springer.

Sass, L. (2013). Jaspers, phenomenology, and the 'ontological difference'. In G. Stanghellini & T. Fuchs (Eds.), *One century of Kal Jaspers' general psychopathology* (pp. 95–106). Oxford: Oxford University Press.

Sass, L. (2014). Self-disturbance and schizophrenia: Structure, specificity, pathogenesis (current issues, new directions). *Schizophrenia Research, 152*, 5–11.

Sass, L., & Parnas, J. (2003). Schizophrenia, consciousness, and the self. *Schizophrenia Bulletin, 29*, 427–444.

Sass, L. A., & Parnas, J. (2007). Explaining schizophrenia: The relevance of phenomenology. In M. Chung, W. Fulford, & G. Graham (Eds.), *Reconceiving schizophrenia* (pp. 63–96). Oxford: Oxford University Press.

Sass, L., Pienkos, E., & Nelson, B. (2013a). Introspection and schizophrenia: A comparative investigation of anomalous self experiences. *Consciousness and Cognition, 22*, 853–867.

Sass, L., Pienkos, E., Nelson, B., & Medford, N. (2013b). Anomalous self-experience in depersonalization and schizophrenia: A comparative investigation. *Consciousness and Cognition, 22*, 430–441.

Schwartz, W. E. (2013). Schizophrenia, cultural marginalization, and dissociation of the body: An application of Ernest Becker's work to psychotherapy. *Psychosis, 5*, 26–35.

Schwartz, M. A., & Wiggins, O. P. (1987). Typifications. The first step for clinical diagnosis in psychiatry. *Journal of Nervous and Mental Disorders, 175*, 65–77.

Skodlar, B., Henriksen, M. G., Sass, L. A., Nelson, B., & Parnas, J. (2013). Cognitive-behavioral therapy for schizophrenia: A critical evaluation of its theoretical framework from a clinical-phenomenological perspective. *Psychopathology, 46*, 249–265.

Stanghellini, J. (2004). *Disembodied spirits and deanimated bodies. The psychopathology of common sense*. Oxford: Oxford University Press.

Stanghellini, G. (2008). Qualitative analysis. Its use in psychopathological research. *Acta Psychiatrica Scandinavica, 117*, 161–163.

Stanghellini, G. (2011). Phenomenological psychopathology, profundity, and schizophrenia. *Philosophy, Psychiatry and Psychology, 18*, 163–166.

Stanghellini, J., & Cutting, J. (2003). Auditory verbal hallucinations—breaking the silence of inner dialogue. *Psychopathology, 36*, 120–128.

Stanghellini, G., & Lysaker, P. H. (2007). The psychotherapy of schizophrenia through the lens of phenomenology: Intersubjectivity and the search for the recovery of first- and second-person awareness. *American Journal of Psychotherapy, 61*, 163–179.

Vallina-Fernández, O., Pérez-Álvarez, M., Fernández-Iglesias, P., Soto-Balbuena, C., Perona-Garcelán, S., & García-Montes, J. M. (2014). Person-based contextual therapy applied to a complex case of schizophrenia. *Psicothema, 26*, 299–307.

Velikonja, T., Fisher, H. L., Mason, O., & Johnson, S. (2015). Childhood trauma and schizotypy: A systematic review. *Psychological Medicine, 45*(5), 947–963. doi:10.1017/S0033291714002086.

Catatonia—Phenomenology, Psychopathology, and Pathophysiology

18

Georg Northoff

Case History

The 27-year-old was admitted to the hospital suddenly in the middle of the night after being found on a park bench, immobile. She did not move or speak a word, and, most bizarrely, she kept her arms in an upright position, defying gravity in a strange posture that should have been exhausting after ten minutes. It wasn't for her, though. When questioned about her whereabouts, she remained silent.

In the hospital emergency room, the doctor in charge did various blood tests but could not find any abnormalities, nor could he detect any sign of neurological disorders with lesions in the brain, like a tumor. The information came through that the patient had been missing for several days. The patient's father arrived and reported that she had been making some strange utterances before she disappeared. The patient had been preparing for her final examination at university, where she was studying biology. As the exam approached, she became more afraid and anxious. Her father had noticed that his daughter appeared depressed; she looked very sad, could not sleep, barely ate, and secluded and detached herself from the usually close and intense family life.

He noticed that his daughter was referring more and more to strange thoughts: she began to say she was unworthy of taking the exam and of becoming a biologist and that she would only bring disaster upon mankind if she proceeded. In fact, she began to think the world would come to an end if she became a biologist and that she would be left to face a tribunal that would condemn her to burn in hell.

The father also noticed that his daughter's speech had become more robot-like before she stopped speaking at all, just before her disappearance. Her movements, too, became more and more sparse and she began to sit in strange postures for hours

G. Northoff (✉)
Mind, Brain Imaging and Neuroethics, University of Ottawa Institute of Mental Health Research, Ottawa, ON, Canada
e-mail: Georg.Northoff@theroyal.ca; georg.northoff@rohcg.on.ca

G. Stanghellini, M. Aragona (eds.), *An Experiential Approach to Psychopathology*,
DOI 10.1007/978-3-319-29945-7_18

in her room, like a fencing position with outstretched arms. She did not respond when he asked what she was doing, and just when he had decided to take her to the hospital, she disappeared. That is when he called the police who, after some hours, got back to him to say that she had been found and admitted to the hospital.

The doctor in charge could not detect any medical or neurological abnormality. He did not know what to do. The state of the patient did not change at all. She was still in the same posture: outstretched arms, wide-open eyes, and an anxious expression. She remained completely mute. The doctor was well trained in internal medicine as well as in neurology. He had worked for years in the emergency room and had seen all kinds of patients. But he had never seen anything as bizarre as this. He called his superior, who was also stumped. "The only thing you can do," he said, "is to call the psychiatrist. When it becomes too bizarre and strange for us, it is usually his territory."

But the psychiatrist, a young resident in his second year, also had no idea what to do with the patient. He did, however, notice some typical psychiatric symptoms. When the patient's father told him about her social withdrawal, her feelings of guilt and unworthiness, and her lack of appetite, the psychiatrist thought of depression that the patient could be suffering from a first episode of depression or a major depressive disorder. Her thoughts about the tribunal and burning in hell, as well as other ideas about saving the world from global warming, were more typical of schizophrenic delusions though, he thought. And the most bizarre of all was the continuous posturing and the complete lack of speaking. He had never seen anything like that, and, to his knowledge, it had never been discussed in his hospital during his time there. So he called his own superior, an older and more experienced clinician nearing retirement whom the resident referred to as "the walking psychiatric encyclopedia."

"That is a really interesting case," the senior psychiatrist said after examining the patient herself. She recognized it as a typical case of catatonia. "When I was as young as you," she told the resident, "in my first and second year of residence, I saw several patients like her but they disappeared and were forgotten. The lack of speech is called mutism or stupor, the bizarre positioning of the extremities is a typical case of posturing or catalepsy, and the muscle tone is low, hypotonic, rather than being rigid and hypertonic, as one would expect."

The senior psychiatrist prescribed an injection of benzodiazepines, like lorazepam, to which the patient could respond within five minutes, she said.

Sure enough, five minutes after the resident followed his superior's instruction, the patient lost her position and posturing; five minutes after that she even started talking. "What a wonder," the young psychiatrist thought when he brought the patient to her father, who was visibly relieved to see his daughter back in a "normal" state.

What did the patient say? She said she was extremely anxious and afraid of the tribunal that she was sure she would bring down the world and mankind and that she would not save it from global warming, which had been the focus of her studies. Various people conveyed this message to her simply by looking at her. Taking the exam and passing, she said, would mean the end of the world. Voices had told that she was in charge of the universe and that responsibility for the world rested with her. She could not escape this burden, which caused her crippling anxiety.

It had all started eight weeks ago when her long-term boyfriend, whom she had intended to marry, suddenly terminated their relationship, sending her into an extreme state of depression. She was very sad, lost her appetite, and locked herself in her room. When asked why she did not move and speak at all in the last days, she was surprised: "Did I not move? Did I not speak? I could have spoken and moved any time, it is just that I was afraid of losing control completely, which would have further aggravated my anxieties."

During subsequent examinations and reports, she still looked anxious, and both her speech and movements began to decline again, becoming more and more sparse until she again receded into the state, catatonia, she had displayed when admitted. The young doctor gave her another shot of lorazepam: "If it helps once why not twice?" he thought. And indeed the injection allowed the patient to retreat again from the catatonic state. She was prescribed lorazepam twice per day, and she also received antidepressant and antipsychotic medication for her depressed and psychotic symptoms.

18.1 What Is Catatonia and How Can We Treat It?

Catatonia was described for the first time by the German psychiatrist Karl Ludwig Kahlbaum (1874). He described various cases like ours and others that all share the absence of speaking, called mutism or stupor, and the bizarre positioning of limbs, described as posturing or catalepsy. In addition, he described several other bizarre behavioral signs. For instance, some patients show too much movement rather than no movement, which is called hyperkinesia. Some patients might also perform the same movement over and over again; this is described as stereotypy. The most bizarre is that some patients show the tendency to do and perform exactly what another person does, mitmachen and mitgehen. I had one patient who, after recovering from his acute mutistic and posturing state, followed me and wanted to do exactly what I did: when I went to the other end of the clinic, he followed me; when I raised my hands and wrote something down (like his notes), he did the same. Most bizarre, he did that only with me, not with other people or nurses. He apparently developed a special relationship with me, probably because he knew me from previous admissions [see also Northoff (1997, 2002a, b) for an overview].

Besides the motor and behavioral symptoms, Kahlbaum also described strong emotional or affective abnormalities. Catatonic symptoms can be associated with depressed affect as it was in the case of our patient. But patients can also show the opposite, a manic or abnormally elated mood, rather than a depressed one. For instance, I recall one patient who became catatonic every time she fell in love with somebody. I saw her five times over a period of 5 years. Each time she came into the hospital in an acute catatonic state with posturing and mutism/stupor occurring over 3–4 days prior to admission. All five times she had met a novel person whom she fell in love with and was elated and excited and finally in a happy mood, which was then followed by the relatively rapid onset of catatonic symptoms. Needless to say, the manifestation of being in love in terms of catatonic symptoms did not help her developing a long-lasting and stable relationship.

Finally, besides motor, behavioral, and affective symptoms, catatonic patients can also show vegetative symptoms like fever. Sometimes these high fevers can lead to the subsequent disintegration of the patient's metabolism, which can ultimately result in death. This form of catatonia has been called "lethal or febrile catatonia" by the German psychiatrist Stauder (1934). At that time, in the first part of the twentieth century, there was not any drug treatment available in psychiatry. Now the situation has changed. Patients with schizophrenia receive what is called "neuroleptics," while patients with depression can be treated with antidepressants like Prozac that target a specific metabolite in the brain, serotonin (Fink 2013).

The neuroleptics can cause stiffness of the body leaving the patients unable to move, which is referred to as akinesia. Neuroleptics can also cause fever. This combination of a lack of movements and fever is called neuroleptic malignant syndrome (NMS) (Caroff 1980; Northoff 1996, 2002a; Fink 2013). Its symptoms overlap with those of febrile catatonia, which also shows fever and lack of movements, i.e., akinesia. This presents the psychiatrist with a dilemma. Febrile catatonia is often associated with strong psychotic symptoms like delusions and hallucinations. Though there was no fever, this was also the case with our patient who exhibited delusions like having to rescue the earth from global warming and the tribunal and who also suffered from hallucinations when hearing voices giving instructions.

These symptoms, delusions, and hallucinations are usually treated with neuroleptics. The very same drugs can lead to akinesia, though, as manifest in NMS. The psychiatrist is then confronted with the question of what comes first and what causes what: are the motor abnormalities caused by the catatonia itself or by the neuroleptics—is this a case of catatonia or NMS? If one treats the symptoms with neuroleptics suspecting catatonia, one would expect remedy and therapeutic effects; however, if the symptoms are due to NMS rather than catatonia, the neuroleptics may make things worse and further aggravate the NMS and its ultimate life-threatening fever (Northoff 1996, 2002a). In other terms, by applying neuroleptics to a case of NMS while suspecting catatonia, the psychiatrist may aggravate the already existing symptoms and, in the worst of all possible cases, cause the death of the patient.

The psychiatrist's dilemma is clear (Northoff 1996, 2010): if he gives neuroleptics, he has to be sure to exclude NMS and to really target delusions and hallucinations that may underlie a catatonic picture. If the motor symptoms are due to catatonia and especially febrile catatonia with underlying delusions and hallucinations rather than NMS, immediate treatment with neuroleptics is necessary to avoid the patient's death. But if the motor symptoms are due to NMS rather than catatonia, he may cause harm. Further complicating matters, the very same patient may develop NMS in response to the neuroleptics, again aggravating the risk of death.

What can we do in the case of fever in either febrile catatonia or NMS? In both instances, the occurrence of fever can be life-threatening and needs to be treated right away. Lorazepam will not help here as it only relieves the acute motor and affective symptoms for some hours but not the underlying cause and the vegetative symptoms. We recall, for instance, that our patient showed some relief of catatonic symptoms for 3–4 h, with gradual reoccurrence of the very same symptoms.

How, then, was our patient treated? Fortunately, she did not develop any fever or other vegetative signs. Due to her depressed symptoms, she received an antidepressant, while her delusions and hallucinations were treated with neuroleptics. That led to gradual recovery over 3 months. She normalized completely and was able to take her exam, which she passed. This is one of the good outcomes. Other outcomes might be more difficult. Patients with fever or febrile catatonia often require electroconvulsive therapy (ECT) where seizures are induced by applying some electric current to the brain. Though it sounds harsh and is usually the last choice, ECT proves quite beneficial in both febrile catatonia and NMS (Northoff 1996, 2002a, 2010; Fink 2013).

18.2 Origin of Catatonia

Where does catatonia come from? Kahlbaum (1874) originally described catatonia as a disease by itself. Catatonia in this sense is like diabetes, a separate disease with its own symptoms and causes. However, others did not agree. German psychiatrists at the beginning of the twentieth century like Emil Kraepelin (1887) and Eugen Bleuler (1911) associated catatonia with schizophrenia. Catatonia, for them, is just a subform of schizophrenia called catatonia schizophrenia, as distinguished from other subforms like paranoid or disorganized schizophrenia. This would mean catatonia is not a disease by itself but a special form of schizophrenia (see Northoff 2002b).

This association of catatonia with schizophrenia is the predominant view of catatonia in our times. This is the case despite the fact that catatonia can also be associated with depression or mania as described above. Severely depressed patients can develop catatonic symptoms and full-blown catatonia even if they do not show delusions and hallucinations, as in schizophrenia. The same applies to patients with mania who show abnormal excitement and happiness, as was the case with the patient who developed catatonia each time she fell in love.

Further complicating matters is the fact that catatonia and its various symptoms can also be associated with various other disorders (Northoff et al. 1996; Northoff 1997, 2002b). Autism can show strong catatonic symptoms, and various neurological and medical disorders can also result in a catatonic picture. Taken in this sense, catatonia is like a fever that can also occur in association with various other underlying disorders. In the same way that various medical and neurological disorders can lead to fever, different kinds of neurological, medical, and psychiatric diseases can result in catatonia. Why and how? We currently do not know.

We also do not know whether catatonia is a separate disorder by itself or just a specific manifestation of another one, like schizophrenia. Resolution of this question is further complicated by the fact that nowadays catatonia is extremely rare. As we saw by the young psychiatrist's confusion in the case study, there are almost no cases of catatonia today, at least in developed countries. Only the older psychiatrist recalled having seen such cases. The reasons for such decline in catatonia are unclear. Many people argue that the introduction of novel drugs like antidepressants and neuroleptics prevented both depression and schizophrenia from going all the way to their final extreme, a catatonic picture [see Northoff (1997) and Fink (2013) for overviews]. Treatment with the drug may thus preempt catatonia.

However, others argue that the disease of catatonia has simply disappeared [Northoff (1997) and Fink (2013) for an overview and history]. As strange as it sounds, psychiatric diseases come and go, depending strongly upon the respective social context. For instance, before being thin became a beauty ideal for women in the middle of the twentieth century in the western countries, spurred by advertising, there were basically no cases of eating disorders. Eating disorders concern obesity and also the opposite, extreme slimness as in anorexia nervosa. The opposite may have happened in the case of catatonia. Some yet unknown change in context may have led to catatonia's disappearance. The exact reasons remain unclear though.

18.3 Catatonia in the Brain

What happens in the brain while the patients no longer speak and move? Obviously, it is rather difficult to investigate catatonia in brain scanning such as fMRI. One cannot scan a patient who does not show any response and postures in bizarre positions. For that reason, we scanned catatonic patients after their acute catatonic symptoms and compared them with depressed and schizophrenic patients who did not show catatonic symptoms but exhibited otherwise similar symptoms, e.g., depression, delusions, or hallucinations.

What did we see in the brains of catatonic patients? We observed that regions involved in emotional processing are strongly abnormal (Northoff et al. 2004; Northoff 2000); these concerned the midline structure, like the perigenual anterior cingulate cortex (PACC) and ventromedial prefrontal cortex (VMPFC). They process emotions and their association with our sense of self. And they also connect both emotions and self to movement and action by their connections to the motor cortex. Our study demonstrated that this connection between PACC/VMPFC and motor cortex was abnormally weak in catatonia patients. They can apparently no longer connect emotions/self with their movements and actions; this mirrors well the subjective experience described in our patients (Northoff et al. 1996, 2004).

Many catatonic patients report afterward that they feel overwhelmed by the intensity of their emotions, whether positive or negative, and that they, their self, can no longer control them (Northoff et al. 1996). Hence, in order to exert some kind of control, they then shut down any movement and action. Standing still and not speaking may be the best defense and reaction against overwhelming emotions and loss of control. Taken in this sense, catatonia may be considered the ultimate defensive reaction, the supergau, the last resort, before everything breaks down and disintegrates (Northoff et al. 2007). One patient, for instance, told me afterward that standing still, not moving, and not speaking gave her at least some relief from the torturing emotions, thoughts, and hallucinations.

Why though does lorazepam show such dramatic effects? We recall in our patient as described above that lorazepam led to almost immediate relief from catatonic symptoms within 5–10 min. Lorazepam acts on a particular metabolite in the brain, GABA, that strengthens and increases inhibition of neural activity. It seems that such inhibition is desperately needed in catatonia since the patient is hyper-excited internally; this transforms into the opposite externally, with catatonia as hypo-excitation (Northoff et al. 1999).

Isn't it strange how the brain can do that? We investigated GABA and its special opening doors, receptors, in the brains of catatonic patients. Indeed, we observed that their number of the so-called GABA-A receptors is much lower and abnormally decreased, especially in PACC and VMPFC (Northoff et al. 1999). There is thus not enough neural inhibition in these regions, which in turn transforms into the abnormally intense experience of positive or negative emotions. How, then, to control and contain the abnormal intensity of these emotions? "The only way to do that," so the brain may say, "is to cut down my connections from PACC/VMPFC to motor cortex. Whether that results in catatonia, as the psychiatrists call it, I do not care, as long as it somehow stabilizes me, the brain, to some degree." Accordingly, catatonia may result from some secondary or compensatory neural mechanisms by means of which it aims to maintain its balance and stability (Northoff 2000, 2002b).

18.4 What Can Catatonia Tell Us About the Brain and Mind?

Catatonia is an extreme state for patients and their brains. The patients experience abnormally intense emotional feelings that they can no longer control with their own self (Northoff et al. 1996). The only way they feel they can have any control is by shutting down completely and avoiding speaking and moving. This results in mutism/stupor and posturing/catalepsy. The brain seems to suffer from abnormally strong excitation with lack of neural inhibition in anterior midline regions like the VMPFC and PACC. That in turn shuts down these regions' connections to the motor cortex and hence to movements.

What can catatonia tell us about the brain? Many of the symptoms we see in psychiatry may not result from primary deficits but may rather be related to secondary and tertiary compensatory mechanisms that aim to stabilize both the brain and the self. This means that the brain is a complex organ that seems to have a variety of different response strategies it can utilize to reply to extreme situations. In order to understand psychiatric symptoms and the brain itself, we need to reveal these various mechanisms and their respective loops. In short, we need to understand the different layers of the brain's neural organization.

That leads us back to the brain itself and its resting state's virtual spatiotemporal structure (Northoff 2014a, b). The different layers of compensatory mechanisms may correspond to different levels or layers of spatiotemporal organization. The ultimate and final level of such spatiotemporal organization consists in stopping time and space altogether, as manifested in the catatonic symptoms. When nothing moves and one does not speak, there is no flow of time anymore, and one can stop time and the changes it imposes upon the respective person and its brain. Catatonic patients can teach us that it is necessary to stop time in at least a mental sense in order to compensate for a too-high intensity of emotions.

What can catatonia tell us about the mind (Northoff 2014b, c)? Catatonia can be regarded as a psychomotor syndrome where psychological or mental changes, felt as abnormally intense emotional feelings, are transformed into body movements and actions (or lack thereof). Mind and body are here closely linked to each other in an almost indistinguishable way. One could even say there is no distinction between the brain and mind anymore, as psychological/mental symptoms are bodily/motor symptoms and vice versa. The distinction between psychological/mental and bodily/motor symptoms is consecutively artificial and more related to us as psychiatrists and investigators than to the brain itself.

Imagine a brain would participate in a discussion about the mind-brain problem between a philosopher and neuroscientist. The brain would probably say that any distinction between the brain and mind is artificial, an illusory figment of our imagination rather than reality itself. One cannot be separated from the other: the brain is not as brainy as we often think, while conversely, the mind is not as mental as we usually assume.

References

Bleuler, E. (1911). *Dementia praecox or the group o schizophrenias* (J. Zinkin, Trans.). New York: International Universities Press, 1950.

Caroff, S. N. (1980). The neuroleptic malignant syndrome. *Journal of Clinical Psychiatry, 41*(3), 79–83.

Fink, M. (2013). Rediscovering catatonia: The biography of a treatable syndrome. *Acta Psychiatrica Scandinavica. Supplementum, 127*(441), 1–47. doi:10.1111/acps.12038.

Kahlbaum, K. (1874). *Die Katatonie oder das Spannungsirresein: Eine klinische Form psychishcer krankheit*. Berlin: Hirshwald. [Translated: Y. Levy & T. Pridon (Trans.). (1973). *Catatonia*. Baltimore: Johns Hopkins Press.]

Krapelin, E. (1887). *Psychiatrie: Ein kurzes Lehrbuch fuer Studierende und Aerzte* (2nd ed.). Leipzig: Ambr Abel.

Northoff, G. (1996). Neuroleptic malignant syndrome and catatonia: One entity or two? *Biological Psychiatry, 40*(5), 431–433.

Northoff, G. (1997). *Katatonie: Einführung in die Phänomenologie, Klinik und Pathophysiologie eines psychomotorischen Syndroms* [Catatonia: Introduction into the phenomenology, clinic, and pathophysiology of a psychomotor syndrome]. Stuttgart: Ferdinand Enke Verlag.

Northoff, G. (2000). Brain imaging in catatonia: Current findings and a pathophysiologic model. *CNS Spectrums, 5*(7), 34–46.

Northoff, G. (2002a). Catatonia and neuroleptic malignant syndrome: Psychopathology and pathophysiology. *Journal of Neural Transmission, 109*(12), 1453–1467. Review.

Northoff, G. (2002b). What catatonia can tell us about "top-down modulation": A neuropsychiatric hypothesis. *Behavioral and Brain Sciences, 25*(5), 555–577. Discussion 578–604. Review.
Northoff, G. (2010). Options for the treatment of febrile catatonia. *Journal of Psychiatry and Neuroscience, 35*(4), E5–E6. No abstract available.
Northoff, G. (2014a). *Unlocking the brain* (Coding, Vol. I). New York: Oxford University Press.
Northoff, G. (2014b). *Unlocking the brain* (Consciousness, Vol. II). New York: Oxford University Press.
Northoff, G. (2014c). *Minding the brain. Introduction to neuroscience & philosophy*. London: Palgrave MacMillan.
Northoff, G., Bermpohl, F., Schoeneich, F., & Boeker, H. (2007). How does our brain constitute defense mechanisms? First-person neuroscience and psychoanalysis. *Psychotheraphy and Psychosomatics, 76*(3), 141–153.
Northoff, G., Kötter, R., Baumgart, F., Danos, P., Boeker, H., Kaulisch, T., et al. (2004). Orbitofrontal cortical dysfunction in akinetic catatonia: A functional magnetic resonance imaging study during negative emotional stimulation. *Schizophrenia Bulletin, 30*(2), 405–427.
Northoff, G., Krill, W., Wenke, J., Travers, H., & Pflug, B. (1996). [The subjective experience in catatonia: Systematic study of 24 catatonic patients]. *Psychiatrische Praxis, 23*(2), 69–73.
Northoff, G., Steinke, R., Czcervenka, C., Krause, R., Ulrich, S., Danos, P., et al. (1999). Decreased density of GABA-A receptors in the left sensorimotor cortex in akinetic catatonia: Investigation of in vivo benzodiazepine receptor binding. *Journal of Neurology, Neurosurgery, and Psychiatry, 67*(4), 445–450.
Richter, A., Grimm, S., & Northoff, G. (2010). Lorazepam modulates orbitofrontal signal changes during emotional processing in catatonia. *Human Psychopharmacology, 25*(1), 55–62. doi:10.1002/hup.1084.
Stauder, K. H. (1934). Die toedliche Katatonie. *Archiv für Psychiatrie und Nervenkrankheiten, 102*, 614–634.

Painful Affect in the Experience and Treatment of Schizophrenia

19

Jay A. Hamm and Paul H. Lysaker

19.1 Introduction

Attending to distressing affective experience has been identified as an important element of a range of approaches to psychotherapy for schizophrenia, including such disparate models as psychodynamic (e.g., Harder and Folke 2012) and cognitive-behavioral therapies (Kingdon and Turkington 2005). Consistent with this are a wide range of theoretical and empirical accounts of emotional experience in schizophrenia (e.g., Sullivan 1927; Kring 1999; Ciompi 1988). Meanwhile, although phenomenology has produced rich accounts of self-experience and the "lived world" of schizophrenia (Stanghellini 2004; Sass 2001; Parnas 2011), at times these models have focused heavily on alterations of perception and cognition (Postmes et al. 2014), potentially at the cost of recognizing the role of emotional distress in the disorder. As a result, phenomenologically informed approaches to treatment may be at risk of neglecting the importance of addressing the persons' emotional distress in treatment and thereby perpetuating the Kraepelinian tradition demarcating "thought" disorders from the "affective" disorders (Moskowitz and Heim 2013). Others have raised these concerns more broadly, with Gumley and colleagues (2013) cautioning: "The separation of affect from experience and meaning by researchers and service providers fails to recognize how these processes together are central to how we can understand and respond to the needs of individuals with psychosis" (p. 7).

Developing an approach to treatment that incorporates the role of affect in the subjective experience of schizophrenia thus seems necessary if we are to recognize

J.A. Hamm, Psy.D. (✉)
Eskenazi Health, Midtown Community Mental Health, 1700 N Illinois St, Indianapolis, IN 46240, USA
e-mail: jay.a.hamm@gmail.com

P.H. Lysaker, Ph.D.
Richard L. Roudebush VAMC, Indiana University School of Medicine, Indianapolis, IN, USA

G. Stanghellini, M. Aragona (eds.), *An Experiential Approach to Psychopathology*,
DOI 10.1007/978-3-319-29945-7_19

and participate in the common human processes involved when people with schizophrenia seek to make sense of their lives and pursue recovery. Accordingly in this chapter, we will explore affective disturbance in schizophrenia first by describing the experience of one man diagnosed with schizophrenia. Following the case description, we will offer a brief overview of a range of different accounts of affect available in the schizophrenia literature, first revisiting classic psychiatry texts of Kraepelin and Bleuler before turning to a range of contributions within psychodynamic, phenomenological, and empirical findings. Following a review of these contributions, we will explore how integration of these views might enrich understanding and offer important implications for phenomenologically informed clinical practice.

19.2 Part 1: Case Illustration—Babbitt

19.2.1 Background Information

Babbitt is an unmarried 30-year-old African-American male who has been involved in mental health services since approximately age 18. He has no brothers or sisters. His unmarried mother and father separated approximately 3 months before Babbitt was born, with Babbitt subsequently having little to no contact with his father during his childhood. Babbitt was raised by his mother with significant involvement from nearby maternal family members. A shy, self-conscious child, Babbitt reports long-standing feelings of social discomfort and depleted confidence in his appearance and capabilities. Babbitt recalls regular mocking of his appearance by peers and emphasizes a period of time in early adolescence involving steadily increasing teasing, bullying, and harassment at school. In addition to these difficulties, when he was approximately 13 years old, Babbitt received a word from a distant paternal family member that Babbitt's estranged father had died suddenly in an automobile accident.

Despite being bright and a generally strong student, Babbitt started frequently skipping classes, using marijuana, and avoiding social events, eventually withdrawing from school with approximately 1 year remaining. Babbitt had two close friends from childhood and adolescence, but following withdrawal from high school, he gradually grew distant and eventually lost contact with these friends, while increasingly spending his time smoking marijuana by himself. Babbitt notes, subjective experiences at the time characterized by prominent feelings of estrangement, particularly when around others. In terms of his emotional experience, Babbitt recalls this time as a period characterized by volatile and intensely negative affects, most notably anger, embarrassment, depression, and loneliness.

At some point, during this period of his life, Babbitt began hearing voices and soon after started developing unusual beliefs about the possibility of being experimented upon by the government. These beliefs escalated over several months into intense and elaborate fears that he and his mother were targets of secret computer technology which placed their lives in imminent danger. These fears were accompanied by heightened emotional distress and erratic behavior, finally prompting family members to bring Babbitt to the hospital. Babbitt was placed on a psychiatric unit, diagnosed with schizophrenia and given medication.

Following release from the hospital was a period of several years of relatively consistent sedentary behavior. Babbitt continued to hear voices, but was less agitated, and followed up with outpatient psychiatry appointments. He stopped smoking marijuana but spent much of his day watching television and smoking cigarettes. He experienced significant weight gain, received disability benefits, and reports having maintained minimal social contacts while also exhibiting a profound cessation of goal-directed behavior. He describes this period of time as "being a fog."

Several years into this phase, Babbitt requested minor changes to his prescribed atypical antipsychotic and noticed this led to increased energy and motivation, as well as renewed interest in pursuing specific goals. He quit smoking cigarettes, returned to school, and received a high school equivalency degree. He developed a small group of new friends and socialized with them in public settings with some regularity. After establishing some temporary part-time work, he was offered a full-time custodial job working nights. He began to experience significant stress related to the adverse effect his work schedule had on his sleep pattern and was shortly thereafter spurned by a potential romantic interest. Following several unexcused absences from work, Babbitt was terminated from his position. These setbacks were followed by increased experience of hearing voices, as well as Babbitt's decision to discontinue using his prescribed medications. A few weeks of intense confusion and distress led to the return of increased erratic behavior, suspiciousness, and a range of grandiose and referential beliefs. During this period, instances of unpredictable and verbally aggressive behavior with neighbors precipitated an interaction with the police, who took Babbitt to the hospital for a short, involuntary psychiatric hospitalization. During his stay in the hospital, Babbitt was reinstated on antipsychotic medications. He subsequently experienced significant reduction in agitation and stopped endorsing the delusional beliefs he had been openly discussing when he was admitted. Babbitt was discharged and with the help of family and social services was able to secure a small apartment where he lived alone.

19.2.2 Therapy

Babbitt was referred for therapy shortly after this hospital admission. At the outset of therapy, Babbitt described his subjective experience as having an unreal quality, noting feeling detached and depersonalized. He gradually was able to articulate a set of complicated beliefs about the nature of his personal reality as human as well as the reality of his world around him. At times this was articulated as belief that he was no longer entirely human, having been turned into a humanoid robot by the government, as well as that the therapy sessions were actually taking place in some form of alternate computerized reality. At other times, he described the felt sense that secret technology had left him de-animated and inert, but that he occasionally could be reanimated in order to either complete routine behaviors (cleaning his apartment, walking to the clinic, etc.). Babbitt also began to view others as automatons rather than living, polyvalent humans with separate agendas and lives from his own.

Babbitt would often express mild perplexity and indicated that the words he was using were not quite accurate descriptions of his thoughts and beliefs, as though his actual subjective experiences were in some ways elusive, ineffable, and uncanny. His overall behavior was characterized by significant withdrawal. He had completely stopped communicating with the group of friends he had established in the previous years, stopped engaging in other enjoyable activities, and began smoking cigarettes again. He spent much of his time sleeping, blankly watching the television, or engrossed in some type of nonverbal engagement with myriad voices that he heard nearly continuously. He reported that engaging with the voices interfered with pursuit of meaningful activities, but he also expressed a loss of interest in previous pastimes and indicated feeling little motivation to pursue these.

As therapy progressed, Babbitt slowly explored aspects of his personal narrative and over time shared with his therapist the autobiographical material detailed above. Reflecting upon the narrative episodes that formed his personal history was accompanied by the emergence of a range of affects in session. Most prominently, embarrassment, anger, discouragement, and hopelessness were routinely encountered. Often these were transient and tended to recede as Babbitt shifted his focus onto efforts to describe his uncanny experiences, interactions with the voices, and his beliefs about de-animated or otherwise depersonalized view of himself. Babbitt began to acknowledge, though, that when in the consulting room with his therapist, he did not feel as detached or devitalized as he did much of the week while at home.

Babbitt would begin to report frequent vacillations in his explanations of his experiences and difficulties. At times, he would entertain the possibility that the voices, his unusual beliefs, and his withdrawal from social life were indicative of mental illness. At other times, though, Babbitt reported strong skepticism of his diagnosis or the concept of mental illness in general. In these moments, Babbitt would endorse belief that the voices were government agents that were using secret technology to control him and the other automatons surrounding him (including his therapist), who only superficially appeared to be human beings.

19.2.3 Outcome

Despite these frequent vacillations in his view of his dilemmas, Babbitt attended therapy sessions regularly and consistently engaged in reflective dialogue with his therapist. Babbitt began to increasingly demonstrate ability to experience and reflect upon subjective emotional states and to describe aspects of the nature of his relationships with family members. Through this process, he slowly began articulating a more coherent personal narrative which could be shared and understood by both him and his therapist and began expressing ideas about life goals and desires, as well as the perceived barriers to enacting behavior toward these goals. Though continuing to demonstrate an overall diminishment in physical activity and goal-directed behavior, Babbitt became increasingly engaged in sessions and has begun making small behavioral steps toward his goals of improving his living situation, acquiring independent means of transportation, and seeking out involvement in personally meaningful pastimes.

19.3 Part 2: Models of Painful Affect in Schizophrenia

Descriptions of emotional experience of affective disturbance can be found in widely ranging texts investigating the nature and treatment of schizophrenia. Although an exhaustive exploration of this topic is well beyond the scope of the current discussion, below we will provide a brief overview of a range of sources in which painful affect is either emphasized as central, or conversely, argued to be diminished, or absent in schizophrenia.

19.3.1 Classic Psychiatry

Kraepelin's descriptions of dementia praecox strongly influenced views of his time and left a lasting impact on subsequent models of schizophrenia. As mentioned above, Kraepelin has been credited for the tradition in which schizophrenia is seen as a "thought" disorder, distinct from the "affective" psychoses (Moskowitz and Heim 2013). Describing affective abnormalities in dementia praecox, Kraepelin (1919) suggested that "very striking and profound damage occurs as a rule in the emotional life of our patients" (p. 32). Kraepelin characterized these disturbances as "singular indifference to former emotional relations" (p. 33), underlining his point by noting that "The patients have no real joy in life, 'no human feelings'; to them 'nothing matters, everything is the same'; they feel 'no grief and no joy'" (p. 33). Even adopting this strong position regarding decrements in emotional experience, Kraepelin acknowledged a certain presence of affective experience, though argued that this was "mostly shallow and of short duration and essentially independent of external influences" (p. 270).

Largely in contrast to these claims, Eugen Bleuler (1911/1950) argued that affect was instead central to the primary difficulties in schizophrenia, describing what he termed "affectively charged complexes" to be at the heart of the condition. Bleuler's positioning of affect as a core element of schizophrenia was at least partially an attempt to reconcile contemporary biomedical models and insights from the burgeoning field of psychoanalysis. He offered a critique of conventional understandings of schizophrenia that had characterized affective experience in schizophrenia as one of indifference or the absence of affect. Bleuler acknowledged the frequent lack of expressed affect; however, pointing to his own clinical work with hospital patients with schizophrenia, Bleuler argued that the observable diminutions in expressed affect were not reflective of a subjective state devoid of affect, noting that "*There can be no doubt at all that the psyche's capacity to produce affects has not disappeared in schizophrenia*" (Bleuler 1911/1950, p. 47, emphasis original).

Bleuler supported these contentions with numerous clinical examples illustrating the emergence of affect in these patients. Of note, Bleuler explicitly applied his view of affective experience to persons in all phases of the disorder, observing "genuine states of melancholic depression even in schizophrenics [sic] of long standing. These patients may be painfully conscious of their sad situation, their inability to act" (Bleuler 1911/1950, p. 209).

19.3.2 Psychoanalytic and Psychodynamic Models of Affect

Psychoanalysis has offered significant contributions to theoretical models of schizophrenia. Additionally, despite Freud's pessimism about the possibilities of therapy in schizophrenia, a number of subsequent psychoanalytic writings report successful treatments of persons with schizophrenia, and drawing from these, successful interventions offered a number of observations regarding emotional experience. These contributions further developed the views of Bleuler and Freud, and importantly many offered detailed descriptions of the subjective experiences of people with schizophrenia, creating a vibrant but often overlooked phenomenology of schizophrenia.

For instance, Sullivan (1927) proposed a model of schizophrenia in which contrary to views positing a loss of affect, persons with this condition instead experience extraordinary distress, though this emotional pain might be obscured due to its disturbed manner of expression.

Sullivan (1927) supported his clinical observations with findings from early laboratory experiments aimed at measuring indicators of affective experience of persons with schizophrenia. Sullivan concluded: "the alleged indifference, apathy, and emotional disharmony of the schizophrenic [sic] patient is more a matter of impression than a correct evaluation of the inner experience" (p. 482).

Also sensitive to the presence and role of painful affect, Harold Searles offered clinical observations from his work with persons with schizophrenia. Consistent with Bleuler and Sullivan, he argued that the expressions of apparent indifference or loss of affect could instead be viewed as a defense against unbearable emotional pain. Searles viewed this emotional pain as understandable as well as a force that influences manifestations of the disorder or symptoms. As a result, recovery was then seen as involving the development of improved ability to acknowledge and reflect upon these painful states. Illustrating this point, Searles observes of a patient that "as she became more and more able to admit freely into awareness her feelings of hostility, disappointment, and grief, the confusion was less and less in evidence" (Searles 1965, p. 100).

Similar observations of painful affect in schizophrenia are found in a range of subsequent psychoanalytic writings. For instance, Eissler (1953) described an inability in schizophrenia to reconcile contradictory emotions or modulate the intensity of experienced affect as underlying certain psychotic experiences in schizophrenia. Eissler's clinical observations emphasize that recovery in schizophrenia at least partially involve the development of an increased capacity to tolerate, name, and understand emotional experience. Additionally, Bak (1954) and Freeman (1962) argued that a central process in schizophrenia involves defensive efforts to manage intense anxiety. Spotnitz (1976) likewise positioned intolerable affect as central in schizophrenia, suggesting that symptoms of schizophrenia emerge as a result of inability to effectively express painful affective states. Stemming from this contention, he viewed developing "the ability to engage in the verbal release of feelings, especially aggressive feelings" (p. 124) as critical for recovery.

19.3.3 Phenomenology

Turning more directly to the phenomenology literature, phenomenological accounts have detailed alterations in schizophrenia in individuals' experience of self as subject (Stanghellini et al. 2011a; Sass 2014; Parnas and Sass 2001). To date, though, these accounts have often described subjective experience in terms of the thoughts and perceptions associated with self-experience rather than affective states (Uhlhaas and Mishara 2007; Parnas and Sass 2001; Postmes et al. 2014). Possibly echoing early claims of Kraepelin, accounts of phenomenological psychopathology have at times explicitly emphasized a loss of normal emotional experience, describing a detached, affectless subjective world (e.g., Sass 1992; McGilchrist 2009).

The prominence of the model of schizophrenia sometimes referred to as the ipseity-disturbance model may further illustrate the apparent tendency within phenomenology toward de-emphasis or negation of the presence of affective pain. This theoretical model argues that persons with schizophrenia experience a core alteration in subjective experience rooted in instability of pre-reflective self-awareness (e.g., Nelson et al. 2014; Sass et al. 2011). These self-disturbances are suggested to involve a form of hypertrophied self-consciousness in which normally tacit phenomena become focal, termed *hyper-reflexivity*, as well as a loss of a sense of agency or "existing as an experiencing entity," referred to as *diminished self-affection* (Sass et al. 2011). Extensive elaboration of these proposed self-disturbances has generally emphasized thought content and qualities of experience (e.g., Mishara 2007; Sass et al. 2011), at times leaving unclear the nature of affectivity assumed within the model. Early writings by Sass characterized schizophrenia as characterized by states of solipsistic fragmentation, alienation, and affectless detachment, an "entrapment in a sort of morbid wakefulness or hyper-awareness" (Sass 1992). Sass (2004, 2007) elsewhere has contended that the affective lives of those with schizophrenia involve concurrent diminishment of normal emotionality and exaggeration of certain kinds of abnormal emotional states, offering the terms "quasi-emotion" and "nonemotional affectivity" to represent intensifications of the form of abstract anxiety previously described in characterizations of the disorder as devoid of affect.

Others have offered alternative phenomenological views of affect in schizophrenia. For instance, Stanghellini and Ballerini (2011a, b) have acknowledged the presence of painful affect, suggesting "emotional flooding" as an important element of what they term disorders of embodiment. They summarize the phenomenological viewpoint as understanding schizophrenia as a "loss of emotional, prereflexive, prelinguistic attunement with other persons." A critical distinction then may be that this loss of emotional attunement with other persons does not necessarily represent a subjective state devoid of affect and in fact may involve at least periods of intense affect.

From a more integrative perspective, but one that certainly bears upon phenomenology, Ciompi has extensively elaborated his view of the interrelatedness of cognition and affect in self-disturbance in schizophrenia. Ciompi emphasizes the importance of the role of instability of emotions and disturbances in associations with other cognitive and communication functions as contributing to the expression of schizophrenia (Ciompi 1988). Like others, Ciompi cites personal clinical experience in which he encounters examples of persons with schizophrenia, who have never lost the capacity for "intense emotional feelings" (Ciompi et al. 2010).

19.3.4 Empirical Findings

Separate from these clinical reports and conceptual models a number of quantitative studies report that persons with schizophrenia experience high levels of physiological arousal commonly linked with emotional distress, including anxiety and depressive symptoms (Kring 1999; Lysaker and Salyers 2007). Persons with schizophrenia have also been found to report the presence of heightened negative affective states including despair and hopelessness (Lysaker et al. 2008; Strauss and Gold 2012). Laboratory studies have further demonstrated that people with schizophrenia report heightened negative emotion in response to exposure to stimuli with a range of emotional valence (Cohen and Minor 2010). More recently, persons with deficit syndrome have been found to produce plasma cortisol levels consistent with high levels of human stress response (White et al. 2014).

Regarding the role played by emotional distress, a number of studies have found that it is not merely a by-product of the illness but contributes to its development. Increased levels of emotional distress have been found to predict later exacerbations in positive (Bentall et al. 2008; Erickson and Lysaker 2012) and negative symptoms (White et al. 2013). Emotional distress has also been observed to trigger disorganized speech and related forms of thought disorder (Docherty et al. 1998; Minor and Cohen 2010; Minor et al. 2011).

Even when considering the concept of anhedonia, a phenomenon typically linked to a sense of reduced presence of pleasure or emptiness in schizophrenia, researchers have suggested that anhedonia is a multicomponent phenomenon involving difficulties in affect regulation, encoding-retrieval problems, and representational deficits (Cohen et al. 2011). Regarding the first identified component, affect regulation, Cohen et al. (2011) suggest a reduced capacity to enhance positive emotions while regulating the presence of distressing emotions, a hypothesis strikingly consonant with theoretical claims of Eissler regarding problems reconciling contradictory emotions in schizophrenia.

19.4 Part 3: Implications for Conceptualization and Clinical Practice

19.4.1 Conceptualization

Drawing from this literature on affect in schizophrenia, our view is that despite periods of diminished expressed affect and his report of feeling detached, Babbitt's subjective experience is one driven by core difficulties related to pain and conflict. In other words, though initially obscured from both Babbitt's own report and his interactions with others, his interpersonal stance and his ideas regarding his existence reflect significant emotional pain. This view is consistent with a number of the sources above, which would suggest that while Babbitt gives the impression of a loss of normal emotional experience, this appears to function as a guard against intense underlying emotional distress and difficulties acknowledging, reflecting upon, and responding to intolerable affective experience.

Importantly, aspects of this view of Babbitt seem at odds with aspects of certain models of schizophrenia. Certainly, these contentions stand in direct contrast with traditional biomedical views of schizophrenia characterized by apathy or indifference. It also at least on the surface seems to contradict certain phenomenological models that emphasize a loss of normal affect and an experience characterized primarily by hyper-reflexivity. One way to reconcile this apparent conflict is by proposing that phenomena such as hyper-reflexivity might in fact serve as a guard against unbearable affect. If intolerable emotional pain is central to schizophrenia, it is possible that phenomena such as hyper-reflexivity and diminished self-affection may represent a form of dissociation in which affect is rendered inaccessible. These phenomena may also function to ward off the emergence of emotional distress by disrupting normal intersubjective processes, thereby inhibiting interpersonal connection that may often serve to provoke affect. In this sense, these phenomena enable an interpersonal stance by the person that leads to a state of apparent unknowability or incomprehensibility. In this sense, Babbitt's expressed unusual beliefs about the nature of his own existence and disruptions in his view of his interpersonal field (as well as his diminished goal-directed behavior and passive avoidance) may function to keep Babbitt from being known. If interpersonal encounters such as those Babbitt has with his therapist or with his family members tend to provoke the emergence of affect, then these aspects of his experience serve to disrupt connections and thereby protect against opportunities for affect to surface.

Adopting this view may have some explanatory power in understanding how therapy with Babbitt unfolded as it did. Initially and superficially, Babbitt presented clinically in a state characterized by flat, devitalized subjective experience, which he described as for the most part detached and devoid of affect. His behavior was characterized by limited goal-directed activity, and he initially appeared to have minimal emotional reactivity to external circumstances. He demonstrated a sort of vague anxiety and perplexed mental state, and his intense inward focus on his experiences might be described nearly exclusively through the lens of phenomenological concepts such as hyper-reflexivity and diminished self-affection. Significant declines in social and occupational role functioning, a profound loss of sense of agency, and decrements in Babbitt's abilities to form complex mental representations of self, others, and his social context also accompanied these periods of apparent affective detachment. Despite this initial clinical presentation, though, intersubjective processes in therapy allowed a range of painful affects to emerge, be named and reflected upon by Babbitt. As Babbitt became increasingly able to allow emotion to emerge and be discussed, he also became better able to articulate a more integrated personal narrative to account for his life circumstances as well as to form ideas about future goals. Our encounters with Babbitt thus seem to parallel clinical observations from Bleuler, Searles, Sullivan, and others who have not only noted the emergence of normal and difficult affects as common in the context of a treatment relationship but have also emphasized the importance of this for recovery.

19.4.2 Treatment Implications

These observations have important implications for treatment. If emotional distress is indeed at the heart of the experience of schizophrenia, treatment that overlooks emotional pain in favor of an exclusive focus on behavioral disturbances or perceived distortions in thought content runs the risk of causing harm by failing to attend to the person's anguish or otherwise potentially aligning with unhealthy processes at work in the disorder. Indeed if painful emotion is obscured by dissociative processes, then ignoring the presence of that pain risks collusion with unhealthy processes and might potentially impede recovery. Also, if persons are knowable but central aspects of the condition contribute to the impression of unknowability, adopting the view that these phenomena are incomprehensible risks contributing to stigmatizing beliefs which position persons with schizophrenia as categorically or essentially different from persons without psychosis. Many now reject this essentialist view of schizophrenia and instead support a model of psychosis as part of a continuum of normal human experience (e.g., van Os et al. 2009). Furthermore, in light of the significant evidence to the contrary, treatment approaches that outright deny the presence of emotional distress in what have been called "thought" disorders are thus founded upon questionable ethical footing. Clinicians should not only be able to incorporate the role of emotional distress into an evolving case conceptualization but should be prepared to respond therapeutically to its emergence.

Recent descriptions of psychodynamic therapies for schizophrenia suggest awareness of this central role of affect in psychosis, highlighting emotional development, affect regulation and dissociative processes as important treatment targets (e.g., Harder and Folke 2012; Garfield and Dorman 2009). Additionally, cognitive treatments of psychosis, despite a strong focus on proposed dysfunctional beliefs also encourage therapists to be attentive and responsive to the emergence of painful affect as the treatment relationship develops (Kingdon and Turkington 2005). Though cognitive and psychodynamic approaches have historically been pitted against one another (e.g., Tarrier et al. 2002), review of recent literature reveals a number of emerging integrative treatment approaches that would appear consistent with the ideas discussed here (Hamm et al. 2013).

19.4.3 Future Directions

These contentions and developing models call attention to particular areas of need for future research. For instance, work exploring the links between the development of complexity of integrative, the mental representations of self and others, and the management of affect needs further exploration. Additionally, as we have suggested that aspects of the experience of schizophrenia are linked with difficulties in intersubjectivity, it may be warranted to further operationally investigate the impact of intersubjective processes in therapy on the development of capacities to form these complex mental representations, sometimes referred to as metacognition (e.g., Lysaker and Dimaggio 2014). As argued elsewhere (Hamm and Lysaker 2016), we see opportunities to synthesize valuable theoretical contributions such as those above with emerging neuroscience research methods to develop operational approaches to many of these lines of inquiry.

19.4.4 Conclusions

A wide range of clinical, theoretical, and empirical reports suggest that emotional distress is present in schizophrenia. Though there remains substantial room for theorizing the role of this distress in the disorder, treatment approaches tied to models of schizophrenia that neglect or negate the emotional pain that persons with schizophrenia experience run the risk of siding with unhealthy aspects of the disorder and impeding recovery processes. We have set forth tentative possibilities regarding the role of painful affect in the subjective experience of schizophrenia. In keeping with the spirit of an individualized experiential approach, what appears most pertinent for assessment and treatment is for the clinician to attend to painful affect in the person's experience while remaining open to a number of conceptual possibilities in their efforts to understand the person. For instance, schizophrenia may indeed involve experiences of a fragmented, alienated subjective world in which painful affect is dissociated. This detachment and lack of exhibited affect may function to protect persons from being known by others, and thereby indirectly guarding against pain, or may be reflective of atrophied capacities associated with extended periods of disappointment, social isolation, and stigma. Certainly these could both be true simultaneously, as appears likely to be the case with Babbitt.

Importantly, we contend that the emotional experience of persons with schizophrenia can be known and their pain grasped and dealt with. Babbitt's seemingly incomprehensible uncanny experiences and shifting beliefs about his own status as human appear fraught with meaning and function. It seems a mistake to view his unusual reports of his experience as incomprehensible. Respectful invitation for Babbitt to share and make sense of his personal narrative has been accompanied by the emergence of emotions that are understandable and coherently linked with the matters of reflection. Our interactions with persons such as Babbitt at all stages of psychosis, who are increasingly able to acknowledge, reflect upon, and discuss painful affects, and to begin to integrate these experiences into a more integrated, complex account of self, have strengthened our conviction that psychotic experience can be understood and that the processes and conditions by which persons confront and make sense of emotional pain are central to recovery.

References

Bak, R. C. (1954). The schizophrenic defense against aggression. *International Journal of Psychoanalysis, 35*, 129–134.

Bentall, R. P., Rouse, G., Kinderman, P., Blackwood, N., Howard, R., Moore, R., et al. (2008). Paranoid delusions in schizophrenia spectrum disorders and depression: The transdiagnostic role of expectations of negative events and negative self-esteem. *Journal of Nervous and Mental Disease, 196*(5), 375–383.

Bleuler, E. (1911/1950). *Dementia praecox or the group of schizophrenias*. New York: International Universities Press.

Ciompi, L. (1988). *The psyche and schizophrenia*. Cambridge, MA: Harvard University Press.

Ciompi, L., Harding, C., & Lehtinen, K. (2010). Deep concern. *Schizophrenia Bulletin, 36*(3), 437–439.

Cohen, A. S., & Minor, K. S. (2010). Emotional experience in patients with schizophrenia revisited: Meta-analysis of laboratory studies. *Schizophrenia Bulletin, 36*, 143–150.

Cohen, A. S., Najolia, G. M., Brown, L. A., & Minor, K. S. (2011). The state-trait disjunction of anhedonia in schizophrenia: Potential affective, cognitive, and social-based mechanisms. *Clinical Psychology Review, 31*, 440–448.

Docherty, N. M., Hall, M. J., & Gordinier, S. W. (1998). Affective reactivity of speech in schizophrenia patients and their nonschizophrenic relatives. *Journal of Abnormal Psychology, 107*(3), 461–467.

Eissler, K. R. (1953). Notes upon the emotionality of a schizophrenic patient and its relation to problems of technique. *Psychoanalytic Study of the Child, 8*, 199–251.

Erickson, M. A., & Lysaker, P. H. (2012). Self-esteem and insight as predictors of symptom change in schizophrenia: A longitudinal study. *Clinical Schizophrenia and Related Psychoses, 6*(2), 69–75.

Freeman, T. (1962). Narcissism and defensive processes in schizophrenic states. *International Journal of Psychoanalysis, 43*, 415–425.

Garfield, D., & Dorman, D. (2009). Strengthening the patient. In D. Garfield & D. Mackler (Eds.), *Beyond medication: Therapeutic engagement and the recovery from psychosis*. New York: Routledge.

Gumley, A., Gillham, A., Taylor, K., & Schwannauer, M. (Eds.). (2013). *Psychosis and emotion: The role of emotions in understanding psychosis, therapy, and recovery*. New York: Routledge.

Hamm, J. A., Hasson-Ohayon, I., Kukla, M., & Lysaker, P. H. (2013). Individual psychotherapy for schizophrenia: Trends and developments in the wake of the recovery movement. *Psychology Research and Behavior Management, 6*, 45–54.

Hamm, J. A., & Lysaker, P. H. (2016). Psychoanalytic phenomenology of schizophrenia: Synthetic metacognition as a construct for guiding investigation. *Psychoanalytic Psychology, 33* (1), 147–160.

Harder, S., & Folke, S. (2012). Affect regulation and metacognition in psychotherapy of psychosis: An integrative approach. *Journal of Psychotherapy Integration, 22*(4), 330–343.

Kingdon, D. G., & Turkington, D. (2005). *Cognitive therapy for schizophrenia*. New York: Guilford.

Kraepelin, E. (1919). *Dementia praecox and paraphrenia* (R. Barclay & G. M. Robertson, Trans.). Edinburgh: Livingstone.

Kring, A. (1999). Emotion in schizophrenia: Old mystery, new understanding. *Current Directions in Psychological Science, 8*(5), 160–163.

Lysaker, P. H., & Dimaggio, G. (2014). Metacognitive capacities for reflection in schizophrenia: Implications for developing treatments. *Schizophrenia Bulletin, 40*(3), 487–491. doi:10.1093/schbul/sbu038.

Lysaker, P. H., & Salyers, M. (2007). Patterns of anxiety symptoms in schizophrenia spectrum disorders: Associations with social function, positive and negative symptoms, and trauma history. *Acta Psychiatrica Scandinavica, 116*, 290–298.

Lysaker, P. H., Salyers, M. P., Tsai, J., Yorkman-Spurrier, L., & Davis, L. W. (2008). Clinical and psychological correlates of two domains of hopelessness in schizophrenia. *Journal of Rehabilitation Research and Development, 45*, 911–921.

Mcgilchrist, I. (2009). Problems of symmetry. *Philosophy, Psychiatry, and Psychology, 16*(2), 161–169.

Minor, K. S., & Cohen, A. C. (2010). Affective reactivity of speech disturbances in schizotypy. *Journal of Psychiatric Research, 44*, 99–105.

Minor, K. S., Cohen, A. C., Weber, C. R., & Brown, L. A. (2011). The relationship between atypical semantic activation and schizotypy across emotionally evocative conditions. *Schizophrenia Research, 126*, 440–448.

Mishara, A. L. (2007). Missing links in phenomenological clinical neuroscience: Why we are still not there yet. *Current Opinions in Psychiatry, 20*, 559–569.

Moskowitz, A., & Heim, G. (2013). Affect, dissociation, psychosis: Essential components of the historical concept of schizophrenia. In A. Gumley, A. Gillham, K. Taylor, & M. Schwannauer (Eds.), *Psychosis and emotion: The role of emotions in understanding psychosis, therapy, and recovery*. New York: Routledge.

Nelson, B., Parnas, J., & Sass, L. A. (2014). Disturbance of minimal self (ipseity) in schizophrenia: Clarification and current status. *Schizophrenia Bulletin, 40*(3), 479–482. doi:10.1093/schbul/sbu034.

Parnas, J. (2011). A disappearing heritage: The clinical core of schizophrenia. *Schizophrenia Bulletin, 11*(6), 1121–1130.

Parnas, J., & Sass, L. A. (2001). Self, solipsism, and schizophrenic delusions. *Philosophy, Psychiatry, and Psychology, 8*(2/3), 101–120.

Postmes, L., Sno, H. N., Goedhart, S., van der Stel, J., Heering, H. D., & de Haan, L. (2014). Schizophrenia as a self-disorder due to perceptual incoherence. *Schizophrenia Bulletin, 152*(1), 41–50.

Sass, L. A. (1992). *Madness and modernism: Insanity in the light of modern art, literature, and thought*. New York: Basic Books.

Sass, L. A. (2001). The phenomenology of self-disturbances in schizophrenia: Some research findings and directions. *Philosophy, Psychiatry, and Psychology, 8*(4), 347–356.

Sass, L. A. (2004). Affectivity in schizophrenia: A phenomenological view. *Journal of Consciousness Studies, 11*(10–11), 127–147.

Sass, L. A. (2007). Contradictions of emotion in schizophrenia. *Cognition and Emotion, 21*(2), 351–390.
Sass, L. A. (2014). Self-disturbance and schizophrenia: Structure, specificity, pathogenesis (current issues, new directions). *Schizophrenia Research, 152*, 5–11.
Sass, L. A., Parnas, J., & Zahavi, D. (2011). Phenomenological psychopathology and schizophrenia: Contemporary approaches and misunderstandings. *Philosophy, Psychiatry, and Psychology, 18*(1), 1–23.
Searles, H. (1965). *Collected papers on schizophrenia and related subjects*. New York: International Universities Press.
Spotnitz, H. (1976). *Psychotherapy of the preoedipal conditions*. New York: Jason Aronson.
Stanghellini, G. (2004). *Disembodied spirits and deanimated bodies: The psychopathology of common sense*. New York: Oxford University Press.
Stanghellini, G., & Ballerini, M. (2011a). What is it like to be a person with schizophrenia in the social world? A first-person perspective study on schizophrenic dissociality. Part 1: State of the art. *Psychopathology, 44*, 172–182.
Stanghellini, G., & Ballerini, M. (2011b). What is it like to be a person with schizophrenia in the social world? A first-person perspective study on schizophrenic dissociality. Part 2: Methodological issues and empirical findings. *Psychopathology, 44*, 183–192.
Strauss, G. P., & Gold, J. M. (2012). A new perspective on anhedonia in schizophrenia. *American Journal of Psychiatry, 169*, 364–373.
Sullivan, H. S. (1927). Affective experience in early schizophrenia. *American Journal of Psychiatry, 6*, 467–483.
Tarrier, N., Haddock, G., Barrowclough, C., & Wykes, T. (2002). Are all psychological treatments for psychosis equal? The need for CBT in the treatment of psychosis and not for psychodynamic psychotherapy: Comment on Paley and Shapiro. *Psychology and Psychotherapy: Theory, Research, and Practice, 75*(4), 365–374.
Uhlhaas, P. J., & Mishara, A. L. (2007). Perceptual anomalies in schizophrenia: Integrating phenomenology and cognitive neuroscience. *Schizophrenia Bulletin, 33*, 142–156.
van Os, J., Linscott, R. J., Myin-Germeys, I., Delespaul, P., & Krabbendam, L. (2009). A systematic review and meta-analysis of the psychosis continuum: Evidence for a psychosis-proneness-persistence-impairment model of psychotic disorder. *Psychological Medicine, 39*, 179–195.
White, R. G., Laithwaite, H., & Gilbert, P. (2013). Negative symptoms in schizophrenia: The role of social defeat. In A. Gumley, A. Gillham, K. Taylor, & M. Schwannauer (Eds.), *Psychosis and emotion: The role of emotions in understanding psychosis, therapy, and recovery*. New York: Routledge.
White, R. G., Lysaker, P. H., Gumley, A. I., McCleery, M., O'Neill, D., MacBeth, A., & Mulholland, C. C. (2014). Plasma cortisol levels and illness appraisal in deficit syndrome schizophrenia. *Psychiatry Research, 220*(3), 765–771.

Phenomenological Psychopathology and Care. From Person-Centered Dialectical Psychopathology to the PHD Method for Psychotherapy

20

Giovanni Stanghellini

20.1 Introduction

We are a dialogue of the person with herself and with other persons. The crisis of the dialogue of the person with the alterity that inhabits her and with the alterity incarnated in the other person (through which we strive to build and maintain our personal identity and our position in the world) is at the heart of mental disorders. Schizophrenia is an exemplary case study of this interrupted dialogue between the person and herself in the general framework of dialectic person-centered psychopathology.

Central to human existence is a yearning for meaning, unity and identity. Yet, this attempt is unfulfilled in the encounter with alterity, that is, with all the powers of the involuntary: perplexing experiences, unwitting drives, uncontrolled passions and automatic habits leading to unintended actions, as well as needs, desires, impulses and dreams. And finally, one may encounter alterity in one's body, the impersonal and pre-individual element that is to each of us the closest and the remotest at the same time (Agamben 2005). One may feel forced to live in intimacy with an extraneous being—one's own body, that is, the a priori determined *Whatness* of *Who* we are. One may feel stuck with one's sheer biological body, its facticity, the raw material that constitutes the unchosen and sedimented part of one's being and sets the boundaries of one's freedom. *Who* one is stems from the fragile, complex and obscure dynamics of the voluntary efforts to make sense of the involuntary *What* inherent in human personhood.

G. Stanghellini (✉)
Department of Psychological, Humanistic and Territorial Sciences, 'G. d'Annunzio' University, Chieti, Italy

'D. Portales' University, Santiago, Chile
e-mail: giostan@libero.it

G. Stanghellini, M. Aragona (eds.), *An Experiential Approach to Psychopathology*,
DOI 10.1007/978-3-319-29945-7_20

All this generates feelings of estrangement. Mental symptoms can be read as miscarried attempts to struggle for a sense of reconciliation, to heal the wounds of disunion. Only when I recognize the alterity that inhabits me as an incoercible datum can I begin to use it in my service. Care is an attempt to re-establish such a fragile dialogue of the soul with herself and with others. Such an attempt is based on one pillar: a dialectic, person-centered understanding of mental disorders. Its aim is to improve both our understanding of mental symptoms and syndromes and our therapeutic practice in mental health care.

20.2 Person-Centered Dialectic Psychopathology

The dialectic understanding of mental disorders acknowledges the vulnerability constitutive of human personhood. It assumes that the person is engaged in trying to cope, solve and make sense of new, disturbing, puzzling experiences stemming from her encounter with alterity. Each patient, urged by the drive for the intelligible unity of her life-construction, with her unique strengths and resources, plays an active role in interacting with these experiences. The product of this yearning for meaning can be establishing a new identity, or producing psychopathological symptoms. These are the outcome of a miscarried attempt to make sense of one's disturbing experiences (Stanghellini and Rosfort 2013). Psychopathological symptoms are not simply the direct outcome of some kind of dysfunction or of a 'broken brain'. A person's symptom is not generated as such—as it was the case with Minerva, who sprang fully armed from Jupiter's head. Rather, it is the outcome of the need for self-interpretation that each person has with respect to her encounter with alterity, that is, with challenging, unusual or abnormal experiences.

The psychopathological configurations that human existence takes on in the clinic are the outcome of a disproportion between the person and her encounter with alterity, including the disturbing experiences that stem from this encounter. Alterity is made manifest as a kind of estrangement from oneself and alienation from one's social environment. Faced with new, puzzling experiences, the person tries to make sense of them. The attempt to achieve a self-interpretation of her perplexing experiences characterizes the person's attitude, alongside a comprehending appropriation, that is, the constant search for personal meaning.

The encounter with alterity may offer the vantage from which a person can see herself from another, often radically different and new, perspective. Thus, otherness kindles the progressive dialectics of personal identity. Narratives are the principal means of integrating alterity into autobiographical memory, providing temporal and goal structure, combining personal experiences into a coherent story related to the Self. Yet, the encounter with alterity is also the origin of mental symptoms. The production of a symptom is the *extrema ratio* for alterity to become discernible. The symptom is the last chance for the person to recognize alterity in herself. The patient, as a self-interpreting agent who interacts with her anomalous experiences, 'works through' them in such a way that they become symptoms. Psychopathological symptoms are the outcome of miscarried attempts to give a meaning to distressing experiences, to explain and to cope with them. Psychopathological symptoms arise when one's tacit background preconceptions and ways of interpreting the world fail to incorporate some kind of anomalous experiences, i.e. to make them into something that makes sense. Preconceptions (in the sense of Gadamer's *Vorurteil*, which can be translated prejudgments, presuppositions and prejudices) 'are conditions whereby we experience something—whereby what we encounter says something to us' (Gadamer 2008, p. 9; Fernandez submitted, Fernandez and Stanghellini, in press). In response to anomalous experiences, new preconceptions are enacted. This results in a fundamentally different conception of the world, in whose framework anomalous experiences are no longer 'anomaly' to the experiencing person—as it is typically the case with people who develop psychotic symptoms.

The main difference between this person-centered dialectic understanding of mental disorders and a reductionist model is that in the latter the patient is conceived as a passive victim of her symptoms, whereas the former attributes to the patient an active role in shaping her symptoms, course and outcome. Urged by the painful tension that derives from the drive for the intelligible unity of life-construction (Mayer-Gross 1920), each patient, as a 'goal-directed being', plays an active role and stamps her autograph onto the raw material of her basic abnormal experiences.

This person-centered, dialectic approach helps us to see the patient as meaning-making entity rather than passive individual (Stanghellini et al. 2013). The patient 'can see himself, judge himself, and mould himself' (Jaspers 1997). His attempts at self-understanding are not necessarily pathological and are potentially adaptive.

This approach contains a theoretical framework and practical resources for understanding the diversity of psychopathological structures, including symptom presentation, course and outcome as a consequence of the different ways patients seek to make sense of and value the basic changes in self and world experiences. It also contains a framework for engaging with human fragility by means of a person-centered, dialectic therapy.

The person-centered, dialectic approach involves two fundamental attitudes to mental illness:

- It is a therapeutic approach that acknowledges the subjective fragility constitutive of human personhood.
- It also insists, however, on our responsibility to care for this fragility for becoming the person that we are.

To become the person that we are, we must become aware of what we care about—or our own values—because being a person is to take upon oneself the responsibility involved in what one cares about. This approach is sensitive to the constitutional fragility of Who and What we are and thus conceives psychopathological structures as the result of a normative vulnerability intrinsic to being a human person. It insists that to help a suffering person is to help that person to responsibly deal with the obscure entanglement of freedom and necessity, the voluntary and involuntary, and with her sufferings as the result of the collapse of the dialectic of selfhood and otherness.

20.3 What Is a Symptom?

Handbooks usually present a list of phenomena that should be assessed and treated. By doing so, they establish a system of relevance concerning what should attract the clinician's attention. These relevant phenomena are called 'symptoms'.

Of course, there are different psychopathological paradigms (among which the biomedical, the psychodynamic, the phenomenological, etc.), and each paradigm has its own hierarchy of priorities (what should be the clinician's focus of attention) as well as its own concept of symptom. As a consequence, the concept of symptom covers a vast array of indexicalities (Stanghellini 2013a). In biological medicine, a symptom is the epiphenomenon of an underlying pathology. Red, itchy and watery eyes, congestion, runny nose and sneezing, sometimes accompanied by itchy ears and a buzzing sound, itchy and sore throat, cough and postnasal dripping are known to be the manifestations of an inflammation of the respiratory apparatus.

But long before we discovered the cause of these disturbing phenomena (namely, rhinovirus infection), we all knew that they were the symptoms of a mild, although distressing and untreatable, disorder called the common 'cold'. Within the biomedical paradigm, a symptom is first of all an index for diagnosis, i.e. it is used by clinicians to establish that the person who manifests that symptom is sick (rather that healthy) and that he or she is affected by a particular illness or disease.

The principal utility of any system of medical taxonomy relies on 'its capacity to identify specific entities to allow prediction of natural history and response to therapeutic intervention' (Bell 2010, p. 1). The biomedical understanding of 'symptom' is clearly coherent with this. Biomedical research aims to sharpen its tools to establish increasingly more reliable and valid diagnostic criteria. Its real ambition is not simply to establish a diagnosis through the assessment of clinical manifestations (i.e. symptoms), but to discover the causes of these symptoms (aetiology) and the pathway that leads from aetiology to symptoms (pathogenesis). 'Ultimately, disease specification should be related to events related to causality rather than simply clinical phenotype' (Bell 2010, p. 1). It is assumed that progress in medicine is dependent on defining pathological entities as diseases based on aetiology and pathogenetic mechanisms—rather than as clinical syndromes based on symptom recognition. In the biomedical paradigm, the truth about a symptom is its cause. The main, more or less explicit, assumptions in the biomedical paradigm are the following: (1) Each symptom must have at least one cause, (2) this cause lies in some (endogenous or exogenous) *noxa* affecting the living organism, and (3) the presence of a symptom causes some kind of dysfunction (cause → symptom → dysfunction). Also, (4) if we want to eliminate a symptom, we should eliminate its cause or interrupt the pathogenetic chain that connects its putative aetiology with the symptom itself. Thus, the biomedical paradigm is a knowledge device based on the concept of 'causality'. In general, causality (in the biomedical paradigm) goes from aetiology (in our example, the presence of a virus), to symptom(s) (breathing difficulties), to dysfunction (poor physical performance due to blood hypo-oxygenation and thus reduced adaptation of the person to his or her environment).

An important, implicit assumption is also that symptoms are considered accidental—i.e. non-essential to the living organism—whereas the absence of symptoms is considered essential—i.e. normal to living organisms. In other terms, health is considered normal, whereas disease is considered abnormal.

Many of these assumptions—if we apply this paradigm to the field of mental pathology—are at least controversial or even counterfactual. What is of utmost interest here is the fact that in the biomedical paradigm, symptoms have causes, not meanings. Also, we can assume that a symptom is not an accident to that person; rather, it displays his true essence. As such, it is the contingent opportunity of a possible encounter between the person and alterity. Symptoms are the via *regia* to recognition as they express the person's vulnerability. Someone's *vulnus* displays what is most personal and intimate to him. 'Come inside—says Eumaeus to Ulysses when he arrives at his hut—and when you have had your fill of bread and wine, tell me where you come from, and *all about your misfortunes*' (Homer 2005, XIV, p. 47). Only after Odysseus had a hearty meal of pork does Eumaeus ask about his story: 'And now, old man, tell me your own story; tell me also, for I want to know, who you are and where you come from. Tell me of your town and parents, what manner of ship you came in, how crew brought you to Ithaca, and from what country they professed to come-for you cannot have come by land'.

The recognition of Ulysses in the episode of Eurycleia—Ulysses' wet nurse—comes with the recognition of his scar. As Eurycleia is putting Ulysses' feet in a basin of water, she notices a scar on one of his feet. She immediately recognizes it as the scar that he received when he went boar hunting with his grandfather Autolycus: 'As soon as Eurycleia had got the scarred limb in her hands and had well hold of it, she recognized it and dropped the foot at once. The leg fell into the bath, which rang out and was overturned, so that all the water was spilt on the ground; Eurycleia's eyes between her joy and her grief filled with tears, and she could not speak, but she caught Ulysses by the beard and said, "My dear child, I am sure you must be Ulysses himself, only I did not know you till I had actually touched and handled you"' (ibid., XIX, p. 392).

This myth has a clear correspondence in Karl Jaspers' concept of 'cypher' (Jaspers 2003). 'Cypher-reading is the primary requisite of manhood' (Jaspers 2003, p. 50). Cypher reading is an essential character of the human being. Cyphers show what without them would remain implicit for us. Symptoms are a special category of cyphers: through them alterity, that is, the hidden yet operative (and perplexing or disturbing) dimension of our existence, is made manifest. Like a patient's symptom, which is not accidental to that patient but is rather the manifestation of his or her true identity, cyphers are the contingent opportunity of recognition, that is, of a possible encounter between the person and the encompassing dimension of her existence.

The cypher must keep on an inexhaustible signification with which no definite interpretation is commensurate (Jaspers 2003, p. 42). If the cypher 'becomes fixed and definite and turns into an object, then it loses its essential force. It collapses into a sign' (Jaspers 2003, p. 49). Cyphers must not be crystallized into a kind of definite, categorical concept. The meaning(s) of the cypher must be kept 'in suspension' (Jaspers 2003, p. 38), i.e. remain *unsaturated*. The defection from the cypher to the pure concept (as occurs when the cypher grows a single meaning), as well as the interpretation of a cypher as if it were a symbol (such as when the cypher is interpreted through an 'other'), destroys the force of the cypher.

20.4 Symptoms in Phenomenological Psychopathology

Phenomenology is essentially concerned with laying bare the structure of the lifeworld inhabited by a person (Stanghellini and Rossi 2014). A symptom is a feature of a person's lifeworld whose meaning will be enlightened by grasping the deep architecture of the lifeworld itself and the person's invisible transcendental structure that projects it. The lifeworld is the original domain, the obvious and unquestioned foundation of our everyday acting and thinking. In its concrete manifestations, it exists as the 'realm of immediate evidence'. Although the majority of people are situated within a shared lifeworld, there are several other frameworks of experience—for example, fantasy worlds, dream worlds and 'psychopathological worlds' (Schutz and Luckmann 1989). Abnormal mental phenomena are the expression of a modification of the ontological framework within which experience is generated. The overall change in the ontological framework of experience transpires through the single symptoms, but the specificity of the core is only graspable at a more comprehensive structural level (Stanghellini and Rossi 2014). The experience of time, space, body, self and others, and their modifications, are indexes of the patient's basic structures of subjectivity within which each single abnormal experience is situated. We can rephrase and extend all this as follows: the non-experienced ontological disturbances of the basic structures of subjectivity, i.e. selfhood, produce anomalous experiences. In response to these alterations of experience, generated by a variation at the ontological level, a new set of preconceptions are enacted. These anomalous experiences act as a catalyst for the shift of the person's background preconceptions about the world since these preconceptions are not sufficient to make sense of the person's experiences. In the framework of this new set of preconceptions, anomalous experiences are 'normalized', become meaningful to the experiencing person and are integrated as part of his personal identity.

Before we proceed in this direction, I need to clear the ground of a possible misunderstanding. To consider phenomenology as a purely descriptive science of the way the world appears to the experiencing subject is a serious mistake, although it is true that phenomenology sponsors a kind of seeing that relates to something already there, rather than to what stands before, beyond or behind what is existent. 'Making the invisible visible' can instead be taken as the motto of phenomenology, just as it was the passion that possessed many of the artists of the twentieth century and the intellectual motor of the major scientists of the 'invisible century', including Einstein and Freud, in their search for hidden universes.

The symptom is conceived as a part of a discourse, to be deployed and analyzed as a text. The issue, then, is how to rescue its invisible and unintended meaning. All human deeds can be produced or reproduced as a text. The text—be it oral or written—is a work of discourse that is produced by an act of intentional exteriorization. One of the main characteristics of a text is that once it is produced, it is no more a private affaire, but is of the public domain. It still belongs to the author, but it also stands independent of the intentions of the author.

The externalization of one's actions, experiences and beliefs via the production of a text implies their objectification; this objectification entails a distantiation from the person herself and an automatization of the significance of the text from the intentions of the author. Once produced, the text becomes a matter for public interpretation. Now, the author's meanings and intentions do not exist simply for himself, but also for another.

This process of objectification and of automatization is nicely described in Hegel's theory of action (Berthold-Bond 1995). Indeed, there is a parallel between a text and an action. Just as every action involves a recoil of unintended implications back upon the actor, every text—including symptoms—implies a recoil of unintended meanings back upon its author.

Whenever we act, via the externalization of our intentions, we experience a kind of alienation and estrangement from ourselves. We discover alterity within ourselves. The symptom deployed as a text exposes its author to this very destiny. A text is the product of an action—a linguistic action. Like all actions, once produced the text shows the disparity between the author's conscious intentions and unintended consequences. The symptom exposed like a text recoils back upon its author, displaying the discrepancy between the private intended sense and its public tangible result. The text, as the tangible result of a linguistic act with its unintended consequences, reflects—in the sense of making visible—the 'mind' of the author much more faithfully than a simple act of self-reflection. To paraphrase Hegel, the 'mind' cannot see itself until it produces a text objectifying itself in a social act. Because all conscious intentions are incomplete, self-reflection is just an incomplete form of self-knowledge. A person cannot discern alterity within himself until he has made of himself an external reality by producing a text and after reflecting upon it.

The production of a symptom is simply a particular case of this general rule. Just as in a text, in the symptom alterity becomes manifest. A symptom is the outcome of an interrupted dialogue between the person and alterity. The symptom is nothing but a text by which an unrecognized alterity is made manifest. When alterity is no more integrated into the narrative the person fabricates about herself, a symptom is produced as an *extrema ratio* for alterity to become discernible. The symptom is the last chance for the person to recognize herself.

This is a kind of understanding that 'seeks to find the logos of the phenomena in themselves, not in underlying subpersonal mechanisms' (Fuchs 2008). The symptom, then, is an anomaly, but not an abnormal, aberrant or insane phenomenon in a strict sense. Rather, it is a salience, a knot in the texture of a person's lifeworld, like a tear in the matrix. It is a place that attracts someone's attention, catches one's eyes and awakens one's care for oneself—as we will see in great detail in the section on the person-centred dialectical (PCD) model. The symptom reflects and reveals alterity in oneself—in it alterity becomes conspicuous. From the vantage offered by the symptom, one can see oneself from another, often radically different and new, perspective.

20.5 Selfhood and Personhood in Schizophrenia

In recent years, schizophrenia has been conceptualized as a disorder of the minimal Self. The self-disorder hypothesis conceives schizophrenia as a basic disturbance of the sense of self. The notion 'selfhood' serves to investigate the pre-reflective structures and dynamics of experience. The Self is the subject of his perceptions, feelings, thoughts, volitions and actions. The phenomenological notion of the Self serves to explore the fact that we live our conscious life in the first-person perspective, as an embodied, self-present, single, temporally persistent and demarcated being. This basic form of self-experience is implicitly, pre-reflexively and non-observationally manifest. It is usually called 'minimal' self or 'core' self, referring to a minimum of what must be the case for an experience to be considered 'subjective' at all and which must be in place in order for an experience to be someone's experience, rather than existing in a free-floating state and only appropriated post hoc by the subject in the act of reflection. The minimal self is the pre-reflective sense of existing as a vital and self-identical subject of experience, which serves as a necessary foundation for the articulation of a richer reflective and narrative representation.

It was noted already at the outset of the modern notion of schizophrenia that these basic aspects of the structure of subjectivity (and not merely a change in the *contents* of experience and action) may become altered in this illness. The complaints of persons affected by schizophrenia point to the disruptions of formal or structural aspects of the minimal self. Abnormal self-experiences in schizophrenia can be divided into three main domains:

Self-presence: This includes a troubled sense of self (e.g. 'I don't feel myself', 'I am losing contact with myself') and an alienated sense of self (e.g. 'I am almost nonexistent'; 'I have a strange ghostly feeling as if I were belonging to another planet').

Perspective: This is mainly the loss of first-person perspective (e.g. 'I have thoughts rather than being thoughts (...) having thoughts [means that] the thoughts are delimited; you can hear or see them').

Phenomenality: This includes loss of 'immersion' in the world (e.g. 'I live only in the head') and hyper-reflexivity (e.g. 'I'm always in the mode of simultaneous introspection', 'Whenever I see something I also think of myself seeing it').

An extended account on this, including the main references, is given by Henriksen and Nordgaard in this book as well as by Sass and his colleagues.

The self-disorder hypothesis provides a very rich and detailed account of the experiential dimension of the schizophrenic condition. Yet one may wonder what is the role of the person who is affected by these abnormal experiences in *reacting* to the experiences themselves.

Focusing on troubled selfhood brings to light the patients' immediate subjective experiences, e.g. their feeling ephemeral and lacking core identity, affected by a diminished sense of existing as a self-present subject. Self-disorders have been conceptualized as the core of the vulnerability to schizophrenia. What may remain out of focus in these descriptions, though, is the person's attitude towards these anomalous experiences. Taking into account the notion of personhood allows for an articulation of the way the suffering person *reflectively responds* to and makes sense of her troubled selfhood (Stanghellini and Rosfort 2015). This can help to develop a person-centred psychopathology of schizophrenia that is concerned not only with the phenomenological description of troubled selfhood, but also with how persons with schizophrenia understand themselves and interpret their own anomalous experiences. By bringing into focus the question of personhood (rather than only selfhood), we draw attention to the person's attitude towards her anomalous experiences and to the active role that the person, as a self-interpreting agent with her individual existential orientation (Stanghellini et al. 2013), has in interacting and coping with these experiences and in the shaping of psychopathological symptoms and syndromes.

In order to give a more comprehensive account of the schizophrenic condition, we must take into account the notion of 'personhood' in addition to the notion of 'selfhood'. The notion of personhood is markedly more comprehensive than the notion of selfhood. 'Selfhood' articulates the phenomenological dimension of our experience of being human. 'Personhood' requires a hermeneutical elaboration of the phenomenological method, bringing into account the *normative* dimensions of human experience. This hermeneutic qualification of phenomenology deals with the fact that first-person experience is not merely concerned with self-awareness and experiential objects but also with *how* the experienced objects and the sense of being a self are experienced as an integral part of a person's life. Hermeneutical phenomenology deals with *how* we respond to and interpret the questions that our self-awareness and phenomenal consciousness give rise to. Whereas phenomenology deals with the *What* of experience, hermeneutical phenomenology deals with the way the *Who* takes care of the *What*.

20.6 A Case Study

An illustration of the vulnerable duplicity inherent in the human condition and of the emergence of symptoms as the cypher of a miscarried dialogue with alterity can be taken from the following case study:

A man in his twenties is very keen to describe the abnormal experiences affecting him:

> I had these strange energies inside. It all started like this. I felt as if my body was sending me messages from another place. I was different from all the others. Distinct from them. Separate from my body and from them. A funny funny feeling, although it made me feel very vulnerable in front of others as it in most cases happened when I was with others.

As one can see, his abnormal experiences include two main categories: abnormal bodily phenomena (coenesthopathies) and disorders of intersubjectivity (dissociality). He feels 'strange energies', a kind of force that to him is hard to explain and make sense of and even to express with an ordinary vocabulary. These energies are 'strange', perplexing and awkward. They are ambiguous as they are 'funny' but they also make him feel 'vulnerable'. They elude ordinary language as well as ordinary evaluation since they are neither good nor bad. One may say that he experiences a kind of bodily arousal, but contrary to what one normally would say about this he does not say that these feelings are part of one (or more) emotions that are elicited in a given situation. Another sense in which these feelings are 'strange' is that these 'energies' are located in some part of his body, but in a space that is outside his self-boundaries, 'as if' they came from without. He feels 'separate' from his body and 'distinct' from these. In short, his feelings are 'other' with respect to ordinary meaning (what are they?), function (what are they for?), language (how can one talk about them?), value judgment (are they good or bad?), origin (do they come from me or not?) and spatial location (are they inside or outside my Self?).

Also, these strange sensations are closely connected to abnormal interpersonal experiences. They mainly take place during social encounters. They make him feel 'different' from other persons and 'distinct' from them. By 'different' he may mean that he feels that he does not belong to the human community, and by 'distinct' he may mean that he feels a kind of separated when he is in social circumstances—a lack of grip or hold in situations that would otherwise involve interpersonal contact or attunement.

Obviously, for him this is all in need of some meaning and of some explanation. He needs to 'work through' these abnormal experiences and makes sense of them:

> At first, I thought someone was poisoning me. Then I realized that I lacked the internal wisdom that leads you in life. And all of sudden there came this intuition: that They had chosen me for the experiment.

In these sentences, there is a *Who* trying to make sense of the *What* of his uncanny experiences. His first 'interpretation' of his strange experiences is quite coarse: he thinks that someone is poisoning him. This explains his feeling of weakness and vulnerability. He feels bad because someone infected him with some toxic substance. He develops an explanation that leads him to a delusion of a paranoid kind. I would call this an 'ontic' (Stanghellini 2009) working-through as if there is really nothing unusual, odd or 'bizarre'. This kind of working-through expresses the rather common-sense, universal fear to be damaged by someone or something.

Later he develops a second kind of interpretation, far more out of touch with common sense than the previous one. His strange feelings derive from a quality that he possesses and the others don't. This quality is that he lacks the 'internal wisdom' that leads all the others in their lives and makes of them ordinary people. He considers this not as a deficit, but rather as a gift—or, as we may say, a *charisma*. Since he was gifted with this charisma, 'They' chose him for the experiment. Let's have a closer look at this gift. It is not the prey of common sense in the way as his other interpretations. Common sense is a kind of 'wisdom' that implies conformity. 'They' appreciate his nonconformity. This is why he has been *chosen*.

Although 'They' are conducting an 'experiment' on him, this is not meant to harm him (as was the case with the first paranoid interpretation). 'Their' intention is radically different from the one expressed in the ontic working-through (poisoning). What 'They' want to do with him is near to creating a 'new' man, a new kind of human being with a special destiny.

Note that 'They' express an impersonal entity—whereas in the previous 'ontic' interpretation the others who poison him are other persons, ordinary people. 'They' are to be imagined as nonhuman, extraterrestrial entities. They are located in a non-time, non-space, that is, they are 'now', 'here' and 'now-here'. They possess extraordinary powers and act and affect reality by means that are not reducible to ordinary causality. In short, 'They' belong to another reality, that is, to a lifeworld or ontological dimension where space, time, body, causality, etc. are different from our own. This extraordinary structure or scaffolding is the 'bizarre' quality of the lifeworld to which 'They' and the patient himself belong.

Also note that this interpretation comes as a sudden intuition, as a kind of 'Ah-ah!' experience that enables the patient to make sense of all strangeness affecting him. It is not the effect of a deductive or inductive process. It is based in his abnormal experiences, but he does not present it as the outcome of reasoning. Rather, his 'new' understanding has the character of a *revelation*. Being for him a revelation, it does not need to be validated or corroborated by some 'facts'. He would not agree to call his understanding an 'interpretation', since his 'intuition' has to him the character of an absolute and indubitable truth, whereas an interpretation has the perspectival character of a subjective belief. Indeed, you cannot find a real development from his first to his second working-through. Although he mentions a first and a second understanding of his abnormal experiences, these are not set in a historical context. History would make of his intuition a relative, rather than absolute truth. For an idea to be absolutely true, it has to be set out of history, and this is what revelation does: it discloses an unhistorical truth uncovering a fact that has always been there.

> I was chosen to incarnate myself in one body and to come to the Earth. This explained why I felt a stranger in my body. And a stranger on the Earth too. It was worthwhile. The Earth is a very élite place to go through to reach a planet that is higher in evolution. Here on planet Earth everything is a task, even drinking a cup of coffee. My destination after this is a place where everything is vibration, a pure state of consciousness, so elevated that everything is peace.

Once he realized that 'They' had chosen him because of his charisma, his abnormal sensations become all of a sudden meaningful to him. Especially his abnormal *bodily* sensations get a new meaning: the body in which he feels so uncomfortable is not his own body; rather, 'They' 'incarnated' him in one body. The body into which he was thrown is an impersonal body—that's why he feels a stranger in it. One can imagine that before 'They' incarnated him in that body he was living as a disembodied spirit. One can also visualize the scenario in which all this took place: his disembodied spirit was deposited by 'They' into one of the soulless bodies stored in some place in the universe. This is obviously reminiscent of Gnostic theories of being imprisoned in a body and being a stranger on the Earth. The important thing here is that after he had his 'intuition', everything—including bodily and world experiences, as well as the difficulties he has in performing everyday tasks ('drinking a cup of coffee')—became parts of a meaningful and coherent lifeworld. His explanation is *ontological* in nature (Stanghellini 2009) since he achieves an understanding of single experiences via framing them into a totally new set of prejudices that radically depart from common sense. Because of this ontological working-through, bizarre as they can be, his experiences are not insignificant to him—and they are not meaningless to us too. He believes he is not a human being that belongs to planet Earth, but a traveller who has to go through the 'lower world' in order to deserve a 'higher' place. The Earth is not his destination, but a stage in his personal evolution.

It's very important to note that his belief is framed within a positive and even euphoric emotional state ('It was worthwhile', 'the Earth is a very elite place'). Also, his understanding of his own condition is coherently embedded in a very well-defined value structure (Stanghellini and Rosfort 2015). What matters for him is reaching his 'destination', no matter how painful or difficult this can be. Disembodiment to him is destiny. He thinks of himself to be a disembodied Self: this is to him not only his point of departure but also his destination as a form of life characterized by being 'pure consciousness' in a planet where 'everything is vibration'.

> Well, I must admit that all this started when that girl refused my 'intentions'. . .

Abnormal experiences are embedded in the patient's life history. They began, or at least became more severe and distressing, when 'that' girl rejected his *advances*. This comes as a confession after his spontaneous long and detailed descriptions of his feelings and beliefs. This admission posits the whole story in a meaningful context. Although it may sound odd that a full-blown psychotic state develops out of one's love being rejected, the revelation of this traumatic experience sets it in a framework that includes some type of psychological continuity, motivation and meaningfulness. Traditional psychopathology has always been sceptical about pathogenic hypotheses linking traumatic events and severe psychopathological states like schizophrenia (Stanghellini 2013b). Jaspers (1997) insists that empathic understanding fails when it comes to certain kinds of abnormal phenomena like, for instance, delusion proper and maintains that the 'primary experiences', i.e. the background metamorphosis of consciousness underlying delusions proper, are beyond the reach of understanding. Yet our patient's 'confession' suggests that we can apply psychological understanding based on meaningful connections in order to shed some light on his uncanny experiences of self- and world transformation. Jaspers' ill-famed 'theorem of incomprehensibility' (Baeyer 1979) applies to the formal aspects of psychotic experiences, not to their contents and meanings (Fernandez and Stanghellini, in press). To make sense of a given phenomenon is finally to posit it in a meaningful context, trying to grasp how psychic phenomena 'emerge' out of each other in the context of the life history of a given person.

20.7 The Person-Centered Dialectical Model

The main characteristic of the PCD model of mental disorders is that it seeks to see clinical phenotypes and abnormal forms of existence as the outcomes of the interaction between the *Who* (the person) and the *What* (her experiences). It emphasizes the importance of the involuntary, a priori determined Whatness of Who we are. But also it emphasizes the importance of the role of the Who in trying to make sense of his experiences. A good way to approximate the meaning of the Whatness of an experience is to see it in the light of Ricoeur's (1966) notion of 'experienced necessity' or the experience of necessity—of what we did not and cannot choose. This notion comes close to that of sheer biological life (Agamben 2005), but also to what Heidegger (2010) called *Geworfenheit*, in the sense of being stuck with the particularity of one's situation. Notions like instinct, emotion, habit, character, unconscious, etc., belong to the circle of the involuntary.

The involuntary dimension of our being the person that we are includes *What* is a priori given in our existence, the raw material that constitutes the sedimented part of our being and sets the boundaries of our freedom: our past (e.g. a traumatic experience), our body (e.g. our emotions and drives) and the world (e.g. its rules and values) in which we are thrown. *Who* we are stems from the fragile, complex and obscure dynamics of the voluntary efforts to make sense of the involuntary *What* inherent in human personhood. Only as I recognize my involuntary as an incoercible datum can I begin to use it in my service.

When a clinical syndrome manifests, the line of the pathogenetic trajectory is the following:

1. An extreme disproportion of vulnerability and person, of experience and understanding, of emotions and rationality, of *pathos* and *logos* and of selfhood and otherness—that is, of the voluntary and involuntary aspects of being a person—bringing about an uncanny metamorphosis of the lifeworld
2. A miscarried auto-hermeneutics of one's abnormal experiences and of the transformations of the lifeworld that they bring about
3. The fixation in a psychopathological structure in which the dialectics between the person and her vulnerability gets lost

The PCD approach helps us to see the patient as meaning-making entity (as the involuntary becomes meaningful only *for* the voluntary), rather than passive individual. The patient 'can see himself, judge himself, and mould himself' (Jaspers 1997). The 'matter' of vulnerability receives explicit form from the intention of the person. His attempts at self-understanding are not necessarily pathological and are potentially adaptive. Pathology is not vulnerability itself. Rather, it is the loss of the dialectics between a person and her vulnerability, the voluntary and the involuntary.

20.8 Advantages of the PCD Model

In our case study, the PCD model provided a theoretical framework to explore self-disorders and the way our patient's position-taking generated his particular schizophrenic phenotype. The PCD model

1. Articulates the *dialectics* of the impersonal and personal aspects of illness
2. Provides a solid framework for the *narrative articulation* of the patient's position-taking to her abnormal experiences and her attempt to cope with those experiences by working through her troubled sense of identity
3. Brings out the fundamental role of *values* that inform and shape a person's attitudes to the disturbance of her sense of selfhood and identity

In this way, it secures the autonomy of the patient by evidencing the importance of the patient's interpretation of her suffering.

The PCD model involves two fundamental attitudes to mental illness:

- It is a therapeutic approach that acknowledges the subjective fragility constitutive of human personhood.
- It also insists, however, on our responsibility for being the person that we are.

To become the person that we are, we must become aware of what we care about because being a person is to take upon oneself the responsibility involved in what one cares about. Health is preserved through the dialectics of the involuntary and the voluntary as the appropriation of the involuntary by the voluntary, as we do not choose our involuntary, but we can decide to appropriate it. This therapeutic approach is sensitive to the constitutional fragility of who and what we are and thus conceives psychopathological structures as the result of a normative vulnerability intrinsic to being a human person. It insists that to help a suffering person is to help that person to responsibly deal with the obscure entanglement of freedom and necessity, the voluntary and involuntary, and with her sufferings as the result of the collapse of the dialectic of selfhood and otherness.

The PCD model has important *diagnostic implications* since it serves to establish a two-tier diagnostics. It integrates the self-disorder model, as it helps to disentangle basic vulnerability (first tier) from personal 'reaction' and emotional tone (second tier). This approach contains a theoretical framework and practical resources for understanding the diversity of psychopathological phenotypes, including symptom presentation, course and outcome as a consequence of the different ways patients seek to make sense of the basic changes in self and world experiences.

The PCD model also has *therapeutic implications*. It enhances insight and awareness of illness by shifting their focus from full-blown symptoms (e.g. delusions and hallucinations) to more basic manifestations of vulnerability. It helps to take a reflective stance with respect to her vulnerability, that is, to articulate it in a better expressive and communicative format and to construe it as situated in a personal-historical as well as a relational-interpersonal context. It enhances efforts to modify position-taking and construing different and more effective narratives of illness and interpretation of anomalous experiences.

This approach, in building on patients' individual values and experiences as key aspects of their self-understanding of their suffering, supports recovery and development of self-management abilities. It also contains a framework for engaging with this fragility by means of a PC, dialectical therapy. The aim of such a therapy is to re-establish the dialectics of a person and vulnerability that will allow the suffering person to become who she is.

20.9 The PHD Method

Building on and extending these principles, the PCD therapeutic interview is based on the integration of three basic dispositives:

- *Phenomenological unfolding* (P): The basic purpose is to empower clinicians and patients with a systematic knowledge of the patient's experiences. This is done through a process of unfolding that aims to open up and lay bare the furrows and layers of the patient's experiences. What comes into sight is the *texture* that is immanent in the patient's style of experience and action, although it may remain prima facie invisible to or unnoticed by her. Unfolding enriches understanding by providing further resources in addition to those that are immediately visible. The aim of this process is sometimes referred to as 'thick description', in contrast to the explanations of causal analyses. It aspires to force the tacit, implicit and opaque structure to the surface of awareness and to collect a range of phenomena that point to multiple facets of a potentially significant construct. The final purpose is to rescue the *logos* of the phenomena in themselves, that is, in the immanent intertwining of phenomena.

- *Hermeneutic analysis* of the person's position-taking towards her experience (H): The central idea of clinical hermeneutics is that there is an active interplay between the person and her basic abnormal experiences. If we assume that a given set of abnormal experiences are the *core Gestalt* of a given type of vulnerable structure, then we can assume that the manifold, fluctuating and state-like phenotypes are the consequence of the vulnerable person's individual position-taking in response to this state-like, structural core anomaly. As self-interpreting animals, we continuously strive to make a *logos* out of *pathos*. In psychotherapy, attention is paid to the active role that the person has in taking a position and interacting with her abnormal, distressing and dysfunctional experiences. Her attempt at self-understanding and coping are determined by her unique strengths and resources as well as needs and difficulties. Hermeneutic analyses aim at rescuing the patient's active role in shaping her symptoms, course and outcome. Although the patient's attempts may generate a miscarried self-understanding, they are not necessarily pathological and potentially resilient.
- *Dynamic analysis* of the life history in which abnormal experiences and position-taking are embedded (D): To make sense of a given phenomenon is finally to posit it in a meaningful context, and this context includes the personal history of the patient. The basic presuppositions of psychodynamics, endorsed by the PHD method, are psychological continuity and psychological determinism. The former assumes that the totality of a person's psychological events (including those that look inconsistent) is lawful and potentially meaningful in a particular way for that person. The latter presumes that all psychic events have at least as one of their 'causes' a psychological motivation and can thereby be understood on a psychological basis. Dynamic analysis tries to grasp how psychic phenomena 'emerge' out of each other in the context of the life history of a given person. More precisely, it tries to approximate how they stem from *involuntary* factors that restrict, enable and form our lives This involuntary dimension of our being the person that we are includes *what* is a priori given in our existence, the raw material that constitutes the sedimented part of our being and sets the boundaries of our freedom: our past (e.g. a traumatic experience), our body (e.g. our drives) and the world (e.g. its rules and values) in which we are thrown. *Who* we are stems from the fragile, complex and obscure dynamics of the voluntary efforts to make sense of the involuntary *What* inherent in human personhood. Through dynamic analysis, 'what sedimentation has contracted, narrative can redeploy' (Ricouer 1966).

20.10 Phenomenological Psychopathology and Care

The challenge facing the clinician is how to offer the patient an insight into her fragile personhood, that is, into the alterity she experiences in herself, as well as helping her to understand the way she tries to make sense of this and, moreover, to acquire the appropriate means to cope with her unease. Hermeneutical phenomenology is a resource when dealing with this challenge of therapy because of three basic features of this philosophical approach to human personhood.

First, the phenomenological character of the approach provides a theoretical framework to assess and explore the patient's experience of troubled personhood. This is an important methodological contribution to therapy, since it is open to an unusual extent in that it reveals aspects of experience that other approaches tend to overwrite or eclipse with their strong theoretical—and sometimes moralistic—claims. In this sense, we can say that the ethics of this approach is based on the principle of letting the patient have his or her say. This principle admonishes the clinician to bracket her own prejudices and let the features of a pathological condition emerge in their peculiar feel, meaning and value for the patient, thus making every effort to focus on the patient's suffering as experienced and narrated by her.

Second, the phenomenological articulation of the dialectics of selfhood and otherness gives the clinician an epistemic tool with which to understand how the struggle with one's involuntary dispositions makes personhood not just a fact but also a problem. The vulnerable character of personhood that is so dramatically expressed in mental disorders is closely connected with the problem of the fragility of human identity, that is, with the problem of our cares and concerns. Making sense of what we care about and how we care about being the particular person we are involves the responsibility for one's being so, that is, for one's vulnerable and troubled personhood. This responsibility implies how to respond to the challenges involved in discovering alterity in one's own Self, how to make sense of one's troubled personhood and how to become the person that one is.

Third, the hermeneutical character of this approach provides a framework by means of which the clinician can make sense of norms and values involved in a person's struggle with her involuntary dispositions. We care about being persons, and the hermeneutical emphasis on both the *What* and *Who* of the person that we care about being and becoming—that is, both the a-rational, biological values and the rational, personal values at work in our care—provides the clinician with a framework with room for the ethical problems involved in being a person.

Acknowledgement A special thanks to Anthony Fernandez for his careful and insightful revision of the manuscript.

References

Agamben, G. (2005). *Profanazioni*. Roma: Nottetempo.

Baeyer, W. V. (1979). *Wähnen und Wahn*. Stuttgart: Enke.

Bell, J. (2010). *Redefining disease: The Harveian oration*. London: Royal College of Physicians.

Berthold-Bond, D. (1995). *Hegel's theory of madness*. New York: State of New York Press.

Fernandez, A. V. (submitted). *The subject matter of phenomenological research: Existentials, modes, and prejudices*.

Fernandez, A. V., & Stanghellini G. (in press). Comprehending the whole person: On expanding Jaspers' notion of empathy. In A. L. Mishara, P. Corlett, P. Fletcher, A. Kranjec, & M. A. Schwartz (Eds.), *Phenomenological neuropsychiatry: How patient experience bridges clinic with clinical neuroscience*. New York: Springer.

Fuchs, T. (2008). Comment: Beyond descriptive phenomenology. In K. S. Kendler & J. Parnas (Eds.), *Philosophical issues in psychiatry; Explanation, phenomenology, and nosology* (pp. 278–285). Baltimore, MD: Johns Hopkins University Press; p. 280.

Gadamer, H.-G. (2008). In D. E. Linge (Ed.), *Philosophical hermeneutics*. Berkeley, CA: University of California Press.

Heidegger, M. (2010). *Being and time*. Albany, NY: The State University of New York Press.

Homer. (2014). *Odyssey*. Oxford: Oxford University Press.

Jaspers K. (1997). *General psychopathology* (J. Hoenig & M. W. Hamilton, Trans.). Baltimore, MD: The Johns Hopkins University Press.

Jaspers, K. (2003). *Truth and symbol*. Lanham, MD: Rowman & Littlefield.

Mayer-Gross, W. (1920). Uber die Stellungnahme zur abgelaufenen akuten Psychose: Eine Studie uber verstandliche Zusammenhange in der Schizophrenie [Concerning the position-taking to past acute psychosis: A study of meaningful connections in schizophrenia]. *Zeitschrift für die Gesamte Neurologie und Psychiatrie, 60*, 160–212.

Ricoeur, P. (1966). *Freedom and nature: The voluntary and the involuntary* (E. V. Kohák, Trans.). Evanston, IL: Northwestern University Press.

Schutz, A., & Luckmann, T. (1989). *The structures of the life-world*. Evanston, IL: Northwestern University Press.

Stanghellini G. (2009). *Psicopatologia del senso comune*. Milano: Cortina (new English edition forthcoming: Oxford, Oxford University Press).

Stanghellini, G. (2013a). Philosophical resources for the psychiatric interview. In K. W. M. Fulford et al. (Eds.), *Oxford handbook of philosophy and psychiatry*. Oxford: Oxford University Press.

Stanghellini, G. (2013b). The ethics of incomprehensibility. In G. Stanghellini & T. Fuchs (Eds.), *One century of Karl Jaspers' general psychopathology*. Oxford: Oxford University Press.

Stanghellini, G., Bolton, D., & Fulford, K. W. M. (2013). Person-centered psychopathology of schizophrenia: Building on Karl Jaspers' understanding of patient's attitude toward his illness. *Schizophrenia Bulletin, 39*, 287–294.

Stanghellini, G., & Rosfort, R. (2013). *Emotions and personhood: Exploring fragility-making sense of vulnerability*. Oxford: Oxford University Press.

Stanghellini, G., & Rossi, R. (2014). Pheno-phenotypes: A holistic approach to the psychopathology of schizophrenia. *Current Opinion in Psychiatry, 27*, 236–241.

Stanghellini, G., & Rosfort, R. (2015). Disordered selves or persons with schizophrenia? *Current Opinion in Psychiatry, 28*, 256–263.

Index

G. Stanghellini, M. Aragona (eds.), *An Experiential Approach to Psychopathology*,
DOI 10.1007/978-3-319-29945-7

MIX
Papier aus verantwortungsvollen Quellen
Paper from responsible sources
FSC® C105338

If you have any concerns about our products,
you can contact us on
ProductSafety@springernature.com

In case Publisher is established outside the EU,
the EU authorized representative is:
Springer Nature Customer Service Center GmbH
Europaplatz 3, 69115 Heidelberg, Germany

Printed by Libri Plureos GmbH
in Hamburg, Germany